# Ethics in Practice

*The Harvard Business Review Book Series*

Designing and Managing Your Career,
Edited by Harry Levinson

Ethics in Practice: Managing the Moral Corporation,
Edited by Kenneth R. Andrews

# Ethics in Practice
# Managing the Moral Corporation

Edited, with an Introduction by
Kenneth R. Andrews
Donald K. David Professor Emeritus
of Business Administration,
Harvard Business School

## Harvard Business School Press

### Boston, Massachusetts

Most of the articles included in this collection are available as individual reprints. For information and ordering call 617-495-6192 or contact Operations Department, Harvard Business School Publishing Division, Boston, MA 02163 (Fax: 617-495-6985).

Printed in the United States of America
93                5 4

---

**Library of Congress Cataloging-in-Publication Data**

Ethics in practice.

(The Harvard business review book series)
Includes bibliographies and index.
1. Business ethics.  I. Andrews, Kenneth
Richmond, 1916-         II. Series.
HF5387.E847   1989        174'.4       88-32878
ISBN 0-87584-207-0

# Contents

# Ethics in Practice

# Introduction

## Managers as Moral Individuals

Public interest in ethics as a critical aspect of business behavior comes and goes. As the 1990s overtake us, this interest is at a historic high. Stimulated by press attention to blatant derelictions in Wall Street, the defense industry, and the Pentagon, and to questionable activities in the White House, the attorney general's office, and the Congress, many people wonder whether our society is sicker than we suspect. Over time, of course, the standards applied to corporate behavior have risen and have in turn raised the average rectitude (observable even to the naked eye) of business persons and politicians. It has been a long time since we could say with Mark Twain that we have the best Senate that money can buy or, with a muckraker like Upton Sinclair, that our large companies are the fiefdoms of robber barons. But illegal and unethical behavior persists even as efforts to expose it often succeed in making its rewards short lived.

This book is a collection of articles from the *Harvard Business Review* addressed over a considerable period of time to corporate ethics as a management problem. The three sections emphasize in turn the problems of the executive as a moral person, the influences of the corporation as a moral environment, and the action needed within the corporation to lay out a high road to economic and ethical performance and the guardrails to keep corporate wayfarers on it.

These articles reflect the best of what business leaders and close observers of business have had to say over the last generation about the difficulties in arriving at ethical decisions and carrying them out in large organizations. Our authors point out that these decisions, large and small, policy guided or instinctive, one after another finally establish what the corporation's ethical level is to be. As managers and management scholars, the authors do not pretend to provide definitive rules for executive choices when right and wrong are confusingly entangled. Judgment-free formulas do not appear here. The writers' wisdom, however, will engage readers of experience in new appraisals of their own situations and indicate courses of action that can convert good intentions into good results.

Why cannot these authors be more definitive? Why is business ethics a problem that snares not just a few mature criminals or crooks-in-the-making but also a host of apparently good people who lead exemplary private lives while concealing information about dangerous or lethal products or falsifying cost records? It used to be said that malfeasance in business is an individual failure. A person of the proper moral fiber, properly brought up, would not cheat. There are enough such people, it is assumed, to fill management ranks if we choose care-fully. But because we are fallible, a few bad apples will appear in any big barrel. These can be scooped out.

It also used to be said that any decline in ethical behavior is chargeable to all the institutions of society that deliver morally weak people to the companies they join. Long before people go to work to make a living, family, church, and school have shaped their moral characters. If so, then the corporation may have to eliminate all unethical persons, or more practicably, look to see what it can do to foster moral development and eliminate corporate practices that bring more pressure than is necessary upon a person's ability to resist temptation.

In any case, universal development of ethical judgment and moral behavior is still an unsolved problem at home, at school, at church, or at work. The fabled instruction in basic principles at Mother's knee, if ever as effective as folklore would have it, is clearly diluted by two-career parentage, day care, television, preschool education, and the virtual disappearance of the dinner table as a forum for the discussion of moral issues. Our battered school systems, under fire for poor performance of their traditional functions, cannot be expected to assume the moral role of the family. Religious instruction is less help than nostalgia suggests it used to be when it was supported by membership in a distinct com-munity that promoted coercive conventions of moral behavior. The increasing secularization of society, the profusion of sects, the divergence of the conservative church from the new life styles that permit birth control, abortion, and alter-natives to marriage and heterosexuality and the pervasive distrust of the religious right mean that we cannot depend on uniform religious instruction to ensure that recruits to business, the odd rotten apple notwithstanding, are armed against the temptations they are about to encounter.

Higher education, particularly in moral philosophy and the humanities, has in the twentieth century deliberately avoided moral indoctrination. Great liter-ature was once considered an obvious source of ethical instruction, for it informs the mind and the heart together of the complexities of moral decision. But professors of literature, as James T. Engell of the Harvard English Department has pointed out, consciously offer no guidance to ethical interpretation, prefer-ring instead to stress technical, aesthetic, or historical analysis. The wish to be noncoercive, to be intellectual rather than moral role models, or to encourage students to think for themselves may explain this aversion to a discussion of the application of literature to contemporary life. Authors themselves usually dis-claim a moral purpose for their art. With dispassionate instruction, however, students can be stirred to apply their personal values to crises they experience vicariously.

Moral philosophy, as an academic discipline, is of course the proper home of ethical instruction, but in departments of philosophy the professors do not often teach applied ethics. In the twentieth century, in Stephen Toulmin's ironic words in *The American Scholar* (Summer 1988), any "attempt to be edifying" has been avoided. A quest for certainty and proof and a distrust of subjectivity have led to the development, for example, of logical positivism, a closed system of thought in which one proposition incontrovertibly leads to another, but to none that can be usefully applied to the complexity of a real-life moral problem.

Kenneth E. Goodpaster, one of the best known philosophers of applied ethics, has usefully classified frameworks developed by philosophers for the careful and systematic examination of questions of right and wrong, virtue and vice, or good and evil. One set of frameworks is concerned with the *results* of conduct, not with any right or wrong that might be inherent in the *means* by which they are achieved. Thus Thomas Hobbes's egoism postulates that persons act only in their self-interest to procure for themselves more good than bad results. An economist might argue that this is the only framework that does justice to the reality of human motivation. That human motivation, in which self-interest must be an important part, excludes any obligation or concern for others, and thus concern for means, however, is not established by research or common sense.

Other philosophers, such as Jeremy Bentham and John Stuart Mill, insist that persons and organizations ought to act only to seek the greatest good for the greatest number. Appealing as is this altruism, which is embodied in what Ralph Waldo Emerson said was the first civic duty of any government, it omits altogether the claims of any minority or the justice owed to the individual. Since the heart of Emerson's philosophy is the sanctity of the individual against any claim by organization or society, he and the utilitarians have a problem. But, as in the case of self-interest, the utilitarian position cannot be abandoned altogether.

We begin to see the problem of submitting to any one school of thought. The conflicting claims of self and others were recognized by Henry Sidgwick, who wrote, sensibly enough, that the two had to be reconciled. We come then to the question we all face: how are we to do that? Whereas Hobbes, the utilitarians, and Sidgwick are concerned with ends that justify the means, another set of frameworks stresses duty and obligation over results. F. H. Bradley's views on self-realization and Jean-Paul Sartre's existentialism maintain that the final arbiter in separating right from wrong is the free will of the decision maker. The authenticity of the decision depends in part on a universal form of morality that keeps a person within reasonable bounds. Purity of motive rather than the good or harm of the outcome is the higher good. No anchor in fixed doctrine is offered. However realistic this self-reliance may be, it does not satisfy those who want a doctrinal directive. The question is: where will they find it?

In John Rawls's development of Locke's contractarianism perhaps. Fairness, or decision making guided by principles anyone and everyone would agree with, is a central value in the unwritten contract people make with society. Social and economic inequalities are just only if they result in compensating benefits for the least-advantaged members of society. Institutions permitting hardships for some cannot be justified on the utilitarian grounds that the aggregate good is greater. What is fair thus becomes highly controversial. Immanuel Kant, like Sidgwick and the latter's dualism, brings together the free will of the rational decision maker and the need to make that will universal. One should act first according to that principle by "which you can at the same time will that it should become a universal law." Second, humanity—oneself and others—must always be treated as an end and never only as a means. The rigidity of the universal law requirement makes it *always* wrong to tell a lie or break a promise. It leaves little room for the details of a complex situation. Complete loyalty to this school is as impractical as rejection of all of it.

Although these fragmentary references cannot do justice to the philosophy summarized, it should be abundantly clear that a person confronting a business decision must draw on all of these conceptions in order to do justice to a thorny real-life case. Some philosophers, like W. D. Ross, have tried to combine them in "intuitionism" with a set of principles as prima facie obligations. Ross at least recognizes the conflict that develops among basic duties and the need to decide which obligation is overriding. This is indeed the manager's dilemma. But even Ross's brave attempt to develop seven principles that embrace ethical egoism, utilitarianism, existentialism, and contractarianism does not come close to embracing all the obligations that appear in the context of an important business decision. It also does not tell people how to decide when specified or acknowledged duties conflict. That managers must decide anyway is clear.

The search by managers for practical instruction in philosophy—if it ever were to begin in earnest—would be further confounded by the disdain of the philosophic community for the managers of corporate affairs. Alasdair MacIntyre, in a widely praised study of ethics entitled *After Virtue*, extends the unhelpfulness of analytical and historical philosophy by arguing that the concept of managerial effectiveness is a moral fiction. In a curious reality-denying argument, MacIntyre holds that the manager cannot possibly "mold, influence and control the social environment" in the corporation because there exists no "factual law-like generalizations" that enable a manager to predict outcomes with certainty. Only such knowledge would justify his authority. *After Virtue* is an impressive history of post-Aristotelian ethics and a challenging attack on moral relativism. It is also a monument to the gulf between formal philosophy and the practice of ethical management.

Responsible moral judgment thus cannot be transferred ready-made from philosophers to decision makers. The process for developing it is described— mostly by nonphilosophers—in the articles constituting the body of this book. In business it turns out to be an administrative process that both reveals the ethical implications of a decision and creates opportunities for different perceptions of ethical issues to surface. Then the tentative decision needs testing for its adequacy to balancing self-interest and consideration of others, its import for future policy, and its consonance with company values. After consideration of these factors, however, if a clear consensus has not emerged, then the executive in charge must decide, drawing on his own intuitions and convictions. Infinitely debatable and rebuttable decisions need to be closed out and defended by those considerations that support rather than argue against the decision. This being the case, the caliber of the decision maker is decisive. This is especially true when an immediate decision must be made without opportunity for reflection, analysis, or discussion.

Consequently, for the mature person obligated to act, philosophical inquiry can only result in a personal choice, dependent for its quality on the experience, intelligence, and integrity of the decision maker. That quality depends upon certain forces that do not diminish but educate subjective judgment—namely, information, experience, good intentions, and careful concern.

This existential resolution requires the would-be moral person to be the final authority in a situation where conflicting ethical principles are joined. It does not rule out prior consultation with others or recognition that in a hierarchical organization such a judgment may be overruled.

Given these requirements, it is not wise for corporate boards of directors and senior managers to assume that recruits are prepared to enter the corporate environment without need for further education. The graduates of MBA programs have had as undergraduates minimum exposure to the liberal arts, however important even that can be. Almost all of them, moreover, in high school and college have been directly instructed (courses) in elementary economics in

a theory of human behavior that relates all human motivation to personal pleasure, satisfaction, and self-interest. It diminishes the significance of ethical judgment to the point sometimes that people are said to behave morally only if it
serves their own economic well-being. Far more business students study economics than literature or philosophy.

Ironically, as recognition of a role for the corporation more complex than
that of a profit-maximizing agent of the shareholders has increased, the MBA
curriculum has moved away from consideration of professional ideals toward
quantification, formal models, and formulas that minimize the application of
judgment and the debate about values. A determined effort to reintroduce
business ethics in elective and required courses is currently being made in response to business and public concern about the education of potential business
leaders. The ethical issues in functional and general management courses are
being rediscovered and introduced into the curriculum. The recent dominant
interest of MBAs in financial economics, however, with its bias toward the neoclassical economics model of the firm, is a strong countervailing force. How to
teach ethics, especially with the biases of the academy blocking the choice of
modest but feasible goals, and how to interest students in the development of
ethical awareness are needs not yet met. In the best of circumstances they represent goals hard to achieve.

The difficulty in fostering moral reasoning in the hostile environment of
economic theory is nowhere more poignant than in the new attempts to analyze
situations requiring identification of ethical issues. Discussion of these issues, in
a situation in which it is inappropriate for the instructor to make authoritarian
calls to virtue, does not excite eager aspirants to executive power and high
compensation. It is likely, however, that more faculty members will attempt even
more creative attacks on the problem.

In any case, the role of any school is to prepare its graduates for a lifetime of
learning from experience that would go better and faster than without formal
education. No matter how much business schools expand their investment in
moral instruction, this limitation persists. Most of the instruction, in business
ethics as in all other aspects of business acumen, will occur in the organizations
in which the graduates of our schools and colleges will spend most of the rest
of their lives.

The stubbornness of the problem of business ethics can be traced, then, to
the diversity of a democratic, multiethnic, pluralistic society, and to the related
difficulties of moral instruction in family, church, and school. The economic
theory that is supposed to explain the workings of a materialistic society enshrines
profit maximization and self-interest as commanding goals, anointing the primacy of self-interest as a natural ethical framework. The Darwinian implications
of conventional economic theory are essentially immoral; self-interest is more
easily served than not by encroaching upon or muscling aside others. Competition produces and requires the will to win. Careerism focuses attention on
advancement. Immature people are prey to the moral flabbiness that William
James said attends exclusive service of the bitch-goddess Success.

Despite all the current obstacles to moral development, it does take place.
Expectations of ethical behavior are rising in society and in business. Ethical
decisions require three qualities that cannot be impossible to find and develop.
These, our authors tell us, are, first, the ability to recognize ethical issues and
to think through the consequences of alternative resolutions. Second is the self-

confidence to seek out different points of view and then decide what is right at a given time and place in a particular set of relationships and combination of circumstances. Third is what William James called tough-mindedness, which in this case is the willingness to make decisions when all that needs to be known cannot be known and the questions that press for answers have no established and incontrovertible solutions. The moral person in the modern corporation is all too often on his or her own. This person cannot be expected to remain autonomous, i.e., acting on his or her own best judgment, no matter how well endowed, without positive organized support. The stubbornness of corporate ethics as a problem obscures the simplicity of the solution that can be found once the leaders of a company decide to do something about their ethical standards. Ethical dereliction, sleaziness, or inertia is not merely an individual failure but a management problem as well.

## The Corporate Environment for the Exercise of Moral Judgment

When the persons whose moral judgment might ultimately determine the ethical character of their companies first come to work, they enter a community whose values will influence their moral judgment. Any person has to be affected, as all our authors will acknowledge, by the economic function of the corporation. Theoretical emphasis on the maximization of shareholders' interest and dedication to the survival and compensation of the management will naturally tend to stress the rewards of achievement over fairness of methods. Ethical policy can be dismissed as irrelevant if the invisible hand of the market is believed to moderate adequately the adverse effects of the pursuit of self-interest. Ethical inquiry does not flourish if individuals are encouraged to pursue their own and their companies' well-being without regard to fairness.

The impact on the moral individual of the need to succeed in competition with his or her fellows is no doubt more direct than the permissive influence of neoclassical economic theory on the conduct of the corporation. The corporation itself is saddled with a necessity to establish competitive advantage over time after reinvestment of what could otherwise be the immediate profit by which the financial community and many shareholders judge its performance. The aspiring manager will also be influenced by the way he or she is judged. As several of our authors point out, the imperative of personal success crystallizes multifaceted temptation to pursue advancement for its own sake at the expense of colleagues, to seek personal credit for group achievement, to hide or misrepresent mistakes.

Under pressures to get ahead, the individual of whose native integrity we are hopeful is tempted to become thoughtless and careless, to cut corners, to seek to win at all costs, to take advantage, in sum, of myopic evaluation of performance. People will do what they are rewarded for doing. The quantifiable results of management activity are much more visible than the quality and consequences of the means by which they are attained.

When the corporation is defined, not primarily as a profit-maximizing agent of the shareholders, but as a socioeconomic institution with responsibilities to other constituencies (employees, customers, and communities, for example), policy is established to regulate the single-minded pursuit of maximum immediate profit. The leaders of such a company speak of social responsibility, promulgate ethical policy, and make their own personal values available for emulation by their juniors. They are respectful of neoclassical economic theory, but find it only partially useful.

When the corporation grows beyond the direct influence of its leader, we must reckon with the ethical consequences of size and geographical deployment. The control and enforcement of all policy, but especially that established for corporate ethics, becomes difficult. The development of layers of responsibility brings with it communications problems. The possibility of penalty engenders a lack of candor. Distance from bureaucratic centers complicates evaluation of performance, driving it to numbers. Where dispersal of operations traverses different cultures and countries, where corruption assumes exotic guises, a consensus about moral values is hard to achieve and maintain.

Decentralization of authority in itself has ethical consequences. It absolutely requires trust and latitude for error. The inability to monitor the performance—especially when measurement of results is the only surveillance—of executives assigned to tasks their superiors cannot know in detail results inexorably in delegation. The leaders of a corporation are accustomed to reliance upon the business acumen of profit-center managers, whose results they watch with a practiced eye. Those concerned with the maintenance of the ethical standards of the corporation are dependent just as much on the ethical judgment and moral character of the manager to whom authority is delegated. Beyond keeping our fingers crossed, what do we do?

## The Exercise of Ethical Leadership in the Corporation

Fortunately for the future of the corporation, this microcosm of society can be, within limits, what its leadership and membership make it. It is an organization in which people influence each other to establish accepted values and ways of doing things. Its leadership has more power than elected officials in the larger society to choose who will join or remain in the association. It is not a democracy, although the authority of its leaders, to be fully effective, must be assented to by their followers. A hierarchical organization has problems of communication and bureaucratic diversion from proper purpose. But even as they threaten resistance to change, its members expect direction. Careless or lazy management will let the organization drift or follow its multiple inclinations here and there as it continues its economic performance along lines previously laid out and leaves its ethics to chance. The resolute management does not find the problems that I have dwelt upon insurmountable—once the problems have been separated from their camouflage.

It appears possible, some of our authors imply, to carve out of a pluralistic, multicultured society a coherent community with a strategy defining its economic purposes and the standards of competence, quality, and humanity that will govern its activities. The character of a corporation may be more malleable than an individual's. Certainly its culture can be shaped. Intractable persons can be replaced or retired. Formal and informal sanctions are generated by those committed to the company's goals to constrain and alienate those who are not.

The approach described in the articles in Parts II and III to make good intentions effective begins with the personal influence of the chief executive and that of his juniors who are heads of business units, staff departments, or any other suborganizations to which authority is delegated. It proceeds with the determination of explicit ethical policy and then to the same management procedures that in effective organizations are applied to the execution of any body of policy.

For reasons that are obvious, the personal deportment of the chief executive in the exercise of moral judgment is universally acknowledged to be more influential than written policy. The CEO who orders the immediate recall of all of a product because of a quality defect affecting a limited number of untraceable shipments at a cost of millions of dollars in sales sends a very different message from the executive who suppresses information about actual or potential defects or tacitly condones overcharging for the repairs of rental cars.

Policy is implicit in behavior. The ethical aspect of product quality, personnel, advertising, and marketing decisions is immediately plain. Chief executive officers say much more than they know in the most casual contacts with those who watch their every move. Pretense is futile. "Don't *say* things," Emerson once wrote. "What you *are* stands over you the while, and thunders so that I can't hear what you say to the contrary." He said on another occasion, "What a man *is* engraves itself upon him in letters of light . . . men know not why they do not trust him, but they do not trust him." It follows that "if you would not be known to do anything, never do it."

The modest person might respond to this attribution of transparency with a "Who, me?" Self-confident sophisticates will refuse to consider themselves so easily read. Executives typically underestimate their power and do not recognize deference in others. One of our authors (Robert Jackall) believes indeed that a superordinate deference to the real or imagined wish of the CEO dominates the bureaucratic organization. No one would deny that a CEO's actions speak louder than words. The import of this aspect of a corporation as a moral environment is of course that CEOs should be conscious of the amplifications their positions give to their most casual judgments, their jokes, and their silences. But if a person cannot conceal his or her character, then an even more important implication is that the selection of a chief executive and indeed of any aspirant to management responsibility should include an explicit estimate of character. If you ask, "How do you do that," Emerson would reply, "Just look!"

Once it has been determined that ethical intention and performance will be managed, rather than left untended in the corrosive environment of unprincipled competition, then it is usual to determine and to make explicit corporate policy in much the same way as in other dimensions of corporate purpose. The need for written policy is especially urgent in companies without a strong tradition or those seeking change after the publication of scandal or internal detection of questionable behavior. Codes of ethics are now commonplace. They are not thought to be effective in and of themselves, especially when the terms in which they are cast are so familiar as to be dismissed as merely cosmetic. Internal policies specifically addressed to industry, company, and functional vulnerability make compliance easier to audit and training easier to conduct. Where particular practices are of major concern—for example, price fixing, procurement practices, or opportunity for bribery of government officials—compliance can be made a condition of employment and certified annually by employees' signatures. But the most pervasive problems cannot be foreseen, nor can the proper procedure be so precisely specified in advance as to tell the person on the line what to do. Unreasonably repressive rules undermine trust, which remains indispensable.

What can be done is to advance awareness of the kinds of problems that are foreseeable. The articulation of policy will not be effective unless it is understood. The problems of applying it are becoming the subject of discussion in corporate training sessions. Judgment in making the leap from general policy statements to situationally specific action can be informed by discussion in difficult situations. Such discussion, if carefully conducted, can reveal the inadequacy or ambiguity of present policy, new areas in which the company must take a unified stand, and new ways in which the individual can be supported in making the right decision.

Identification of sensitive issues prospers only when discussion can be open and all points of view can be explored without penalty. The details of such training programs, which should be fully customized, are not discussed in the articles that follow. Consultants in ethics training are available, however, to research company needs, develop cases for discussion, and follow up on the impact (via attitude surveys) of training programs. The aim is to develop through exercise the ability to identify and balance the conflicting interpretations of obligation. Such is the analytical element of judgment.

As in all policy formulation and implementation, the personal deportment of the chief executive officer, the development of relevant policy, and training in its meaning and application are not enough. In companies determined to sustain or raise ethical standards, the information system is extended to illuminate the pressure points—rate of manufacturing defects, product returns and warranty claims, special instances of quality shortfalls, results of competitive benchmarking inquiries, or whatever makes good sense in the circumstances of the company.

Trust is indispensable, as I have said, in decentralized organizations. Corporate ethical aspirations, it becomes evident, must be accompanied by information that serves not only to inform but also to control. Control need not be so much coercive as customary. It need not so much represent suspicion as a normal interest in the quality of operations. The worldly wise do not substitute trust for an awareness that policy undergoes distortions in practice. Ample information, like full visibility, is a powerful deterrent.

The traditional sphere of external and internal audits—wherever fraud may occur—is expanded in purposefully ethical organizations to include compliance, to be sure, with corporate ethical standards. More important is attention to obstacles to intended levels of performance and to problems that need airing before help can be brought.

To obtain information deeply guarded to avoid penalty, internal auditors—long since taught not to prowl as policemen or detectives—must be people of enough management experience to be sensitive to the needs of managers for economically viable decisions. The auditors also should have imagination enough to envision ethical outcomes from bread-and-butter profit and pricing or equal opportunity and payoff dilemmas and downsizing crunches. The trend of operational audits over recent years has been to include problem-solving assistance to managers at intermediate levels in lieu of censorious exposure. To establish an audit and control climate that assumes as normal the open exchange of information between the operating and policy-setting levels of a company is not difficult. Once, that is, as in most other matters of corporate ethics the need to do so is recognized and persons of adequate experience and respect are assigned to the work.

No matter how much empathy is exhibited by audit teams, discipline ultimately requires action. The otherwise loyal secretary who steals petty cash, the successful salesman who falsifies his expense account, the accountant and his boss who alter the record of costs, and more problematically the chronically sleazy operator who never does anything actually illegal must be dealt with cleanly, with minimum attention to alleged extenuation. It is true that hasty punishment may be unjust and improperly absolve superiors of secondary responsibility for the wrongdoing. But long delay or waffling in the effort to be humane obscures a message needed by the organization at large whenever violations occur. Trying to conceal a major lapse or safeguarding the names of persons dismissed is kind to the offender but blunts the salutary impact of disclosure.

The administration of discipline incurs one ethical dilemma after another. A reasoned position on the weight assigned to consideration for the offending individual and for the future of the organization must be taken and protected. A company dramatizes its uncompromising commitment to lawful and ethical comportment when it severs the relationship with offenders whose offense is incontestable and has been classified in advance as critical. When such a decision is fair, its equity becomes clear in the grapevine when more formal publicity is inappropriate. Tough decisions, we are told by Sir Adrian Cadbury, among others, should not be postponed simply because they are painful. The steady support of corporate integrity is never without pain.

In a large decentralized organization, consistently ethical performance requires difficult decisions not only from the current chief executive officer but also from a succession of chief executives. Here the board of directors enters the scene. The board has the opportunity to provide for a succession of CEOs whose personal values and character are consistently adequate for sustaining and developing whatever traditions for ethical conduct may have been established. Once in place, CEOs must rely on two resources for getting done what they cannot do personally: the character of their associates and the influence of policy and the measures taken to make it effective.

As I reflect on these articles—on what they do and do not say—I conclude again that an adequate corporate strategy must include noneconomic goals. An economic strategy is the optimum match of a company's product or market opportunity and its resources and distinctive competence. (That both are continually changing is of course true.) An economic strategy is humanized and made attainable in a living organization by deciding on the character the company is to have, the values it espouses, and its relationships to its customers, employees, communities, and shareholders. The personal values and ethical aspirations of the company leaders, though probably not specifically stated, are implicit in all strategic decisions. They show through the choices made and reveal themselves as the company goes about its business. The importance of this fact of life means that communication should be deliberate and purposeful rather than random.

Although codes of ethics, ethical policy for specific vulnerabilities, and disciplined enforcement are important, they do not contain in themselves the final emotional power of commitment. Commitment to quality objectives—among them compliance with law and high ethical standards—is an organization achievement. It is inspired by pride more than by the profit that rightful pride produces. Once the scope of strategic decision is thus enlarged, its ethical component is no longer at odds with a decision right for many reasons.

## Editor's Note

An obvious feature of this book should be acknowledged and placed in context. Some articles included in this book were written before researchers, writers, and editors began to take into consideration the role of women in management. These articles have been included because their insights far outweigh their anachronistic qualities. Nevertheless, the archaic use of the masculine gender and the assumption that a manager is necessarily male are regrettable. The editor and the publisher hope outdated assumptions about gender will not undermine otherwise cogent and relevant essays.

# The Executive as Moral Individual

## Introduction

We are dependent for ethically adequate business decisions, it is clear, on judgments made by individuals. Men and women in positions of responsibility are ordinarily well educated and of considerable intelligence. They are unguided, as we have seen, by universally accepted criteria for distinguishing right from wrong in situations clouded by ambiguity, incomplete information, and multiplicity of point of view. The seven articles in this section imply that persons contributing to an important decision have a lot to learn about who they are, how much importance should be assigned to fairness, respect for others, reconciliation of conflicting claims in the pursuit of corporate profit, and how to make their conclusions effective. "Ethical managers make their own rules," Sir Adrian Cadbury tells us.

In the face of some difficulty, to be sure. We are told of the need for individual competence, awareness, and concern in even *recognizing* the ethical element in virtually every business decision, to say nothing of appraising accurately the conflict among competing ethical and economic claims. Illegal and unethical steps are often taken by people who mean more or less well. The reasons are many. Rationalizing away the ethical and legal doubts in the prospect of clear corporate gain, compartmentalizing material and spiritual aspirations, living by outmoded precepts of economic theory defining the corporation and indeed the business person as only a profit-maximizing entity—these three easy evasions leave the central problem untouched. The elusiveness of the correct weighting of conflicting considerations—these authors (writing separately) seem to agree —puts the insight, integrity, and moral judgment of the chief executive and the people to whom responsibility is delegated to a tough test.

In the absence of established prescriptions, each problem must be resolved, even after consideration of all affected interests and wide consultation, in the light of the values held by the person making the decision. Those values should not be taken for granted. They are developed by one person, who can be influenced but not compelled to think as somebody else thinks he or she should. In a way, then, people looking for useful moral instruction find themselves at sea. But at least they are free to make their own way to shore. If they work in companies where the ethical ground is untended, they must first escape the corporate influences that stunt the development of an independent capacity to cope with ethical dilemmas. Then in positions of responsibility for others, they can make it easier for their subordinates to avoid the hazards of rationalization and narrow conception of corporate interest. Ethical sophistication makes them realize that the message of ethically consistent decisions will be much clearer, as all behavior is, than codes, credos, or sheaves of written policy.

Saul Gellerman identifies four rationalizations to explain why good managers so often make bad ethical choices. The course of conduct being considered is judged to be within reasonable limits — not "really" wrong. Or because it is in the corporation's best interests, it is to be expected. Or anyway it never will be found out. Or the company will protect the person responsible because the company has benefited. That such shallow justification accounts for the startling behavior associated with the asbestos, the Dalkon shield, and bogus apple juice scandals as well as those long associated with the defense industry and the Pentagon is testimony to the vulnerability of ambitious managers to the perversion of incentives. Middle managers misinterpret senior managers' intent; senior managers, pressed to produce results, do not themselves escape pervasive rationalization. Gellerman's recommended remedial audit and disclosure actions foreshadow the fuller prescriptions of the articles in Part III.

For the individual manager, this article might help harden resistance to what the company demands when those demands imply crossing the wavy line between right and wrong or between sharp and shady. But Albert Z. Carr in "Can an Executive Afford a Conscience?" almost says no to his own question. The company with "a competitive team of managers, a board of directors, and a pride of stockholders" cannot operate in a way that satisfies an active conscience. This is not good news for people seeking to strengthen claims to integrity.

Carr's belief that a company defining right and wrong to "satisfy a well-developed contemporary conscience" could not survive is consistent with the even more astringent views he expresses in "Is Business Bluffing Ethical?" in Part II. But even though the corporate environment he sees is hostile, the plight of the ethically motivated executive, he admits, is not hopeless. It is true that inability to control policy in a company that fails in the ethics of responsibility cannot relieve a person of blame. "He is guilty, so to speak, by employment," for "the ethic of corporate advantage invariably silences and drives out the ethic of individual self-restraint."

Nevertheless, executives in search of a personal policy by which they can maintain their desire for success without serious moral reservation can take a longer-range view of the problems that are the subject of their proposals for achieving their companies' prospective competitive advantage. Nonethical practice is shortsighted, Carr thinks, if for no other reason than it exposes the company to reprisals. "I would go so far as to say," he continues, "that almost anything an executive does, on whatever level, to extend the range of thinking of his superior tends to affect an ethical advance." To connect the "long economic view with the socially aware outlook" is the opportunity of the individual executive with a "contemporary" conscience.

This emphasis on the net advantage of the long-term point of view versus taking immediate profits at the expense of future returns was written in 1970. Much has been said since then about greater attention to future development in the context of our problems of competitiveness with Japan, where pressures for immediate profit are less than ours. We now hear an early note of what will eventually become a chorus proclaiming that when good management is by definition oriented to the long term, it is likely to be ethical. Obversely, short-term management that neglects the imperatives of quality in all dimensions is inherently unethical. Those of you who hope, as I do, that discussion of ethics will merge into, rather than remain apart from, the definition of effective management (and a conception of the role of the corporation broader than the one observed by Carr) should look for this strand of thought woven into the articles that follow.

"Moral Hazards of an Executive," by Louis William Norris, has, like early music, a quaint sound. Its picture of the executive as a cultivated moral person recalls the idealism of the 1950s and what were once conspicuous teachings at the Harvard Business School. Integrity is unblushingly here asserted as the *chief requirement* of executives. Cultural development through education, reading, travel, and conversation with leaders in other walks of life prepares a person to deal with such moral hazards of corporate life as the control of truth. The idea that the chief executive should seek to be a man of thought as well as a man of action is at odds with the contemporary image of the CEO as reorganizer, meeting-goer, report-reader, and organization-joiner in a way that may be useful. Ultimately, Norris's chief executive finds himself searching for principles where his judgment alone is required: "the fulcrum of his judgment comes at least to be a scheme of values." He is big enough for his office when he can deal with the moral issues put before him. Agreeing with this statement again raises the question of how and whether the quality of person required is developed or recognized. This question is of particular importance, I should note, to boards of directors choosing a chief executive officer, planning executive succession, or monitoring the course of management development in a company.

"Personal Values and Business Decisions" by Edmund P. Learned, Arch R. Dooley, and Robert L. Katz—the product in 1959 of the "current upsurge of businessmen's interest in questions of ultimate values"—is another article of more than a generation ago that illuminates truths sometimes lost to sight. The conflict of the materialism and immorality of business life with the spirituality that gives the individual's life meaning has led to an unfortunate compartmentalization of corporate and spiritual values. One school of thought excludes any reference to spiritual values from business decisions; the other adopts the dubious proposition that good ethics *is* good business. The authors propose a process that is essentially an open and forthright interchange among people, however divergent their values. Like Norris with his perception of ethical advance in long-term, future-oriented proposals, Professor Learned and his colleagues argue that seeking and respecting the views of others augments anybody's fragmentary grasp of "God's reality." That reality is the order in the universe never fully understood because of man's imperfections. Here we have the first extended reference to the idea that openness in discussion and inquiry into differences in values are the keys to recognition of ethical issues and then to ethical decisions in business.

For me the most interesting part of this article is its criticism of the proposition that good ethics is good business. Although this saying can neither be proved nor disproved, its plausibility troubles the authors. They think it eliminates the need for painful choices between mutually incompatible alternatives. They think it is of no help in making short-term decisions. As an easy way out of excruciatingly complex situations, the aphorism deadens sensibility to recurring ethical challenges. Because success or failure in business occurs frequently in the presence and absence of the conscious pursuit of ethical values, the slogan is dangerously vulnerable. It also leads to the statement that good business is good ethics. This latter formulation in turn brings with it the untenable assumption that "men of good will will automatically and without conflict serve ultimate values in their actions."

This discussion is still relevant today. In the councils of the Business Roundtable and similar groups of prominent business leaders, the belief that good ethics is indeed good business is often expressed, perhaps as a way of avoiding denigration of the profit-maximizing function of the corporation. The proposition is, after all, a way of justifying acceptance of good intentions as unsentimental or hardheaded. To say that ethics makes money serves as a verbal bridge between self-interest and respect for others, however much it distorts cause and effect. Whether what is meant by the word *business* in the slogan is the hurly-burly of highly competitive trading and cutthroat competition or the management of a corporation with a long tradition of ethical concern for all its constituencies (to call up two extremes) makes a considerable difference. In the latter case, "good ethics is good business" constitutes a tautology; in the former it is nonsense. These authors think the slogan disguises the painful conflict referred to in all the articles so far discussed: choosing between alternative courses of action reflecting different values. The wise choice can be found only in a process of inquiry resulting ultimately in decisions that are better than any one person could contrive alone.

"Skyhooks," by O. A. Ohmann, is the most famous and oldest article in this collection. Constantly in print since 1955, it began the discussion of a kind of leadership appropriate to the demise of economic man — a concept finished off, except among economists and the corporate bar, by the Western Electric experiments and the interest that followed in human behavior in organizations. In a sense, this appeal to the need for a spiritual rebirth in industrial leadership began the challenge to the profit-maximizing model of the corporation and to the techniques that have subsequently occupied more and more of the curricula of business schools. "The concept of economic man as being motivated by self-interest . . . fails to appeal to the true nobility of spirit of which we are capable." The idealized portrait of a successful executive of sound values, with a stewardship conception of his role as boss and the philosophy that attracts good people and repels the shoddy may now (more than thirty years later) be in the process of reconsideration. Some companies use selective recruiting for compatibility of values as a principal means of shaping the future of a company. If the ethical quality of a company's leadership depends upon the character of the leader, then — this article implies — the character of candidates for high office should be closely examined. This article, like those by Norris, and Learned, Dooley, and Katz, embodies in part the approach to action of what used to be taught in the Harvard Business School course called "Administrative Practices." "Skyhooks" has reached and moved thousands of executives. Its influence has not gone so far, however, as to eliminate the underweighting of the intangibles of an art that academics have since tried to convert to a science.

The Learned and Ohmann articles are the last in which God's will is invoked. God has dropped out of the discussion of business ethics in the *Harvard Business Review* and elsewhere, by a choice manifested through its contributors rather than a policy of the editors. A deeper reason may be the increasing diversity of religious belief among the religious, the rejection of the narrow strictures of born-again fundamentalism, the growth of the secularization that finds God in man without talking much about it. No necessary connection unites formal religion and ethics in any case. No specific answer to conflicts of ethical interpretation emerges from the tenets of any religious sect.

We come then to Sir Adrian Cadbury, who as chairman of Cadbury Schweppes addresses in "Ethical Managers Make Their Own Rules" the resolution of clashes of principle. He believes, with his fellow authors, that most business decisions involve a degree of ethical judgment. He joins the authors in this part by stressing that executives must individually assess the economic and social consequences of their actions as best they can and come to their conclusions on limited information in a limited time. Like Learned and his colleagues, Sir Adrian finds it essential in searching for the optimally ethical economic decision to think through who else will be affected by the decision and how to weight their interests. The alliance between openness and ethics is indeed one of the major themes of this collection. Actions that will not stand open scrutiny from the interests affected are probably unethical. Openness in arriving at any decision not only gives those with an interest in the outcome the opportunity to express their views but also exposes to argument the bases upon which the developing decision rests.

Often in the case of a chief executive recording his beliefs, it is not the originality of what he thinks that is of primary interest, but that he thinks it and makes it work for him. Sir Adrian is no exception. He runs a successful company with a long history of ethical concern. His position, experience, and conviction carry enough weight to persuade other executives that they can and must work out their own codes of conduct within the standards that society has a responsibility of supplying. Sir Adrian does not add that it is extremely unlikely that society will be very clear about what it wants. The business person is likely to be thinking of what society *should* want when he or she contemplates the world outside the corporation.

Robert Coles's account of his experience in teaching ethics through the reading and discussion of fiction, in "Storytellers' Ethics," relates to the central problem I alluded to earlier: how to educate people for moral autonomy and awareness. As a psychiatrist, he takes on what the professors of literature are said to have suspended — inquiry into the implications in fiction for the moral imagination of the reader. The observation of character in works of fiction can influence the character of the reader. The idea that an executive can remain active in moral inquiry throughout a lifetime of reading recalls Norris's portrait of the thoughtful executive. Fiction as a moral source, Coles tells us, may reach the heart as well as the mind and thus be more influential than systematic analysis.

So much then for the individual as a moral person — his or her vulnerability to rationalization and betrayal by the apparent (but surely not inevitable) incompatibility of economic and moral values. This series of articles is not a deeply philosophic and definitively useful guide to resolving the moral dilemmas of business leadership. Such a guide is not to be found anywhere. Useful clues, however, to an agenda for productive reflection here await the attention of anyone ready to work out an approach to achieving in an endless series of unique situations consistent quality in the reconciliation of divergent demands. As if speaking for all these authors, Sir Adrian Cadbury tells us that it is the outcome of our choices that makes us who we are.

# 1

# Why "Good" Managers Make Bad Ethical Choices

## SAUL W. GELLERMAN

How could top-level executives at the Manville Corporation have suppressed evidence for decades that proved that asbestos inhalation was killing their own employees?

What could have driven the managers of Continental Illinois Bank to pursue a course of action that threatened to bankrupt the institution, ruined its reputation, and cost thousands of innocent employees and investors their jobs and their savings?

Why did managers at E.F. Hutton find themselves pleading guilty to 2,000 counts of mail and wire fraud, accepting a fine of $2 million, and putting up an $8 million fund for restitution to the 400 banks that the company had systematically bilked?

How can we explain the misbehavior that took place in these organizations—or in any of the others, public and private, that litter our newspapers' front pages: workers at a defense contractor who accused their superiors of falsifying time cards; alleged bribes and kickbacks that honeycombed New York City government; a company that knowingly marketed an unsafe birth control device; the decision-making process that led to the space shuttle Challenger tragedy.

The stories are always slightly different; but they have a lot in common since they're full of the oldest questions in the world, questions of human behavior and human judgment applied in ordinary day-to-day situations. Reading them we have to ask how usually honest, intelligent, compassionate human beings could act in ways that are callous, dishonest, and wrongheaded.

In my view, the explanations go back to four rationalizations that people have relied on through the ages to justify questionable conduct: believing that the activity is not "really" illegal or immoral; that it is in the individual's or the corporation's best interest; that it will never be found out; or that because it helps the company the company will condone it. By looking at these rationalizations in light of these cases, we can develop some practical rules to more effectively control managers' actions that lead to trouble—control, but not eliminate. For the hard truth is that corporate misconduct, like the lowly cockroach, is a plague that we can suppress but never exterminate.

## Three Cases

Amitai Etzioni, professor of sociology at George Washington University, recently concluded that in the last ten years, roughly two-thirds of America's

500 largest corporations have been involved, in varying degrees, in some form of illegal behavior. By taking a look at three corporate cases, we may be able to identify the roots of the kind of misconduct that not only ruins some people's lives, destroys institutions, and gives business as a whole a bad name but that also inflicts real and lasting harm on a large number of innocent people. The three cases that follow should be familiar. I present them here as examples of the types of problems that confront managers in all kinds of businesses daily.

### Manville Corporation

A few years ago, Manville (then Johns Manville) was solid enough to be included among the giants of American business. Today Manville is in the process of turning over 80% of its equity to a trust representing people who have sued or plan to sue it for liability in connection with one of its principal former products, asbestos. For all practical purposes, the entire company was brought down by questions of corporate ethics.

More than 40 years ago, information began to reach Johns Manville's medical department—and through it, the company's top executives—implicating asbestos inhalation as a cause of asbestosis, a debilitating lung disease, as well as lung cancer and mesothelioma, an invariably fatal lung disease. Manville's managers suppressed the research. Moreover, as a matter of policy, they apparently decided to conceal the information from affected employees. The company's medical staff collaborated in the cover-up, for reasons we can only guess at.

Money may have been one motive. In one particularly chilling piece of testimony, a lawyer recalled how 40 years earlier he had confronted Manville's corporate counsel about the company's policy of concealing chest X-ray results from employees. The lawyer had asked, "Do you mean to tell me you would let them work until they dropped dead?" The reply was, "Yes, we save a lot of money that way."

Based on such testimony, a California court found that Manville had hidden the asbestos danger from its employees rather than looking for safer ways to handle it. It was less expensive to pay workers' compensation claims than to develop safer working conditions. A New Jersey court was even blunter: it found that Manville had made a conscious, cold-blooded business decision to take no protective or remedial action, in flagrant disregard of the rights of others.

How can we explain this behavior? Were more than 40 years' worth of Manville executives all immoral?

Such an answer defies common sense. The truth, I think, is less glamorous—and also less satisfying to those who like to explain evil as the actions of a few misbegotten souls. The people involved were probably ordinary men and women for the most part, not very different from you and me. They found themselves in a dilemma, and they solved it in a way that seemed to be the least troublesome, deciding not to disclose information that could hurt their product. The consequences of what they chose to do—both to thousands of innocent people and, ultimately, to the corporation—probably never occurred to them.

The Manville case illustrates the fine line between acceptable and unacceptable managerial behavior. Executives are expected to strike a difficult balance—to pursue their companies' best interests but not overstep the bounds of what outsiders will tolerate.

Even the best managers can find themselves in a bind, not knowing how far is too far. In retrospect, they can usually easily tell where they should have drawn the line, but no one manages in retrospect. We can only live and act today and hope that whoever looks back on what we did will judge that we struck the proper balance. In a few years, many of us may be found delinquent for decisions we are making now about tobacco, clean air, the use of chemicals, or some other seemingly benign substance. The managers at Manville may have believed that they were acting in the company's best interests, or that what they were doing would never be found out, or even that it wasn't really wrong. In the end, these were only rationalizations for conduct that brought the company down.

### Continental Illinois Bank

Until recently the ninth largest bank in the United States, Continental Illinois had to be saved from insolvency because of bad judgment by management. The government bailed it out, but at a price. In effect it has been socialized: about 80% of its equity now belongs to the Federal Deposit Insurance Corporation. Continental seems to have been brought down by managers who misunderstood its real interests. To their own peril, executives focused on a single-minded pursuit of corporate ends and forgot about the means to the ends.

In 1976, Continental's chairman declared that within five years the magnitude of its lending would match that of any other bank. The goal was attainable; in fact, for a time, Continental reached it. But it dictated a shift in strategy away from conservative corporate financing and toward aggressive pursuit of borrowers. So Continental, with lots of lendable funds, sent its loan officers into the field to buy loans that had originally been made by smaller banks that had less money.

The practice in itself was not necessarily unsound. But some of the smaller banks had done more than just lend money—they had swallowed hook, line, and sinker the extravagant, implausible dreams of poorly capitalized oil producers in Oklahoma, and they had begun to bet enormous sums on those dreams. Eventually, a cool billion dollars' worth of those dreams found their way into Continental's portfolio, and a cool billion dollars of depositors' money flowed out to pay for them. When the price of oil fell, a lot of dry holes and idle drilling equipment were all that was left to show for most of the money.

Continental's officers had become so entranced by their lending efforts' spectacular results that they hadn't looked deeply into how they had been achieved. Huge sums of money were lent at fat rates of interest. If the borrowers had been able to repay the loans, Continental might have become the eighth or even the seventh largest bank in the country. But that was a very big "if." Somehow there was a failure of control and judgment at Continental—probably because the officers who were buying those shaky loans were getting support and praise from their superiors. Or at least they were not hearing enough tough questions about them.

At one point, for example, Continental's internal auditors stumbled across the fact that an officer who had purchased $800 million in oil and gas loans from the Penn Square Bank in Oklahoma City had also borrowed $565,000 for himself from Penn Square. Continental's top management investigated and eventually issued a reprimand. The mild rebuke reflected the officer's hard work and the fact that the portfolio he had obtained would have yielded an average return of nearly 20% had it ever performed as planned. In fact, virtually all of the $800 million had to be written off. Management chose to interpret the incident charitably; federal prosecutors later alleged a kickback.

On at least two other occasions, Continental's own control mechanisms flashed signals that something was seriously wrong with the oil and gas portfolio. A vice president warned in a memo that the documentation needed to verify the soundness of many of the purchased loans had simply never arrived. Later, a junior loan officer, putting his job on the line, went over the heads of three superiors to tell a top executive about the missing documentation. Management chose not to investigate. After all, Continental was doing exactly what its chairman had said it would do: it was on its way to becoming the leading commercial lender in the United States. Oil and gas loans were an important factor in that achievement. Stopping to wait for paperwork to catch up would only slow down reaching the goal.

Eventually, however, the word got out about the instability of the bank's portfolio, which led to a massive run on its deposits. No other bank was willing to come to the rescue, for fear of being swamped by Continental's huge liabilities. To avoid going under, Continental in effect became a ward of the federal government. The losers were the bank's shareholders, some officers who lost their jobs, at least one who was indicted, and some 2,000 employees (about 15% of the total) who were let go, as the bank scaled down to fit its diminished assets.

Once again, it is easy for us to sit in judgment after the fact and say that Continental's loan officers and their superiors were doing exactly what bankers shouldn't do: they were gambling with their depositors' money. But on another level, this story is more difficult to analyze—and more generally a part of everyday business. Certainly part of Continental's problem was neglect of standard controls. But another dimension involved ambitious corporate goals. Pushed by lofty goals, managers could not see clearly their real interests. They focused on ends, overlooked the ethical questions associated with their choice of means—and ultimately hurt themselves.

### E.F. Hutton

The nation's second largest independent broker, E.F. Hutton & Company, recently pleaded guilty to 2,000 counts of mail and wire fraud. It had systematically bilked 400 of its banks by drawing against uncollected funds or in some cases against nonexistent sums, which it then covered after having enjoyed interest-free use of the money. So far, Hutton has agreed to pay a fine of $2 million as well as the government's investigation costs of $750,000. It has set up an $8 million reserve for restitution to the banks—which may not be enough. Several officers have lost their jobs, and some indictments may yet follow.

But worst of all, Hutton has tarnished its reputation, never a wise thing to do—certainly not when your business is offering to handle other people's money. Months after Hutton agreed to appoint new directors—as a way to give outsiders a solid majority on the board—the company couldn't find people to accept the seats, in part because of the bad publicity.

Apparently Hutton's branch managers had been encouraged to pay close attention to cash management. At some point, it dawned on someone that using other people's money was even more profitable than using your own. In each case, Hutton's overdrafts involved no large sums. But cumulatively, the savings on interest that would otherwise have been owed to the banks was very large. Because Hutton always made covering deposits, and because most banks did not object, Hutton assured its managers that what they were doing was sharp—and not shady. They presumably thought they were pushing legality to its limit without going over the line. The branch managers were simply taking full advantage of what the law and the bankers' tolerance permitted. On several occasions, the managers who played this game most astutely were even congratulated for their skill.

Hutton probably will not suffer a fate as drastic as Manville's or Continental Illinois's. Indeed, with astute damage control, it can probably emerge from this particular embarrassment with only a few bad memories. But this case has real value because it is typical of much corporate misconduct. Most improprieties don't cut a corporation off at the knees the way Manville's and Continental Illinois's did. In fact, most such actions are never revealed at all—or at least that's how people figure things will work out. And in many cases, a willingness to gamble thus is probably enhanced by the rationalization—true or not—that everyone else is doing something just as bad or would if they could; that those who wouldn't go for their share are idealistic fools.

## Four Rationalizations

Why do managers do things that ultimately inflict great harm on their companies, themselves, and people on whose patronage or tolerance their organizations depend? These three cases, as well as the current crop of examples in each day's paper, supply ample evidence of the motivations and instincts that underlie corporate misconduct. Although the particulars may vary—from the gruesome dishonesty surrounding asbestos handling to the mundanity of illegal money management—the motivating beliefs are pretty much the same. We may examine them in the context of the corporation, but we know that these feelings are basic throughout society; we find them wherever we go because we take them with us.

When we look more closely at these cases, we can delineate four commonly held rationalizations that can lead to misconduct:

A belief that the activity is within reasonable ethical and legal limits— that is, that it is not "really" illegal or immoral.

A belief that the activity is in the individual's or the corporation's best interests—that the individual would somehow be expected to undertake the activity.

A belief that the activity is "safe" because it will never be found out or publicized; the classic crime-and-punishment issue of discovery.

A belief that because the activity helps the company the company will condone it and even protect the person who engages in it.

The idea that an action is not really wrong is an old issue. How far is too far? Exactly where is the line between smart and too smart? Between sharp and shady? Between profit maximization and illegal conduct? The issue is complex: it involves an interplay between top management's goals and middle managers' efforts to interpret those aims.

Put enough people in an ambiguous, ill-defined situation, and some will conclude that whatever hasn't been labeled specifically wrong must be OK—especially if they are rewarded for certain acts. Deliberate overdrafts, for example, were not proscribed at Hutton. Since the company had not spelled out their illegality, it could later plead guilty for itself while shielding its employees from prosecution.

Top executives seldom ask their subordinates to do things that both of them know are against the law or imprudent. But company leaders sometimes leave things unsaid or give the impression that there are things they don't want to know about. In other words, they can seem, whether deliberately or otherwise, to be distancing themselves from their subordinates' tactical decisions in order to keep their own hands clean if things go awry. Often they lure ambitious lower level managers by implying that rich rewards await those who can produce certain results—and that the methods for achieving them will not be examined too closely. Continental's simple wrist-slapping of the officer who was caught in a flagrant conflict of interest sent a clear message to other managers about what top management really thought was important.

How can managers avoid crossing a line that is seldom precise? Unfortunately, most know that they have overstepped it only when they have gone too far. They have no reliable guidelines about what will be overlooked or tolerated or what will be condemned or attacked. When managers must operate in murky borderlands, their most reliable guideline is an old principle: when in doubt, don't.

That may seem like a timid way to run a business. One could argue that if it actually took hold among the middle managers who run most companies, it might take the enterprise out of free enterprise. But there is a difference between taking a worthwhile economic risk and risking an illegal act to make more money.

The difference between becoming a success and becoming a statistic lies in knowledge—including self-knowledge—not daring. Contrary to popular mythology, managers are not paid to take risks; they are paid to know which risks are worth taking. Also, maximizing profits is a company's second priority, not its first. The first is ensuring its survival.

All managers risk giving too much because of what their companies demand from them. But the same superiors who keep pressing you to do more, or to do it better, or faster, or less expensively, will turn on you should you cross that fuzzy line between right and wrong. They will blame you for exceeding instructions or for ignoring their warnings. The smartest managers already know that the best answer to the question, "How far is too far?" is don't try to find out.

Turning to the second reason why people take risks that get their companies into trouble, believing that unethical conduct is in a person's or corporation's best interests nearly always results from a parochial view of what those interests are. For example, Alpha Industries, a Massachusetts manufacturer of microwave equipment, paid $57,000 to a Raytheon manager, ostensibly for a marketing report. Air force investigators charged that the report was a ruse to cover a bribe: Alpha wanted subcontracts that the Raytheon manager supervised. But those contracts ultimately cost Alpha a lot more than they paid for the report. After the company was indicted for bribery, its contracts were suspended and its profits promptly vanished. Alpha wasn't unique in this transgression: in 1984, the Pentagon suspended 453 other companies for violating procurement regulations.

Ambitious managers look for ways to attract favorable attention, something to distinguish them from other people. So they try to outperform their peers. Some may see that it is not difficult to look remarkably good in the short run by avoiding things that pay off only in the long run. For example, you can skimp on maintenance or training or customer service, and you can get away with it — for a while.

The sad truth is that many managers have been promoted on the basis of "great" results obtained in just those ways, leaving unfortunate successors to inherit the inevitable whirlwind. Since this is not necessarily a just world, the problems that such people create are not always traced back to them. Companies cannot afford to be hoodwinked in this way. They must be concerned with more than just results. They have to look very hard at how results are obtained.

Evidently, in Hutton's case there were such reviews, but management chose to interpret favorably what government investigators later interpreted unfavorably. This brings up another dilemma: management quite naturally hopes that any of its borderline actions will be overlooked or at least interpreted charitably if noticed. Companies must accept human nature for what it is and protect themselves with watchdogs to sniff out possible misdeeds.

An independent auditing agency that reports to outside directors can play such a role. It can provide a less comfortable, but more convincing, review of how management's successes are achieved. The discomfort can be considered inexpensive insurance and serve to remind all employees that the real interests of the company are served by honest conduct in the first place.

The third reason why a risk is taken, believing that one can probably get away with it, is perhaps the most difficult to deal with because it's often true. A great deal of proscribed behavior escapes detection.

We know that conscience alone does not deter everyone. For example, First National Bank of Boston pleaded guilty to laundering satchels of $20 bills worth $1.3 billion. Thousands of satchels must have passed through the bank's doors without incident before the scheme was detected. That kind of heavy, unnoticed traffic breeds complacency.

How can we deter wrongdoing that is unlikely to be detected? Make it more likely to be detected. Had today's "discovery" process — in which plaintiff's attorneys can comb through a company's records to look for incriminating evidence — been in use when Manville concealed the evidence on asbestosis, there probably would have been no cover-up. Mindful of the likelihood of detection, Manville would have chosen a different course and could very well be thriving today without the protection of the bankruptcy courts.

The most effective deterrent is not to increase the severity of punishment for those caught but to heighten the perceived probability of being caught in the first place. For example, police have found that parking an empty patrol car at locations where motorists often exceed the speed limit reduces the frequency of speeding. Neighborhood "crime watch" signs that people display decrease burglaries.

Simply increasing the frequency of audits and spot checks is a deterrent, especially when combined with three other simple techniques: scheduling audits irregularly, making at least half of them unannounced, and setting up some checkups soon after others. But frequent spot checks cost more than big sticks, a fact that raises the question of which approach is more cost-effective.

A common managerial error is to assume that because frequent audits uncover little behavior that is out of line, less frequent, and therefore less costly, auditing is sufficient. But this condition overlooks the important deterrent effect of frequent checking. The point is to prevent misconduct, not just to catch it.

A trespass detected should not be dealt with discreetly. Managers should announce the misconduct and how the individuals involved were punished. Since the main deterrent to illegal or unethical behavior is the perceived probability of detection, managers should make an example of people who are detected.

Let's look at the fourth reason why corporate misconduct tends to occur, a belief that the company will condone actions that are taken in its interest and will even protect the managers responsible. The question we have to deal with here is, How do we keep company loyalty from going berserk?

That seems to be what happened at Manville. A small group of executives and a succession of corporate medical directors kept the facts about the lethal qualities of asbestos from becoming public knowledge for decades, and they managed to live with that knowledge. And at Manville, the company—or really, the company's senior management—did condone their decision and protect those employees.

Something similar seems to have happened at General Electric. When one of its missile projects ran up costs greater than the air force had agreed to pay, middle managers surreptitiously shifted those costs to projects that were still operating under budget. In this case, the loyalty that ran amok was primarily to the division: managers want their units' results to look good. But GE, with one of the finest reputations in U.S. industry, was splattered with scandal and paid a fine of $1.04 million.

One of the most troubling aspects of the GE case is the company's admission that those involved were thoroughly familiar with the company's ethical standards before the incident took place. This suggests that the practice of declaring codes of ethics and teaching them to managers is not enough to deter unethical conduct. Something stronger is needed.

Top management has a responsibility to exert a moral force within the company. Senior executives are responsible for drawing the line between loyalty to the company and action against the laws and values of the society in which the company must operate. Further, because that line can be obscured in the heat of the moment, the line has to be drawn well short of where reasonable men and women could begin to suspect that their rights had been violated. The company has to react long before a prosecutor, for instance, would have a strong enough case to seek an indictment.

Executives have a right to expect loyalty from employees against competitors and detractors, but not loyalty against the law, or against common morality, or against society itself. Managers must warn employees that a disservice to customers, and especially to innocent bystanders, cannot be a service to the company. Finally, and most important of all, managers must stress that excuses of company loyalty will not be accepted for acts that place its good name in jeopardy. To put it bluntly, superiors must make it clear that employees who harm other people allegedly for the company's benefit will be fired.

The most extreme examples of corporate misconduct were due, in hindsight, to managerial failures. A good way to avoid management oversights is to subject the control mechanisms themselves to periodic surprise audits, perhaps as a function of the board of directors. The point is to make sure that internal audits and controls are functioning as planned. It's a case of inspecting the inspectors and taking the necessary steps to keep the controls working efficiently. Harold Geneen, former head of ITT, has suggested that the board should have an independent staff, something analogous to the Government Accounting Office, which reports to the legislative rather than the executive branch. In the end, it is up to top management to send a clear and pragmatic message to all employees that good ethics is still the foundation of good business.

# 2

# Can an Executive Afford a Conscience?

ALBERT Z. CARR

Ask a business executive whether his company employs child labor, and he will either think you are joking or be angered by the implied slur on his ethical standards. In the 1970's the employment of children in factories is clearly considered morally wrong as well as illegal.

Yet it was not until comparatively recently (1941) that the U.S. Supreme Court finally sustained the constitutionality of the long-contested Child Labor Act, which Congress had passed four years earlier. During most of the previous eight decades, the fact that children 10 years old worked at manual jobs for an average of 11 hours a day under conditions of virtual slavery had aroused little indignation in business circles.

To be sure, only a few industries found the practice profitable, and the majority of businessmen would doubtless have been glad to see it stopped. But in order to stop it the government had to act, and any interference with business by government was regarded as a crime against God, Nature, and Respectability. If a company sought to hold down production costs by employing children in factories where the work did not demand adult skills or muscle, that was surely a matter to be settled between the employer and the child's parents or the orphanage.

To permit legitimate private enterprise to be balked by unrealistic do-gooders was to open the gate to socialism and anarchy — such was the prevailing sentiment of businessmen, as shown in the business press, from the 1860's to the 1930's.

Every important advance in business ethics has been achieved through a long history of pain and protest.[1] The process of change begins when a previously accepted practice arouses misgivings among sensitive observers. Their efforts at moral suasion are usually ignored, however, until changes in economic conditions or new technology make the practice seem increasingly undesirable.

Businessmen who profit by the practice defend it heatedly, and a long period of public controversy ensues, climaxed at last by the adoption of laws forbidding it. After another 20 or 30 years, the new generation of businessmen regard the practice with retrospective moral indignation and wonder why it was ever tolerated.

A century of increasingly violent debate culminating in civil war had to be lived through before black slavery, long regarded as an excellent business proposition, was declared unlawful in the United States. To achieve laws forbidding racial discrimination in hiring practices required another century. It took 80 years of often bloody labor disputes to win acceptance of the principle of collective bargaining, and the country endured about 110 years of flagrant financial abuses before enactment of effective measures regulating banks and stock exchanges.

In time, all of these forward steps, once bitterly opposed by most businessmen, came to be accepted as part of the ethical foundation of the American private enterprise economy.

## Jesse James versus Nero

In the second half of the twentieth century, with the population, money supply, military power, and industrial technology of the United States expanding rapidly at the same time, serious new ethical issues have arisen for businessmen — notably the pollution of the biosphere, the concentration of economic power in a relatively few vast corporations, increasing military domination of the economy, and the complex interrelationship between business interests and the threat of war. These issues are the more formidable because they demand swift response; they will not wait a century or even a generation for a change in corporate ethics that will stimulate businessmen to act.

The problems they present to business and our society as a whole are immediate, critical, and worsening. If they are not promptly dealt with by farsighted and effective measures, they could even bring down political democracy and the entrepreneurial system together.

In fact, given the close relationship between our domestic economic situation and our military commitments abroad, and the perils implicit in the worldwide armaments buildup, it is not extreme to say that the extent to which businessmen are able to open their minds to new ethical imperatives in the decade ahead may have decisive influence in this century on the future of the human species.

Considering the magnitude of these rapidly developing issues, old standards of ethical judgment seem almost irrelevant. It is of course desirable that a businessman be honest in his accountings and faithful to his contracts — that he should not advertise misleadingly, rig prices, deceive stockholders, deny workers their due, cheat customers, spread false rumors about competitors, or stab associates in the back. Such a person has in the past qualified as "highly ethical," and he could feel morally superior to many of those he saw around him — the chiselers, the connivers, the betrayers of trust.

But standards of personal conduct in themselves are no longer an adequate index of business ethics. Everyone knows that a minority of businessmen commit commercial mayhem on each other and on the public with practices ranging from subtle conflicts of interest to the sale of injurious drugs and unsafe automobiles, but in the moral crisis through which we are living such tales of executive wrongdoing, like nudity in motion pictures, have lost their power to shock.

The public shrugs at the company president who conspires with his peers to fix prices. It grins at the vice president in charge of sales who provides call girls for a customer. After we have heard a few such stories, they become monotonous.

We cannot shrug or grin, however, at the refusal of powerful corporations to take vigorous action against great dangers threatening the society, and to which they contribute. Compared with such a corporation or with the executive who is willing to jeopardize the health and well-being of an entire people in order to add something to current earnings, the man who merely embezzles company funds is as insignificant in the annals of morality as Jesse James is compared with Nero.

The moral position of the executive who works for a company that fails in the ethics of social responsibility is ambiguous. The fact that he does not control company policy cannot entirely exonerate him from blame. He is guilty, so to speak, by employment.

If he is aware that the company's factories pollute the environment or its products injure the consumer and he does not exert himself to change the related company policies, he becomes morally suspect. If he lends himself to devious evasions of laws against racial discrimination in hiring practices, he adds to the probability of destructive racial confrontations and is in some degree an agent of social disruption. If he knows that his company is involved in the bribery of legislators or government officials, or makes under-the-table deals with labor union officials, or uses the services of companies known to be controlled by criminal syndicates, he contributes through his work to disrespect for law and the spread of crime.

If his company, in its desire for military contracts, lobbies to oppose justifiable cuts in the government's enormous military budget, he bears some share of responsibility for the constriction of the civilian economy; for price inflation, urban decay, and shortages of housing, transportation, and schools; and for failure to mitigate the hardships of the poor.

From this standpoint, the carefully correct executive who never violates a law or fails to observe the canons of gentlemanly behavior may be as open to ethical challenge as the crooks and the cheaters.

## "Toxins of Suppressed Guilt"

The practical question arises: If a man in a responsible corporate position finds that certain policies of his company are socially injurious, what can he do about it without jeopardizing his job?

Contrary to common opinion, he is not necessarily without recourse. The nature of that recourse I shall discuss in the final section of this article. Here, I want to point out that unless the executive's sense of social responsibility is accompanied by a high degree of realism about tactics, then he is likely to end in frustration or cynicism.

One executive of my acquaintance who wrote several memoranda to his chief, detailing instances of serious environmental contamination for which the company was responsible and which called for early remedy, was sharply rebuked for a "negative attitude."

Another, a successful executive of a large corporation, said to me quite seriously in a confidential moment that he did not think a man in a job like his could afford the luxury of a conscience in the office. He was frank to say that he had become unhappy about certain policies of his company. He could no longer deny to himself that the company was not living up to its social responsibilities and was engaged in some political practices that smacked of corruption.

But what were his options? He had only three that he could see, and he told me he disliked them all:

If he argued for a change in policies that were helping to keep net earnings high, he might be branded by his superiors as "unrealistic" or "idealistic" — adjectives that could check his career and might, if he pushed too hard, compel his resignation.

Continued silence not only would spoil his enjoyment of his work, but might cause him to lose respect for himself.

If he moved to one of the other companies in his industry, he would merely be exchanging one set of moral misgivings for another.

He added with a sigh that he envied his associates whose consciences had never developed beyond the Neanderthal stage and who had no difficulty in accepting things as they were. He said he wondered whether he ought not to try to discipline himself to be as indifferent as they to the social implications of policies which, after all, were common in business.

Perhaps he made this effort and succeeded in it, for he remained with the company and forged ahead. He may even have fancied that he had killed his conscience — as the narrator in Mark Twain's symbolic story did when he gradually reached the point where he could blithely murder the tramps who came to his door asking for handouts.

But conscience is never killed; when ignored, it merely goes underground, where it manufactures the toxins of suppressed guilt, often with serious psychological and physical consequences. The hard fact is that the executive who has a well-developed contemporary conscience is at an increasing disadvantage in business unless he is able to find some personal policy by which he can maintain his drive for success without serious moral reservations.

## Distrustful Public

The problem faced by the ethically motivated man in corporate life is compounded by growing public distrust of business morality.

The corporation executive is popularly envied for his relative affluence and respected for his powers of achievement, but many people deeply suspect his ethics — as not a few successful businessmen have been informed by their children. Surveys made in a number of universities across the country indicate that a large majority of students aiming at college degrees are convinced that business is a dog-eat-dog proposition, with which most of them do not want to be connected.

This low opinion is by no means confined to youngsters; a poll of 2,000 representative Americans brought to light the belief of nearly half of them that "most businessmen would try anything, honest or not, for a buck."[2] The unfairness of the notion does not make it less significant as a clue to public opinion. (This poll also showed that most Americans are aware of the notable contributions of business to the material satisfactions of their lives; the two opinions are not inconsistent.)

Many businessmen, too, are deeply disturbed by the level of executive morality in their sphere of observation. Although about 90% of executives in another survey stated that they regarded themselves as "ethical," 80% affirmed "the presence of numerous generally accepted practices in their industry which they consider unethical," such as bribery of government officials, rigging of prices, and collusion in contract bidding.[3]

The public is by no means unaware of such practices. In conversations about business ethics with a cross-section sampling of citizens in a New England town,

I found that they mentioned kickbacks and industrial espionage as often as embezzlement and fraud. One man pointed out that the kickback is now taken so much for granted in corporations that the Internal Revenue Service provides detailed instructions for businessmen on how to report income from this source on their tax returns.

The indifference of many companies to consumers' health and safety was a major source of criticism. Several of the persons interviewed spoke of conflicts of interest among corporation heads, accounts of which had been featured not long before in the press. Others had learned from television dramas about the ruthlessness of the struggle for survival and the hail-fellow hypocrisy that is common in executive offices.

Housewives drew on their shopping experience to denounce the decline in the quality of necessities for which they had to pay ever-higher prices. Two or three had read in *Consumer Reports* about "planned obsolescence."

I came to the conclusion that if my sample is at all representative—and I think it is—the public has learned more about the ways of men in corporate life than most boards of directors yet realize.

These opinions were voiced by people who for the most part had not yet given much thought to the part played by industrial wastes in the condition of the environment, or to the inroads made on their economic well-being by the influence of corporation lobbyists on military decision makers. It is to be expected that if, as a result of deteriorating social and economic conditions, these and other major concerns take on more meaning for the public, criticism of business ethics will widen and become sharper.

If the threats of widespread water shortage in the 1970's and of regional clean air shortages in the 1980's are allowed to materialize, and military expenditures continue to constrict civilian life, popular resentment may well be translated into active protest directed against many corporations as well as against the government. In that event, the moral pressure on individual executives will become increasingly acute.

Regard for public opinion certainly helped to influence many companies in the 1950's and 1960's to pledge to reduce their waste discharges into the air and water and to hire more people with dark skins. Such declarations were balm for the sore business conscience.

The vogue for "social responsibility" has now grown until, as one commentator put it, "pronouncements about social responsibility issue forth so abundantly from the corporations that it is hard for one to get a decent play in the press. Everybody is in on the act, and nearly all of them actually mean what they say!"[4] More than a few companies have spent considerable sums to advertise their efforts to protect a stream, clean up smokestack emissions, or train "hardcore unemployables."

These are worthy undertakings, as far as they have gone, but for the most part they have not gone very far. In 1970 it has become obvious that the performance of U.S. corporations in the area of social responsibility has generally been trivial, considering the scope of their operations.

## Behind the Boardroom Door

No company that I have ever heard of employs a vice president in charge of ethical standards; and sooner or later the conscientious executive is likely to come up against a stone wall of corporate indifference to private moral values.

When the men who hold the real power in the company come together to decide policy, they may give lip service to the moral element in the issue, but not much more. The decision-making process at top-management levels has little room for social responsibilities not definitely required by law or public opinion.

Proposals that fail to promise an early payoff for the company and that involve substantial expense are accepted only if they represent a means of escaping drastic penalties, such as might be inflicted by a government suit, a labor strike, or a consumer boycott. To invest heavily in antipollution equipment or in programs for hiring and training workers on the fringe of employability, or to accept higher taxation in the interest of better education for the children of a community—for some distant, intangible return in a cloudy future—normally goes against the grain of every profit-minded management.

It could hardly be otherwise. In the prevailing concept of corporate efficiency, a continual lowering of costs relative to sales is cardinal. For low costs are a key not only to higher profits but to corporate maneuverability, to advantage in recruiting the best men, and to the ability to at least hold a share of a competitive market.

Of the savings accruing to a company from lowered costs, the fraction that finds its way into the area of social responsibility is usually minuscule. To expend such savings on nonremunerative activities is regarded as weakening the corporate structure.

The late Chester I. Barnard, one of the more enlightened business leaders of the previous generation and a man deeply concerned with ethics, voiced the position of management in the form of a question: "To what extent is one morally justified in loading a productive undertaking with heavy charges in the attempt to protect against a remote possibility, or even one not so remote?"[5] Speaking of accident prevention in plants, which he favored in principle, he warned that if the outlay for such a purpose weakened the company's finances, "the community might lose a service and the entrepreneur an opportunity."

Corporate managers apply the same line of reasoning to proposals for expenditure in the area of social responsibility. "We can't afford to sink that amount of money in nonproductive uses," they say, and, "We need all our cash for expansion."

The entrepreneur who is willing to accept some reduction of his income—the type is not unknown—may be able to operate his enterprise in a way that satisfies an active conscience; but a company with a competitive team of managers, a board of directors, and a pride of stockholders cannot harbor such an unbusinesslike intention.

Occasionally, statesmen, writers, and even some high-minded executives, such as the late Clarence B. Randall, have made the appeal of conscience to corporations. They have argued that, since the managers and directors of companies are for the most part men of goodwill in their private lives, their corporate decisions also should be guided by conscience.

Even the distinguished economist A.A. Berle, Jr., has expressed the view that the healthy development of our society requires "the growth of conscience" in the corporation of our time.[6] But if by "conscience" he meant a sense of right and wrong transcending the economic, he was asking the impossible.

A business that defined "right" and "wrong" in terms that would satisfy a well-developed contemporary conscience could not survive. No company can be expected to serve the social interest unless its self-interest is also served, either by the expectation of profit or by the avoidance of punishment.

### "Gresham's Law" of Ethics

Before responsibility to the public can properly be brought into the framework of a top-management decision, it must have an economic justification. For instance, executives might say:

"We'd better install the new safety feature because, if we don't, we'll have the government on our necks, and the bad publicity will cost us more than we are now saving in production."

"We should spend the money for equipment to take the sulfides out of our smokestacks at the plant. Otherwise we'll have trouble recruiting labor and have a costly PR problem in the community."

It is worth noting that Henry Ford II felt constrained to explain to stockholders of the Ford Motor Company that his earnest and socially aware effort to recruit workers from Detroit's "hard-core unemployed" was a preventive measure against the recurrence of ghetto riots carrying a threat to the company.

In another situation, when a number of life insurance companies agreed to invest money in slum reconstruction at interest rates somewhat below the market, their executives were quick to forestall possible complaints from stockholders by pointing out that they were opening up future markets for life insurance. Rationally, the successful corporate manager can contemplate expense for the benefit of society only if failure to spend points to an eventual loss of security or opportunity that exceeds the cost.

There can be no conscience without a sense of personal responsibility, and the corporation, as Ambrose Bierce remarked, is "an ingenious device for obtaining individual profit without individual responsibility." When the directors and managers of a corporation enter the boardroom to debate policy, they park their private consciences outside.

If they did not subordinate their inner scruples to considerations of profitability and growth, they would fail in their responsibility to the company that pays them. A kind of Gresham's Law of ethics operates here; the ethic of corporate advantage invariably silences and drives out the ethic of individual self-restraint.

(This, incidentally, is true at every level of the corporate structure. An executive who adheres to ethical standards disregarded by his associates is asking for trouble. No one, for example, is so much hated in a purchasing department where graft is rife as the man who refuses to take kickbacks from suppliers, for he threatens the security of the others. Unless he conforms, they are all too likely to "get him.")

The crucial question in boardroom meetings where social responsibility is discussed is not, "Are we morally obligated to do it?" but, rather, "What will happen if we don't do it?" or, perhaps, "How will this affect the rate of return on investment?"

If the house counsel assures management that there will be no serious punishment under the law if the company does not take on the added expense, and the marketing man sees no danger to sales, and the public relations man is confident he can avoid injury to the corporate image, then the money, if it amounts to any considerable sum, will not be spent—social responsibility or no social responsibility.

Even the compulsion of law is often regarded in corporate thinking as an element in a contest between government and the corporation, rather than as a description of "right" and "wrong." The files of the Federal Trade Commission, the Food and Drug Administration, and other government agencies are filled with records of respectable companies that have not hesitated to break or stretch the law when they believed they could get away with it.

It is not unusual for company managements to break a law, even when they expect to be caught, if they calculate that the fine they eventually must pay represents only a fraction of the profits that the violation will enable them to collect in the meantime. More than one corporate merger has been announced to permit insiders to make stock-market killings even though the companies concerned recognized that the antitrust laws would probably compel their eventual separation.

## What Can the Executive Do?

One can dream of a big-business community that considers it sound economics to sacrifice a portion of short-term profits in order to protect the environment and reduce social tensions.

It is theoretically conceivable that top managers as a class may come to perceive the profound dangers, for the free-enterprise system and for themselves, in the trend toward the militarization of our society, and will press the government to resist the demand for nonessential military orders and overpermissive contracts from sections of industry and elements in the Armed Services. At the same level of wishfulness, we can imagine the federal government making it clear to U.S. companies investing abroad that protection of their investments is not the government's responsibility.

We can even envisage a time when the bonds of a corporation that is responsive to social needs will command a higher rating by Moody's than those of a company that neglects such values, since the latter is more vulnerable to public condemnation; and a time when a powerful Executive League for Social Responsibility will come into being to stimulate and assist top managements in formulating long-range economic policies that embrace social issues. In such a private-enterprise utopia the executive with a social conscience would be able to work without weakening qualms.

In the real world of today's business, however, he is almost sure to be a troubled man. Perhaps there are some executives who are so strongly positioned that they can afford to urge their managements to accept a reduced rate of return on investment for the sake of the society of which they are a part. But for the large majority of corporate employees who want to keep their jobs and win their superiors' approbation, to propose such a thing would be inviting oneself to the corporate guillotine.

### He Is Not Powerless

But this does not necessarily mean that the ethically motivated executive can do nothing. In fact, if he does nothing, he may so bleach his conception of himself as a man of conviction as to reduce his personal force and value to the company. His situation calls for sagacity as well as courage. Whatever ideas he advocates to express his sense of social responsibility must be shaped to the company's interests.

Asking management flatly to place social values ahead of profits would be foolhardy, but if he can demonstrate that, on the basis of long-range profitability, the concept of corporate efficiency needs to be broadened to include social values, he may be able to make his point without injury—indeed, with benefit—to his status in the company. A man respected for competence in his job, who knows how to justify ethically based programs in economic terms and to overcome elements of resistance in the psychology of top management, may well be demonstrating his own qualifications for top management.

In essence, any ethically oriented proposal made to a manager is a proposal to take a longer-range view of his problems—to lift his sights. Nonethical practice is shortsighted almost by definition, if for no other reason than that it exposes the company to eventual reprisals.

The longer range a realistic business projection is, the more likely it is to find a sound ethical footing. I would go so far as to say that almost anything an executive does, on whatever level, to extend the range of thinking of his superiors tends to effect an ethical advance.

The hope and the opportunity of the individual executive with a contemporary conscience lie in the constructive connection of the long economic view with the socially aware outlook. He must show convincingly a net advantage for the corporation in accelerating expenditures or accepting other costs in the sphere of social responsibility.

I was recently able to observe an instance in which an executive persuaded his company's management to make a major advance in its antipollution policy. His presentation of the alternatives, on which he had spent weeks of careful preparation, showed in essence that, under his plan, costs which would have to be absorbed over a three-year period would within six years prove to be substantially less than the potential costs of less vigorous action.

When he finished his statement, no man among his listeners, not even his most active rivals, chose to resist him. He had done more than serve his company and satisfy his own ethical urge; he had shown that the gap between the corporate decision and the private conscience is not unbridgeable if a person is strong enough, able enough, and brave enough to do what needs to be done.

It may be that the future of our enterprise system will depend on the emergence of a sufficient number of men of this breed who believe that in order to save itself business will be impelled to help save the society.

### NOTES

1. For amplifications of this view, see Robert W. Austin, "Responsibility for Social Change," HBR July–August 1965, p. 45; and Theodore Levitt, "Why Business Always Loses," HBR March–April 1968, p. 81.
2. Louis B. Harris and Associates, in a survey reported at a National Industrial Conference Board meeting, April 21, 1966.
3. Raymond C. Baumhart, S.J., "How Ethical Are Businessmen?" HBR July–August 1961, p. 6.
4. Theodore Levitt, "The Dangers of Social Responsibility," HBR September–October 1958, p. 41.

5. *Elementary Conditions of Business Morals* (Berkeley: Committee on the Barbara Weinstock Lectures, University of California, 1958).

6. *The Twentieth Century Capitalist Revolution* (New York: Harcourt, Brace, 1954), pp. 113–114.

# 3

# Moral Hazards of an Executive

## LOUIS WILLIAM NORRIS

No business, educational, or political executive today would be so foolhardy as to reiterate Cornelius Vanderbilt in saying, "Let the public be damned." He knows he would not be able to market his product or gain public support on such a platform. Nor would he be caught muttering even under his breath, "Let the employees be damned." His success depends too much on their contentment for any such invective, even when he is positively sure their wage demands are preposterous. His shiny office intercom may, on the other hand, bring in a detectable, "Let the president be damned." For the executive is knowingly involved in the private lives of more people than ever before in history. They let him know what they think of *his* policies.

For an executive, the chief crises are moral. Since his job is so rarely impersonal, his principal problems are what he does about people. He may have started out as a master craftsman, teacher, or production expert, but as an executive he is daily putting into action plans for people to carry out, which will in turn affect other people. The criteria that guide his actions—his morals, in short—are therefore the most important features of his term of service as an executive. He is continuously on the radarscope of public judgment.

It is my thesis in this article that one of the key tests of an executive is his capacity to face the hazards and problems of:

1. Living with the necessity of compromise—but never compromising too much.

2. Being free to disclose only parts of the truth on many occasions, yet needing to see the whole truth.

3. Having to make final decisions but on the basis of incomplete facts.

4. Accepting responsibility for the mistakes of subordinates while not allowing them to make *too many* mistakes.

5. Living up to the image that the public and his associates demand of a man in high office, but not becoming the victim of it.

6. Succeeding as a man of thought as well as a man of action.

## No Recipes

Many have taken pity on the harried executive and tried to show him how to succeed. For example:

In *The Executive Life*,[1] the editors of *Fortune* get down to fundamentals of how to become an executive, how to avoid getting fired, how to manage raises, control the threat of overwork, and similar questions, but they do not identify or provide guidance through the crucial tests of the executive. These tests are moral, for they concern not only what the executive *does*, but what he *should* do.

Others have looked to the education of the executive. The Fund for Adult Education compiled some essays under the title, *Toward the Liberally Educated Executive*.[2] These have been reprinted by popular demand. We are told here that the executive must have a cultivated mind, but not that he must have a cultivated set of morals.

David Lilienthal's *Big Business: A New Era*,[3] shows that America's destiny will be best realized through big organizations and, therefore, through the aid of big executives. Their social, political, and economic influence is enormous, to be sure. He does not, however, show the moral import of such a condition.

The big executives belong to *The Power Elite*,[4] as C. Wright Mills notes. But while the moral standards of the power elite constitute the crux of their social function, that fact remains to be elaborated.

William H. Whyte, Jr., in *The Organization Man*[5] and Alan Harrington in *Life in the Crystal Palace*[6] warn of the hazards in bureaucracy. But what of the moral hazards?

### Moral Maze

Success is demanded of an executive, whether of a distillery or a college. He must stay in office to exercise his functions. He does not become prime minister to preside over the dissolution of his majesty's empire. Even if he and his family own the company, he must succeed in the competitive whirl, or there will be no company over which he may reign as an executive. Hence, a standard of success, which must derive ultimately from moral issues, becomes inevitable. The thoughtful businessman may wonder what test measures his success. Is it

Growth of his organization?

Development of efficiency in production?

Gain in goodwill toward the corporation?

Extension of service to the public?

If any or all these criteria figure in the executive's mind, should they? Does his business *need* to grow? Is there any point to improving production? Suppose the public comes to think better of his organization? Is this change worth the executive's ulcers? Does the public deserve to have the services an executive makes available to them? Or is a supposed service really a luxury that has become a necessity, or even a threat to health and emotional well-being?

Let it not be affirmed with fine disdain that such moral questions are impertinent, impractical, or ephemeral. Some standard of values is assumed or expressed in all thought and action. The executive thinks and acts in the interest of a "better" alternative. He is all wrapped up in moral hazards before he gets into his clothes in the morning. He puts them aside only with the skillful aid of Morpheus again that night—though if Freud is right, they even cling to him in his dreams.

What are the hazards which no executive can bypass, jump over, or wave out of his way?

## Living with Compromise

First of all, the executive in any organization, even of modest complexity, must live on a diet of compromise. Democracy has come to be expected in business, education, and nearly every form of administration, as well as in politics. Leadership rests on an amalgamation of opinion, a fusion of standards. A healthy administrative organization encourages differences and originality of judgment. All this is to the good, but it makes for everyday aches and pains. To illustrate:

The junior executive must be a "comer"—an idea man. Not always will he see eye to eye with senior, more experienced men. Whose counsel shall the chief executive take?

The judgment of the public served is a potent force to be considered in product styling, community relations, and other areas. Shall the policy of the company agree with, educate, or ignore the public? Usually a combination of these factors is chosen.

Every school and college seeks to educate its students to avoid the errors of their elders. To secure the support of these elders, while their youth are being set 25 years ahead of them, takes some doing. Typically it requires compromise of ideals. At least they must be indirectly sought or delayed. The school administrator in large areas of the country, including some districts north of the Mason-Dixon Line, must let integration remain an ideal, while the real feelings of his community play themselves out in some form of intolerance.

Woodrow Wilson found it impossible to compromise on the location of the graduate school at Princeton, or on America's entry into the League of Nations. In the one case, it was expedient for him to resign from Princeton; and, in the other, he brought on the break in his health which was to shorten his life. Was he merely a poor diplomat, or was he illustrating that some issues do not lend themselves to compromise? He had to act, as every executive must, whether his constituents were ready to move with him or not.

### Conflicts of Interest

Let the executive be alert to the kinds of compromise he inevitably makes.

For one thing, he must choose between present and long-term values. Shall the dividends be higher or the capital improvements greater? Is a curriculum change to meet the needs of the time as important as one that fulfills the needs that are timeless? Secondly, a conflict between individual and institutional values must often be resolved. Loyalty to an institution is fundamental to the institution's success. Yet an individual can hinder its success in spite of his loyalty. It might be better for the company for the vice president to be dismissed, though this could ruin his health and reputation. A student might be better off to be permitted continuance in college, though forgiveness of his offense would smirch the honor of old Siwash.

Again, shall decisions be made in the interests of few or many? Democratic morality commonly holds its nose when legislative or executive action is taken or threatened that favors the few. Witness Teapot Dome, or the Dixon-Yates contract. Yet who can say with certainty that F.D.R. should not have run for a third or fourth term? Would anyone else have brought the war to a close sooner? As pressure mounts for admission to college, should a college plan to concentrate its efforts on the intellectual elite, or serve a cross section of the masses?

Unquestionably the most significant compromises are those that balance material and nonmaterial values. Although advertising that plays on the vanity, fear, craving for status, and pride of purchasers may sell the product, the advertising executive may do well to resist trying to win his promotion by performance on these keys alone. And a trade union executive may emphasize the economic needs of his union to such an extent that other and more spiritual advantages already possessed dim out of sight in the eyes of members.

There are benefits in compromise. Often it is the only way to secure group action. The price of diverse wisdom among differing people may be mutual adjustment before action is possible. Further, such compromise educates differing individuals, who try out hypotheses urged by their opponents. In the end, compromise may be the way ideals actualize themselves. Executives of the church found it necessary to compromise with the Roman Empire, property owners, and social leaders to prevent its ideals from remaining a kingdom of heaven, found only in heaven.

Perhaps the chief evil in compromise lies in its apparent disregard of universal principle. An executive undermines his own influence if he becomes motivated largely by expediency. The great executives have been considered "men of principle," no matter how much they may have trimmed their sails on minor points. Virtue remains largely a habit of the will to follow principle, as Aristotle and Kant emphasized. Members of any institution want the security supplied by the knowledge that their executive is "unpurchasable," to use a term made prominent by William Ernest Hocking.[7] Deviation from principle may become habit forming. Fear of mediocrity, shortsightedness, or unpredictability sets in when principle falls out.

### Implications for Action

Every executive must calculate the strength in the tension between the values of compromise and adherence to principle. He will safeguard himself if he seeks to become clearly conscious of the compromises made in nearly every important decision. Choices between black and white are easy. But they never come to a top executive! He is also well advised to keep a chronic idealist in his organization. His conscience should be pricked by this trusted aid every time matters of principle are brought down into the dusty flats of earthy action.

## Control of Truth

Another moral hazard besetting the executive resides in his control of truth on many occasions. It is rare that an executive has the privilege of telling the truth, the whole truth, and nothing but the truth. To take a common illustration, truth, bluntly told, may hurt a subordinate who is incompetent or misguided. When improvement by this subordinate is possible, tactful treatment of the fault to be corrected will involve adroit selection of truths that can be told. So far, so good. But if the executive withholds truth on this occasion, he will on others. Can he be trusted to withhold the *right* truths?

And let us not delude ourselves about the frequency with which these occasions occur in and out of the office. No manager can escape all of them:

A college executive who pointed out to a prospective benefactor, even though truly, that his wealth was accumulated through exploitational labor practices or questionable marketing policies, would soon be looking for another job. He would, in this case, hold to the theory of transubstantiation as far as wealth given to his institution is concerned. The truth about his benefactor would have to wait!

Would a successful sales executive counsel his staff not to sell to those who could not afford to buy? Certainly not very often, and probably never at all.

If an executive consoles himself by saying that even marital bliss requires him not to tell all to his wife when he returns from a business trip, he must realize that he gambles regularly one truth against another, and there is danger in such gambling.

Timing the release of information to the public may involve manipulation of the truth. For instance, though it has been known for some time, figures about the stockpiling of surpluses may be released just before a labor contract runs out; a rise in college fees may be announced at Christmastime when good cheer neutralizes the chilling news that more dollars are needed for education; and a political executive may advise against additional taxes in an election year, knowing they will be necessary the next year.

Obviously, no executive tells all he knows as soon as he knows it!

Emphasis on the value of one's own product or service may suggest the idea (sometimes false, sometimes not) that other products or services are inferior or even nonexistent. An executive of nearly any organization serves as a promoter of it. The ever-present possibility exists that his special pleading will be too successful. In *The Hidden Persuaders*,[8] Vance Packard has shown vividly (even if exaggeratedly) how controllable the public is. The moral issue for the executive consists in whether his organization deserves to control the public in such measure as it seeks to do. For control usually results from withholding some truths while emphasizing others. One need only recall that this has been the avowed means of propaganda used by dictators, if he wants to recognize the gravity of such an issue.

### The Test of Integrity

Of course, to possess partial truth about a subject, or to give out partial truth to others, does not invalidate necessarily the truth as far as it goes. Indeed, it is rarely possible to set forth the whole truth about anything in a single sentence. For truth is a whole system of propositions, values, and relations, and only part of a system can be handled at a time.

The crux of the matter lies in how much importance is attached to that part of the whole which is mentioned, and in how much implied significance is assigned to the remainder that is unmentioned. And how plain is it made that there is a larger whole of truth within which a given proposition or plan of action rests? This must be taken as crucial also. The executive has to look to the orientation of the truth he chooses to emphasize. An advertising statement like "More people are buying one" *could* mean that only three have bought one, as long as just two did last year!

It may be asked whether an executive must be responsible if the publics with which he deals lack powers of critical thought. The answer lies in the fact that every man is responsible in some measure for his actions *and for their effects*.

Surely if a man were idolized as a public hero, he would scarcely think of his position as an accident, but as a consequence of his actions. So, too, must he recognize responsibility for those of his actions that are not considered noble, or might not be so considered if all the facts were recognized.

Integrity becomes the chief requirement for the executive. He can be trusted with the direction of his organization only if he is able to interrelate in one whole all of its affairs. He must see the whole truth about the operations of his institution, and handle the partial truths called for on each occasion by reference to this whole. A man of integrity is a fully integrated man. He can become so and remain so only by constant regard for the whole system of facts he knows — those he does not disclose as well as those he does.

## Finality of Decisions

A third moral dilemma for the executive arises from the many occasions when his judgment alone must be taken as final. Broad matters of policy are usually set by a board of directors, but these are often recommended by the chief executive and, when approved, they are interpreted and applied by him. Often responsibility for a decision can be lodged nowhere else. Some subordinates relish freedom from basic decisions and delight in passing them up the line of command. The president is indeed "the recipient of the ultimate buck." Democracy is more fun for subordinates than it is for top executives!

Time often requires decisions before all the facts are in, or can be obtained. General Eisenhower rightly chose to invade Normandy during bad weather. He counted on the Nazis' belief that the Allied Powers would not risk such weather. He did not *know* they would leave some positions thinly guarded for this reason, but he judged correctly. This is essentially the definition of genius given by the late Justice Holmes. "Genius," he said, "is the capacity to reach the proper conclusion before all the facts are in." The executive is often called on to be a genius. He dare not be wrong, though it may be his own judgment alone he can trust. If he is wrong, the disaster may be overwhelming.

A responsible executive seeks counsel where possible. But some problems cannot be discussed with others. For instance, financial and personnel questions are sometimes so confidential as to require complete secrecy. Besides, no one else has the point of view or responsibility of the chief executive, and rarely the relevant experience. Friendships with associates must remain temperate, for the executive cannot avoid sitting in judgment on the work of his colleagues. He must avoid bias, both seeming and real. A measure of aloofness becomes the price of objectivity.

### Perspective through Values

A certain unavoidable loneliness is attached, consequently, to administrative leadership. The executive may vacillate between overconfidence and underconfidence in his own judgment. Persistent success may breed overconfidence, while too many failures crack morale. If this loneliness becomes apparent to colleagues, the boss finds himself an object of pity and a cause of hushed conversations on his approach. He must like his job, however severe the discipline of issues he must handle alone.

Presumably the executive is one of the best informed men about his organization, else he would not be put in office. He must demand of every subordinate information, in relevant form, about his business, and he must call on "idea men" for help in making changes. But his chief need is for help on problems no one else knows much about. He will find himself searching for principles to guide him where his judgment alone is required. And the fulcrum of his judgment comes at last to be a scheme of values.

What are the aims of my organization? What values does it contribute to my generation, and to those yet to come? What satisfactions should my employees derive from their work? And when I die, what do I hope to be my life's chief accomplishment?

These are questions whose answers serve as a base line for proceeding to handle problems where the boss's judgment alone prevails. Aristotle's *Ethics*, "The Sermon on the Mount," and Whitehead's *Science and the Modern World*[9] should provide perspective. A diet of these discerning analyses of value helps to remove an executive from worry about "his" problems, keep him fresh and humble, and set him on the road to the discovery that there are solutions. All of his problems have been faced before.

An organization of complexity usually succeeds in providing the executive with enough failures to make him quit, if he does nothing to counteract them. Let him use the best judgment he can muster; but when his judgment fails, he needs to do something in which he wins or finds pleasure. This may be a game in which he excels, a hobby he has mastered, or a family outing in which he counts as a necessary feature. Thromboses, ulcers, suicides, and neurasthenia should not invade the executive's office if he has the support of values in the office and of achievements outside.

## Responsibility for Errors

Some hazards come in the form of responsibility for the mistakes of a subordinate. For instance, Sherman Adams's involvement with Bernard Goldfine became a serious moral problem for President Eisenhower. He remained loyal to Adams though the latter's acceptance of gifts for apparent political favors suggested that the President approved of this practice. Had Eisenhower repudiated Adams, he would have withdrawn the support which a subordinate must be allowed to presuppose if he is to do his best work.

Originality and initiative are essential in the subordinates of a healthy organization. Experimentation brings fresh values. A dean who has no new ideas about how a college can improve its instruction is a liability to his president. Conversely, a dean who is not allowed to experiment should resign. Delegated authority implies that a subordinate has the right to make mistakes—and the duty to accept responsibility for his mistakes.

Responsibility given to subordinates obviously matures their judgment. They may learn from their failures. The moral issue enlarges when those failures mount to such proportions that they become expensive or harmful to the prestige of the institution and to the welfare of colleagues. It may be profitable to allow subordinates to annoy each other with their mistakes. Friction, up to a point, defines issues and tests the resourcefulness of colleagues. If a finance vice president will not recommend approval of requests by a production vice president, both are likely to have taken a careful measure of each other.

### Extent of Involvement

How far should the executive go in assuming responsibility for the serious errors of his subordinates? Certainly there are limits. The manager of a baseball team usually gets fired when his team consistently fails to win; there was a shake-up of top executives in the Edsel Division of the Ford Motor Company when the Edsels failed to sell in expected numbers; and the president of a midwestern university was recently dismissed because a strong alumni group felt, among other things, that he was not interested in a winning football team. A board of directors is bound to hold an executive accountable for what goes wrong in his organization. If he tolerates failure too often on the part of subordinates, he becomes a failure himself. His duty lies in cultivating conditions that prevent his subordinates' failure. If they win, he wins.

No executive can administer his organization on an atomistic theory of morals. While he cannot be his brother's keeper, especially if the brother makes too many serious errors, he can be his brother's brother. John Dewey would doubtless say, "If my neighbor steals, I, too, am a thief."[10] That overstates the case, though it emphasizes the mutual involvement of all men in moral questions. It is both right and expedient, therefore, that the executive assume some responsibility for the errors of his subordinates. If they cannot be corrected, his obligations cease, and a new man must be put on the payroll.

Democratic administration depends for its success on common aims individually shared. The democratic administrator stands in a position of mutual influence with his subordinates. He profits from their joint wisdom. He may judge and discipline them when they err, if he has developed for himself sufficiently reliable standards of private judgment. Note, however, that his judgment will consist largely in continuously setting before them high standards of excellence with which they cannot fail to compare themselves. Their ability or inability to reach these standards will generally become so apparent to themselves and their colleagues that they will respond with better effort, or resign.

This means that the executive is a leader, not a boss. Rigid discipline, which once meant enforced obedience, only results in fear, suspicion, hatred, resistance, and similar negative reactions. The executive must be a morale builder who engenders willingness to work, to cooperate, and to improve.

## Images and Mirages

Some interesting issues arise from the nature of a top executive's office. Let us examine just a few of them.

### Picture of Success

For one thing, the chief executive — or possibly the man aspiring to succeed to that position — is called on to live up to, or fit into, an image of the head of his organization that is preestablished in most cases. For example:

The "success" impression must be maintained. A bank, college, retail store, or political office rests on public confidence. The chief office holders must manifest present success and confidence in the future. Credit ratings and sales are related to the "success" atmosphere they generate. Philanthropists and investors are most often interested only in a going concern. Hence the dress, home and furnishings, car, vacations, and general approach of the executive to life all assume basic importance.

Whether or not the executive lives up to the public image expected of him may become a critical question. He may support the image sincerely (else he should not support it at all), but sincerity does not solve his problem. "The good of the company" often comes ahead of his personal pleasures or convenience. He must be the life of the party, whether he feels like it or not. If his fatigue, indigestion, boredom, or even disagreement on moral questions become too evident to his friends, there is something wrong with the company, or he must be a bad choice for the office. The test is a hard one. Any Dr. Jekyll, when he is honest, will want to be a Mr. Hyde at least once a month, and particularly after the annual board meeting!

### Illusions of Praise

Another problem, strange as it may seem, is that the office of the executive often receives a great deal of recognition and praise. The danger is that the executive may be deceived into receiving this recognition for himself rather than for his office. The president presides at all meetings, actually or by implication, and leads all processions, receptions, and delegations. He sometimes forgets that his office requires this prominence, not his personal eminence apart from the office. As awards, citations, and publicity come to the executive for his organization, as if he had done the work himself, it is a subtle temptation to forget that he is the mouthpiece only of his institution, not of the whole body.

Politeness and official protocol may so obscure the true nature of an executive's work as to prevent him from ever securing a true appraisal of what he does. The most reliable judges of his work are not likely to be his subordinates. If they believe themselves unappreciated, they may seek recognition either by excessive praise or by too severe condemnation. As for members of the board of directors, they are likely to represent other interests and to occupy positions far removed from the executive's daily task. Acquaintances outside the firm may not be helpful, either.

There are always some well-meaning friends who praise a well-known figure if he merely stays out of jail. The executive needs to remember the caution Charles Reynolds Brown, formerly dean of the Yale Divinity School, was wont to give young theologues before they received their diplomas: "You will always have about you some kind old ladies, both male and female, who will tell you you are the greatest prophet since Amos. But that won't make it so!"

The executive is, therefore, in a quandary. If he accepts too facilely the public image of his office, he becomes insincere. If he departs too radically from it, he may disturb his constituents. If he accepts the recognition and achievements of his office as his own, he may remove himself from discriminating critics, and ride unjustly on the shoulders of his colleagues' achievements. He must, therefore, come back once more to his own scheme of professional and moral values. His recourse lies in developing for his own use a public image for his office and a private image for himself. This will deliver him from the strait jacket of public opinion. It will also deliver him from the cynicism that he might develop if he tried to stay completely detached from the role of his company and public demand.

## Cultural Development

Another dilemma lies in the relation of personal development to official activity. An executive continually carries out plans of action, and he must do so intelligently. At the same time, however, he wants to give time and attention to self-cultivation. He wants to be fresh and original. How far should he defer appointments at the office while he studies his problems, or defer decisions while he attends professional conferences, or takes a vacation?

As the cold war drags on, it becomes more and more evident that the battle of the century is for men's minds. An executive who ignores this fact may find himself administering an operation of vanishing importance. The involvement of his institution in the changing social, political, and economic conditions of the time requires him to know much about other managers' jobs as well as his own. He serves his own company as he studies conditions not directly related, but nonetheless surely related, to his own post. He must know what his organization is heading for.

In Europe, *the* American philosophy has often been considered pragmatism. The go-getting, successful American, particularly the businessman, is supposed to live by the doctrine that what is true is that which works. But this is a case where we do not want to see ourselves as others see us—or, at least, only as others see us. For in reality the thoughtful American executive has in his mind many a plan that has not worked, but that he knows must be true. He finds himself seeking more satisfactions than mere success. He discovers, too, that many of his employees have other goals than mere financial success.

The Institute for Executives at Aspen, Colorado, like the seminars at the University of Pennsylvania sponsored by the Bell Telephone Company, are interesting efforts to fill the void of cultural ideas and ideals that many an executive has begun to feel.[11] Doubtless the late Justice Holmes was right in saying, "It is required of a man that he share the action and passion of his time at peril of being judged not to have lived."[12] But all action and passion make Jack a dangerous, even if not a dull, boy. I find it significant, for example, that early American life was led by men who were able to unite thought and action in an admirable way. The John Cottons were ministers as well as cultural and political leaders. Thomas Jefferson was a scholar of prodigious practical accomplishment too. Woodrow Wilson was too academic for some, but his ideas are still demanding world acceptance.

## The Ultimate Question

The executive must manage his life so that he can fill up his mind with interesting ideas that supply a context and guide for his actions. He is entitled, even obligated, to read books, to travel, and to confer with leaders outside his line of work so that life can be richer for him.

The thoughtful leader comes at last to face the ultimate question of whether he is big enough for the office. If he is, it will be in a large measure because he is adequate to deal with the moral issues put before him.

### NOTES

1. Garden City, New York: Doubleday, 1956.
2. Robert A. Goldwin, editor (White Plains, New York: Fund for Adult Education, 1957).

3. New York: Harper & Brothers, 1953.
4. New York: Oxford University Press, 1956.
5. New York: Simon and Schuster, 1956.
6. New York: Alfred A. Knopf, 1959.
7. See *Experiment in Education* (Chicago: Henry Regnery, 1954).
8. New York: David McKay, 1957.
9. Alfred North Whitehead (New York: Macmillan, 1925).
10. See *Human Nature and Conduct: An Introduction to Social Psychology* (New York: Henry Holt, 1922), part I, section I.
11. See Charles A. Nelson, "The Liberal Arts in Management," HBR May–June 1958, p. 91.
12. Memorial Day Address, Keene, New Hampshire, May 30, 1884; published in *The Mind and Faith of Justice Holmes*, edited by Max Lerner (Boston: Little, Brown, 1946), p. 10.

# 4

# Personal Values and Business Decisions

EDMUND P. LEARNED, ARCH R. DOOLEY,
AND ROBERT L. KATZ

Among thoughtful businessmen there is growing concern with the spiritual implications of their everyday activities. Some of these men are seeking greater meaning in their business lives than the accumulation of profits for the enterprise or of wealth, power, and prestige for themselves. Others are struggling with the problem of squaring their corporate responsibilities with their personal religious beliefs. Still others are attempting to define their personal values in the context of their business experience.

Symptoms of this concern are to be found everywhere. A tremendous number of speeches and articles on "religion and business" are receiving eager and enthusiastic response. In the pages of this magazine over the last two years, as just one example, every issue has contained at least one article dealing with ethical or moral problems. And, even more significant, the demand for reprints of these articles has held its own with groups of articles on such timely topics as statistical decision making, human relations, marketing, and executive development.

## Why This Concern?

What has caused this current upsurge of businessmen's interest in questions of ultimate values? By tracing the roots of the trend, it will perhaps be more nearly possible to determine its nature and probable hardiness. A variety of partial answers have been advanced. Thus:

Some suggest that the development merely reflects the concessions that have been wrung from businessmen by the pressure of circumstances. The strength of organized labor, the fear of communism, the memories of the recent past in which business emerged as a political whipping boy—all have been cited to explain the growing introspection evidenced by businessmen.

Some push this analysis further and suggest that business has become conscious of its opportunities and responsibilities in other than purely economic affairs because of a guilty conscience. There is, for example, a persistent hard core of opinion that suggests that all manifestations of interest in ultimate values (particularly those which have been associated with outstandingly successful business careers) are an attempt to "buy respectability"—that is, to atone for the accumulation of great wealth and economic power through practices which cannot measure up to the highest ethical standards.

A variation on this basic theme is the suggestion that actually there has been no genuine change in the ethical standards of business or of businessmen. Any evidence to the contrary, it is suggested, is merely carefully mounted public relations campaigns—window dressing to conceal the fact that business motives and tactics remain what they always have been.

On the other hand, some commentators offer a far less cynical interpretation. Some, for example, suggest that the period of uncertainty through which the world has recently passed and the period of equal uncertainty in which it now lives have forced each thoughtful individual, in business or in any other form of human endeavor, to give increasing thought to ultimate values and to seek certain unyielding premises on which he can fix his convictions.

Other opinion centers upon a quite different characteristic of the contemporary era. It has been, these men suggest, a time that has lent itself to the "luxuries of conscience." Satisfying the basic needs for food, shelter, and so on has been increasingly easy for a broad section of the population. For the man of genuine ability in business, the challenge has often been not that of finding an adequate job but that of choosing among a variety of promising alternatives. In increasing numbers, men are able to ask themselves what they would like to do with their lives, with reasonable expectation of being able to move tangibly toward fulfillment of their goals.

### Unavoidable Conflict

It is probable that each of these various explanations contains some element of truth. To the writers of this article, however, neither singly nor in combination do any of these reasons provide as meaningful an explanation as is to be found in the very fact that the businessman is, first of all, a *man*. As a man, he shares the universal trait of wanting to be certain that his life has meaning and purpose. But the nature of his role as a businessman places him continuously in a position of conflict. It forces him constantly to choose between alternative courses of action reflecting differing priorities of values.

In his analysis of these alternatives, and in his consideration of the values they represent, the businessman inevitably finds himself in a state of inner conflict. He wants to do the right thing, but he does not always find it easy to know what that right thing is. Efforts to deny the existence of such conflict, however persistently pursued, offer only temporary and superficial relief. Like all men, the businessman inevitably returns to the questions of ultimate values and to the question of whether his total life is serving those values in the way he would wish.

## Evidence of Concern

A particularly cogent example of the nature and the strength of business's growing concern with spiritual values was evident in the Harvard Business School Association's Fiftieth Anniversary Conference in September 1958, which had as its theme, "Management's Mission in a New Society." It is significant that every major speaker stressed the importance of more attention to spiritual values, and that no fewer than one fourth of the panel discussions, set up to consider topics of major importance to the participants, were directly concerned with these issues.[1]

Erwin D. Canham, editor of *The Christian Science Monitor*, had this to say:

The only valid social goal is improvement of the lot of man and the better relationship of men to one another and to God, to fundamental truth. . . . This thesis is incontrovertible, and once we tended to live by it. . . .

There is nothing inherently wrong with the satisfaction of man's material wants. . . . In fact, the attainment of a better standard of living is itself a spiritual victory, insofar as it exemplifies man's mastery of his physical environment. Behind all our technological, industrial, or mercantile attainments lies this kind of true victory. But we do not often recognize it as such, nor have we made any progress in explaining to the rest of the world that the real American achievement is spiritual instead of material.

Charles S. Malik, formerly Minister of Foreign Affairs of Lebanon and President of the General Assembly of the United Nations, discussed "The Businessman and the Challenge of Communism." After raising the question of the meaning men attach to their work, he went on to say:

The businessman is judged by more than his product and his performance: his humanity is at stake. Rising above his individual interests to the proper consideration of the common good and soaring even beyond the common good to the spiritual significance of his wondrous material civilization, the businessman can clothe his humanity with a shining new splendor. He will put to shame every culture that ends in boredom, self-sufficiency, and human pride. His spiritualized materialism will have something profound to say and give to all men. He will identify himself with their human state. He will be proud of his business and its achievements, but he will be even prouder of that which is beyond business in his culture. He will say, "Let others compete with me in material things and let them even excel, but there is one thing in which they cannot excel because they do not know it and are not even seeking it. That is the power and depth and freedom of the spirit in which man is fully himself." In this way Communism's challenge to the businessman will turn into the businessman's challenge to Communism.

Later in the same program, Stanley F. Teele, dean of the Harvard Business School, described the requirements for "The Businessman of the Future" as being "more rational, more responsible, more religious." He said:

> Personally, I am troubled by our apparent continued emphasis on material progress alone as the measure of success or failure in this kind of competition [with the Soviet Union]. . . . We are falling into a trap of our own making; we have become so impressed by the world's reaction to our tremendous material progress that there is risk that we shall consider this the true measure of our greatness and the most important contribution which we have made and can make to the world. In our hearts we know better; we know that the demonstration of how 170 million people can live together in peace, with basic goals of human dignity, morality, and justice, is our real contribution.

### Mission versus Material Progress

These and many other distinguished men who participated in the program were all pointing at the same thing: the need to place stronger emphasis on spiritual goals, not only so that each man may find greater meaning in his work and in his life, but, even more dramatically, so that our nation and our way of life may survive in the international battle for men's hearts and minds.

As Arnold J. Toynbee, the distinguished historian, pointed out at the conference, no society has ever flourished without a spiritual mission; the quest for material progress alone is insufficient to spur men on to the achievements which are required to create an enduring, dynamic, progressive nation. In fact, his conclusion is that all through history material progress as a national goal has led to stagnation, boredom, and moral decay.

It is significant that the great concern for more spirituality in business comes at a time when our material progress has achieved extraordinary heights. The high level of satisfaction of material wants, taken as a goal, threatens stagnation and destruction of our society; but, at the same time, it provides an unparalleled opportunity for freeing men's minds and ambitions for loftier goals.

## What Is Spirituality?

When we talk about seeking loftier goals and about finding "spirituality" in our business lives, what do we really mean? There is nothing mysterious in the word spirituality. Spirituality in business, as we see it, is the process of seeking to discover, however imperfectly, God's law in each everyday work situation, and of trying to behave in each situation as nearly in accord with that law as we are able to. Perhaps this broad generalization will be clearer and more meaningful if we define our terms.

We conceive of God as that force in the universe which has created and maintained all that is real and true. We believe that God's creation has an order and symmetry which relates all things to one another. We consider the ultimate fulfillment of man, *as man*, to be his comprehension of reality and truth, so that he becomes one with God in his understanding of the relationships of all things and his behavior comes to be in harmony and accord with this orderly reality.

We also believe that man—imperfect in his comprehension and perspective, and burdened with sins and shortsightedness of his own making—is inevitably unable to sense the full reality. To survive in his environment, he makes judgments and evaluations which, because of his limited comprehension, are admittedly imperfect. He arms himself with personal values which, while enabling him to function in the world, may prevent him from seeing the ultimate reality, the truth which actually exists. To us, spirituality means making a continuing, conscious effort to rise above these inevitable human limitations—a maximum endeavor to comprehend the ultimate values, the truth and the reality of the orderliness of the universe—and to live in accordance with this reality.

We cannot prove the point of view we have stated. Neither can it be disproved. It is simply an act of faith. It is comforting to note, however, that research in both the physical and the social sciences has suggested the existence of order in the universe and has indicated that all things are related to one another in a nonrandom way. Moreover, none of these validated findings has in any way contradicted the teachings of the great prophets. One is justified in believing that both prophets and researchers are pointing at the same truth.

Within this view of reality we deal with *personal* values, which are the goals and criteria unique to each individual. We shall talk about ethics or morality, not as ideas necessarily sacred or "right" in themselves, but merely as widely held values which, rightly or wrongly, receive widespread sanction and approval. We will hold as *ultimate* values those goals and criteria which seem to us to be most closely in accord with what is real. These ultimate values, which are held by every great religion and which have been advanced by each of the great prophets and religious leaders throughout recorded history, are: love of fellow man, justice in all acts among men, and the self-fulfillment of the individual through understanding and through actions that bring him closer to living in accord with reality.

## Guides to Action

Systems of values (implicit or explicit) are inherent in the behavior of all persons. Also, each individual's personal values—the standards he uses in making evaluations and the goals he chooses for action—are different, in greater or lesser degree, from anyone else's set of values.

Moreover, not only do values differ from individual to individual, but also each individual's values change from one situation to the next, whether he is aware of it or not. Specific facts, persons, and events cannot be talked about or dealt with without considering the values that different persons, including ourselves, place on them. Two managers are discussing what went wrong in a production schedule. Do they trust the foreman or not? Are they interested or disinterested in the aspirations of production workers? Is their sole concern with making a good profit showing this month? And so on.

For each individual, reality is whatever his values allow him to recognize. And since each person's values are unique, his conception of the "right" thing to do will differ from others'. Nonetheless, many men assume that other persons of good intentions will see things the same way they do and brand those who disagree with them as unethical, immoral, or just plain stupid. By assuming that they can bring a set of absolute values to bear on any situation and thus reveal a course of action, they drastically over-simplify the situation, missing its impact on their interpretation of their values as well as the impact of their values on what they see before them—all of which tends to make them victims of the situation, not masters over it.

On the other hand, just recognizing that values differ from person to person and situation to situation does not provide a satisfactory guide to action either. The world we live in is so complex, and man's capacity so finite, that complete pragmatism can lead only to confusion, inconsistency, or a philosophy of expediency and caprice. What is needed is for each man to try to hold as criteria a very few ultimate values which for him represent essential truths and to cling to these criteria tenaciously and absolutely in every situation. He can then deal highly pragmatically with the inevitable conflicts of *personal* values inherent in any situation and work out the range of action uniquely appropriate to it, using his *ultimate* values as standards for judging the reality of the various courses of action.

This approach is not easy—far from it. It requires living with tremendous personal discomforts and conflicts, with a gnawing, inescapable admission of one's own fallibility and inadequacy. To be consciously aware of the inadequacies of his perceptions and still be able to take action is perhaps the most difficult position that a person can maintain.

With these assumptions and beliefs stated, we can proceed to discuss two questions of great practical importance: What values commonly held by businessmen block the growth of spirituality in business behavior? What do beliefs like those just stated mean for executive action?

## Unrealistic Dreaming

Businessmen have a variety of ways of thinking about the relationships between spiritual and business considerations. For instance, some persons, including many who clearly endeavor to serve the highest concepts of spiritual values in their personal activities, contend that spiritual considerations simply cannot be given a position of major importance in business decisions. To these individuals, the suggestion that such values can be, or are, given a prominent role by management seems unrealistic dreaming at best, or, at worst, hypocritical distortion or misrepresentation. A few go even further to suggest that even if it were realistically possible to do so, it would be inappropriate (perhaps even immoral) for a businessman to employ his business position as a means to the achievement of his individual spiritual concepts.

This general view is documented in a multitude of ways. Central to each of these ways is the belief that most of the problems encountered in business can be dealt with as purely business problems without directly encountering the spiritual values that may be involved. The spiritual ramifications of a situation are not denied; they are simply not treated as factors with which the businessman can or should concern himself as an executive.

### Typical Attitudes

Men who subscribe to this view back it up with statements like these:

"I believe in behaving responsibly; but when the chips are really down (i.e., when the financial stakes are high and the competitive pressures are pronounced), then business profits, and hence long-term business survival, are often incompatible with spiritual considerations. The businessman has no choice but to treat the former as the dominant consideration."

"Business requires competition. That's what private enterprise is all about. And the tougher the competition, the better the service that business can give and the more valuable the contributions it can make. But competition means that someone's going to be hurt. If you *really* worried about spiritual values, you couldn't bring yourself to be truly competitive."

"Look, I wouldn't last six months in this business if I really asked myself whether everything I do really meets acceptable spiritual standards. Now you understand I don't prefer it this way; and, if the time ever comes when things are different, why I'll be the first to go along. But as long as my competitors think it's all right to do this, as long as my customers expect me to do that, as long as my boss tells me such-and-such, and as long as our stockholders demand what they do, and so forth and so forth, why, then I'll just have to...."

"A businessman is supposed to run his business profitably. A successful business in itself can be a tremendous contributor toward 'good.' But if the businessman spends his time worrying about 'doing good,' he'll divert his attention from his real purpose—he'll lose his effectiveness as a businessman. Remember what they say, 'Shoemaker, stick to your last.' A businessman should stick to business and leave to others (the government, the church, the individual) the job of setting right all of mankind's problems."

"Spiritual questions involve value judgments. They hinge on questions of what's right and what's wrong—what's good and what's bad. Business has no right to exercise its power to try to further its own particular answers to such considerations. There's nothing in my company's corporate charter about trying to push my own ideas of social, cultural, or political considerations, and certainly nothing about furthering ultimate values as such. We shouldn't get involved in this sort of thing. And certainly we shouldn't try to force our views on others."

"Only a handful of companies are big enough to exert any real influence insofar as spiritual values are concerned. Even in those companies, there are only a handful of men at the very top who can make any difference. The average fellow would just be committing business suicide if he were to try. He'd lose his value to the organization."

"Do you know what it is to meet a payroll? It's damn tough, and there are plenty of times when you can't take time to worry about whether a saint would approve of everything you've done...."

We are all familiar with similar examples, and many more could be given. What is significant here is that few people find that such a framework gives them much real satisfaction from their work. Most adherents—particularly those to whom their religion is a deep and serious commitment—grant that they wish business life *could* be different; but they believe that, in fact, business is amoral, and they have resigned themselves to it. Many of these people find that participation in church activities, community affairs, charity work, and so on gives their lives some of the meaning which they feel is denied in their work activities, but this compartmentalization tends to add to their frustration rather than diminish it.

## "Just Good Business"

Another familiar framework or rationale is that, over the long run, good ethics *is* good business. Elaboration and support of this proposition fall into a number of subdivisions. Certain of these are so closely related as to overlap. By contrast, some of the arguments advanced in support of the proposition are mutually incompatible. But for each subdivision proof can be (and usually is) advanced in the form of personalized experiences or observations.

### Practical Incentives

One view is that good ethics is good business because of readily understandable *quid pro quo* concepts: a business that behaves ethically induces others to behave ethically toward it. Supporters document this with episodes (actual or hypothetical) drawn from all sectors of the business scene. For example:

A firm exercises particular care in meeting all responsibilities to its employees. As a result, it is rewarded with an unusual degree of employee loyalty, application, and productivity. (In a familiar variation on this theme, such a firm is rewarded by a spirit of militant antiunionism on the part of its loyal, appreciative work force.)

A supplier refuses to exploit his advantage during a sellers' market and thereby retains the loyalty (and continued business) of customers when conditions change to those of a buyers' market.

A firm that employs handicapped persons discovers that they are actually more productive, hardworking, loyal, and so on than the nonhandicapped persons normally employed.

Another view supports the proposition that "good ethics is good business" by stressing the dangers and probable penalties inherent in unethical business behavior. This view is documented with such examples as:

A customer is dealt with unfairly and thereafter refuses to deal with the supplier in question. Other firms, learning of the situation, also refuse to deal with the supplier because "he has shown he cannot be trusted."

A firm allows its salesmen to disseminate misleading information about its competitors' products. This invites open retaliation by competing salesmen (who perhaps prove even more effective in their use of this technique).

A union whose reasonable demands are rejected during a period of union weakness vengefully wrests unreasonable concessions from the company when the balance of bargaining power shifts in its favor.

Advocates of this viewpoint frequently observe that if the entire business community fails to meet the standards and the desires of society, punitive legislation will be enacted which will be far more severe than warranted. Ethical behavior on the part of business is thus advocated as a form of insurance against retaliatory acts.

### Virtue Triumphs

A third view supporting the proposition that good ethics is good business explains itself in essentially mystical terms drawing on empirical evidence. For advocates of this view, the concepts of "good ultimately rising above evil" and of "right making might" (both deeply engrained in human consciousness and buttressed by legend and literature) are seen to be fully operative in business settings. A "good man" who steadfastly tries to be ethical, i.e., "to do the right thing" somehow always overtakes his immoral or amoral counterpart in the long run. Bread cast upon the waters *is* returned, even if the process is sometimes an indirect one and the waiting period is extensive.

Documentation of this view is again drawn from a variety of quarters. Frequently it is characterized by the unexpected, the unforeseen, the mysterious. To illustrate:

A man unjustly discharged from a position in which he has given faithful service finds even greater success and satisfaction in the new job he has been forced to take.

An associate who had persisted in hostility and obstructionism toward a "good man" suddenly sees the error of his ways, apologizes, and becomes a staunch ally.

A firm loses an important account rather than enter into a form of reciprocity that it considers unethical. Then it unexpectedly obtains a new customer whose business fully compensates for the abandoned account.

Or the "Executive Suite" theme — an individual who steadfastly refuses to further his career by the use of unethical tactics wins out (usually at the last split second) over those who do.

For some advocates of this school of thought, the explanation for such occurrences rests in the operation of some divine force that ultimately assures a happy ending. Its operation is not to be analyzed or understood. Rather, it is to be accepted and confidently anticipated by those who put their faith in ethical behavior.

An alternative explanation of the view that virtue ultimately triumphs suggests that when an individual operates with a sense of certainty regarding the ethical soundness of his position, his mind and energies are freed for maximum productivity and creativity. On the other hand, when practicing what he knows to be unethical behavior, an individual finds it necessary to engage in exhausting subterfuge. Furthermore, in a violent battle of conscience, his energies are diluted, his effectiveness is diminished, and his chances of ultimate success are destroyed.

Thus, given any situation in which basic capabilities and tangible resources are in even approximate balance, the individual with a sense of ethical certainty will invariably be more productive than the individual who has elected to pursue his goals unethically.

### Wide Appeal of Concept

Regardless of which explanation is considered, it is not difficult to understand why the concept that good ethics is good business has won for itself so wide a following among those who advocate conscious consideration of spiritual dimensions.

It is, in the first place, a concept that seemingly avoids any painful choice between appealing but mutually incompatible alternatives. Instead it professes to offer the vastly attractive prospect of desirable goals compounded. The businessman, it suggests, really can have "all this and heaven too." Actually, it seems to imply, the two may be more surely achieved jointly than separately. Spiritual values are not attained at the cost of business success; instead, conscious pursuit of them helps create business success.

If this is true, here, indeed, is a merchandisable product!

The appeal of the proposition is further intensified by the fact that it bypasses the troublesome question of the separability of spiritual considerations from all the other elements of a business decision. Once it is accepted that good ethics is good business, it is neither necessary nor germane to ponder whether the two can be separated. If good ethics is good business, no effective businessman would endeavor to isolate spiritual considerations from the other elements in a business situation, even were it possible to do so.

Still further appeal arises from the fact that if good ethics is good business, then spiritual behavior can be frocked in the apparently appealing garb of "hard-headed," "practical" business expediency. No longer need the businessman fear (consciously or subconsciously) that considering spiritual values in business decisions will indicate to "practical men" that he is unwilling to meet the stern realities of the business world. He need never fall into the apparently vulnerable role of an advocate of spiritual values for their own sake. Instead, he can fly the banner of the "practical man" and can stress the goal of business success as the real motive underlying his acts.

The proposition that good ethics is good business also has the important advantage of being difficult, if not impossible, to disprove. By the same token it is, of course, almost impossible to prove. But it is apparent that many businessmen find intuitive support of this proposition to be a more gracious, more comfortable, and more affirmatively human position than its rejection.

## New Approach Needed

To us, neither the proposition that business and spiritual considerations are separable nor the view that good ethics is good business is a fully adequate or satisfying guide for action. Both, we feel, represent oversimplified attempts to find an easy way out of an excruciatingly complex situation.

To us, the thesis that business decisions need not reflect spiritual considerations contains the fatal flaw of unrealism. We believe that in business, as in all other human endeavors, the spiritual values of each individual involved are inextricably linked to all the other elements in the situation, including the often differing value perceptions held with equal sincerity by other people concerned. Businessmen, whether they want to or not, cannot escape involvement with spiritual values in any segment of their activities. Instead, by the very act of responding to the total context of whatever situation confronts them, they either serve or disavow spiritual values held by themselves or by others.

For us, then, the question is not *whether* a businessman must deal with spiritual values. Instead, the question is *how* the businessman can broaden his perception of reality to assure that the spiritual implications which inevitably attend his actions conform as closely as is humanly possible with his ultimate values.

The answer to this question does not lie merely in the assertion that "good ethics is good business." In our judgment, this too is an inadequate framework, and is marred by major shortcomings.

### Uncertainty of Reward

We are troubled, first of all, with the implied certainty of material reward which permeates the proposition and which, we feel, constantly threatens its usefulness to those who embrace it. We grant that furtherance of spiritual values over the long run does often lead to successful business results. But does it follow that such results invariably can or ought to be anticipated, or that they should be interpreted as even partial justification for the pursuance of spiritual goals? None of the major religions says that ultimate values may always be served without cost, sacrifice, or hardship, even in the long run. Insofar as material satisfactions are concerned, man, as man, is not promised "all this and heaven too," even in exchange for the most devout human behavior. And does not the totality of business experience reveal numerous situations in which success or failure emerges both in the *presence* and in the *absence* of conscious pursuit of ethical values?

For us, therefore, the suggestion that there is some close, causal connection between business success and spiritually oriented behavior seems, at best, deceptively superficial and fraught with dangers of disillusionment for those who follow it. At worst, there may even be a danger that, through its appealing simplicity, the proposition could deaden one's sensitivity to the ethical challenges each of us continually faces. If embraced wholeheartedly and employed indiscriminately as the rationale for business decisions, the concept that good ethics is good business could lead unwittingly to acceptance of the reverse corollary that good business is good ethics—and to the deceptive assumption that men of goodwill somehow will, automatically and without conflict, serve ultimate values in their actions.

Even more devastating is the possibility that spiritual values might come to be viewed as a *means* to business success, rather than as a *goal* in themselves. If given such an interpretation, the whole proposition becomes irreverent and irreligious.

### Facing Up to Conflict

We are troubled, too, by the thought that the proposition offers no helpful guidance for a businessman's conduct in the short-term decisions that continually confront him, whatever his rank or status in an enterprise. How can the belief that in the long run good ethics is good business help the manager who is responsible for immediate results, particularly if attention to spiritual values entails a risk of financial loss or even immediate failure for the individual himself, the enterprise, or both?

To us, every decision involves a conflicting set of forces. This is particularly true in business, where the individual often finds himself forced to choose among personal values and ultimate loyalties that may be in sharp conflict with each other, with the values held by others (which look "right" from their points of view), or with urgent organizational considerations. The terrible task of leadership is to live with conflicts and tensions, to make discriminating judgments where necessary, and to find mutual relationships where possible. What is crucial is that the administrator realize that he always has a *choice* of what his behavior or decisions will be—(at least, if he is willing to accept the inevitable discomforts entailed by different courses of action).

There are always a multitude of forces in any organizational framework which make conflict inevitable and negative consequences unavoidable. Someone will always be placed under tensions or restrictions, or denied things that he believes to be rightly his. Individual interests must frequently be sacrificed for the good of the larger organization.

For these reasons we do not believe that it is satisfactory either to ignore spiritual considerations in business or to try to make spiritual and business considerations identical. Both approaches are oversimplifications: the former because it requires a man who wants to serve God to compartmentalize his life; the latter because it offers no way of dealing with the conflicts which occur in every decision-making situation. Neither recognizes the inevitability of conflict or the complexity of the situation in which business decisions must be made. What, then, is a more adequate framework?

## Faith in a Process

To us, a third frame of reference offers a more adequate and realistic basis for facing the awesome complexities that are invariably encountered in industry, and for bearing the inner human tensions that are inevitably experienced when an individual stands at the juncture between his own spiritual values and the demands of his daily business activities.

We do not pretend to know the ultimate course of action in any specific situation. Nor do we believe in the existence of easy, generalized solutions: each situation requires its own unique resolution. But we do have faith in a *process* by which men can perceive and act on as much of God's answer to each situation as is within their limited power of discernment.

### Underlying Assumptions

This process is based on assumptions — some of them cited earlier — which we acknowledge are not within the scope of human proof. But, for us, they require no proof. They are our articles of faith.

We believe that there is an *order* to the universe. We have faith that this order is God's law and that it represents the ultimate *reality*. But we also believe that man's imperfections prevent him from ever fully comprehending this reality in each specific situation that confronts him.

We believe that as a result of this limited perception, finite man is constantly violating God's law in some way. Inevitably, each of us is always inadequate to the full demands of whatever situation we encounter. From each of us, then, is demanded a continuing, profound humility concerning the spiritual adequacy of our own ideas and actions.

We believe that ultimate values — love of fellow man, justice in all dealings among men, and opportunity for self-fulfillment for all persons — although known to man throughout his civilized history and embraced by many of his historical religious and ethical systems, do not provide direct answers for specific situations. Instead, they must be employed as criteria by which man discerns the implications of the alternative courses of action that are available to him.

We believe that every business situation, in common with all other forms of human endeavor, inevitably involves conflicts of values among the men concerned. Wherever possible, men must strive with good will for an integration of these divergent values, even though that integration may involve compromises which frustrate the individual because what he sees as right varies so sharply from what he realizes is attainable. Men must also be willing to face the tensions that result from those conflicts which prove irreconcilable, knowing that these tensions, too, are part of God's process.

We believe that God works through men — others as well as ourselves. We believe that a forthright interchange of views between men, however divergent their values, provides an opportunity for more complete comprehension of God's reality than any one man can achieve alone, however sincere his motivation or intense his application. Men working together, sharing perceptions, and respecting the intrinsic worth of each other's contributions often find integrated solutions to even the most difficult situations.

Even when the conflicts of value prove irreconcilable and integration is, at least for the moment, impossible, comparisons of divergent points of view can help illuminate the probable consequences of alternative courses of action and suggest the interim solution that most effectively preserves an opportunity for integration at some future date. Men's answers will be nearer to God's reality when they emanate from a free and open exchange of views and when they embrace the broadest possible perspective of the values held by all the men involved.

Each of us, therefore, faces the obligation to seek and respect the ideas of others. Only in this way can we augment our own inevitably fragmentary grasp of God's reality. But the ultimate responsibility for decision—and for its consequences, favorable and unfavorable—must be our own.

In short, the essence of the process we advocate is that man should possess complete faith in the omniscience of the Creator and in the existence of order in His universe and constantly strive to comprehend and to act in accord with more and more of the reality in each situation, relying on free discussion with other men as a means through which he may perceive reality more fully.

Implicit in this process is the recognition that there is a spiritual significance to every phase of a man's work, be it in business or any other calling. The businessman who embraces this process must do so knowing that the way of faith is hard, rigorous, and filled with continuously humbling evidences of man's imperfection, and realizing that even when seeking to do good, finite man, with his limited perception of reality, is always inflicting some measure of evil.

### Background for Decision

Those who place their faith in the process described—i.e., men who steadfastly attempt to augment their own fragmentary perception of reality by seeking and comprehending the values held by others, men who honestly attempt to integrate even the most intense value conflicts, men who accept as a normal fact of existence the personal tensions inherent in compromise and in problems yet unresolved—can forthrightly face the spiritual implications and tensions of their daily activities. Although burdened by the knowledge that their efforts have been imperfect, they will nevertheless possess the reassurance that they have tried, within the limits of human capabilities, to do God's work in the everyday world. And even more importantly, they will possess a spiritual reservoir that will enable them to continue unceasingly toward the ultimate, though unattainable, goal of perceiving and fulfilling God's reality.

Such men can bring their faith to every situation they encounter, saying:

I need not fear any situation, any conflicts, any difference in values, or the burden of responsibility. The fact that I have not yet decided what the real problem in the particular circumstances is or that I do not have a ready-made, preconceived solution need not discourage me, for down deep in my heart I know I can draw on the resources of other men's expertness, points of view, and values to assist in reaching a balanced conclusion or plan of action.

All I need to do is to reach out for these resources, have imagination to comprehend who might have interests or points of view to consider, possess a genuine desire to listen to their contributions with an open mind, have a capacity to articulate the other person's point of view to facilitate exchange of ideas and the consideration of potential solutions or new integrations.

I will recognize that the foregoing sets a standard of perfection. While I do not expect perfection either in myself or in others, and realize that all of us are less than perfect, I shall be able to live with my imperfect self and my imperfect answers while endeavoring to achieve the perfect goal. I will try to avoid the sin of pride or self-righteousness. I have faith in the process, and in my ability to participate in it in an open-minded way. I have faith that through the exchange of ideas of men with different views it is practicable to achieve better answers than I can achieve alone. I will attempt to fulfill my own personal destiny and do my share of God's work in this world in this way.

For better or for worse, I, like everyone, must realize my spiritual destiny in connection with my work. I will not find it in some ideal world, detached from reality.

### NOTE

1. See *Management's Mission in a New Society*, edited by Dan H. Fenn, Jr. (New York: McGraw-Hill, 1959).

# 5

# "Skyhooks"

## O.A. OHMANN

During the last several years, while my principal job assignment has been management development, I have become increasingly impressed with the importance of intangibles in the art of administration. With the managerial revolution of the last generation and the transition from owner-manager to professional executive, there has appeared a growing literature on the science and art of administration. A shift in emphasis is noticeable in these writings over the past 30 years.

Following the early engineering approach typified by the work of Frederick Taylor and others, there next developed a search for the basic principles of organization, delegation, supervision, and control. More recently, as labor relations became more critical, the emphasis has shifted to ways of improving human relations. The approach to the problems of supervisory relationships was essentially a manipulative one. Textbooks on the techniques of personnel management mushroomed. Still later it became more and more apparent that the crux of the problem was the supervisor himself, and this resulted in a flood of "how to improve yourself" books. Meanwhile the complexities of the industrial community increased, and the discontents and tensions mounted.

It seems increasingly clear, at least to me, that while some administrative practices and personnel techniques may be better than others, their futility arises from the philosophical assumptions or value judgments on which this super-structure of manipulative procedure rests. We observe again and again that a manager with sound values and a stewardship conception of his role as boss can be a pretty effective leader even though his techniques are quite unorthodox. I am convinced that workers have a fine sensitivity to spiritual qualities and want to work for a boss who believes in something and in whom they can believe.

This observation leads me to suspect that we may have defined the basic purposes and objectives of our industrial enterprise too narrowly, too selfishly, too materialistically. Bread alone will not satisfy workers. There are some in-dications that our people have lost faith in the basic values of our economic society, and that we need a spiritual rebirth in industrial leadership.

Certainly no people have ever had so much, and enjoyed so little real satis-faction. Our economy has been abundantly productive, our standard of living is at an all-time peak, and yet we are a tense, frustrated, and insecure people full of hostilities and anxieties. Can it be that our *god of production* has feet of clay? Does industry need a new religion—or at least a better one than it has had?

I am convinced that the central problem is not the division of the spoils as organized labor would have us believe. Raising the price of prostitution does not make it the equivalent of love. Is our industrial discontent not in fact the expression of a hunger for a work life that has meaning in terms of higher and more enduring spiritual values? How can we preserve the wholeness of the personality if we are expected to worship God on Sundays and holidays and mammon on Mondays through Fridays?

I do not imply that this search for real meaning in life is or should be limited to the hours on the job, but I do hold that the central values of our industrial society permeate our entire culture. I am sure we do not require a bill of par-ticulars of the spiritual sickness of our time. The evidences of modern man's search for his soul are all about us. Save for the communist countries there has been a world-wide revival of interest in religion. The National Council of Churches reports that 59% of our total population (or 92 million) now claim church af-filiation. The November 22, 1954, issue of *Barron's* devoted the entire front page to a review of a book by Barbara Ward, *Faith and Freedom*.[1]

Perhaps even more significant is the renaissance in the quality of religious thought and experience. Quite evidently our religion of materialism, science, and humanism is not considered adequate. Man is searching for anchors outside himself. He runs wearily to the periphery of the spider web of his own reason and logic, and looks for new "skyhooks"—for an abiding faith around which life's experiences can be integrated and given meaning.

### Why "Skyhooks"?

Perhaps we should assume that this need for "skyhooks" is part of man's natural equipment—possibly a function of his intelligence—or, if you prefer, God manifesting Himself in His creatures. It seems to me, however, that the recent intensification of this need (or perhaps the clearer recognition of it) stems in part from certain broad social, economic, political, and philosophical trends. I shall not attempt a comprehensive treatment of these, but shall allude to only a few.

**Abundance without satisfaction.** I have already indicated that on the economic front we have won the battle of production. We have moved from an economy of scarcity to one of abundance. We have become masters of the physical world and have learned how to convert its natural resources to the satisfaction of our material wants. We are no longer so dependent and so intimately bound to the world of nature. In a way we have lost our feeling of being part of nature and with it our humble reverence for God's creation.

While the industrialization of our economy resulted in ever-increasing production, it also made of individual man a production number—an impersonal, de-skilled, interchangeable production unit, measured in so many cents per hour. For most employees, work no longer promotes the growth of personal character by affording opportunities for personal decision, exercise of judgment, and individual responsibility. A recent issue of *Nation's Business* quotes the modern British philosopher, Alexander Lindsay, on this point as follows:

> Industrialism has introduced a new division into society. It is the division between those who manage and take responsibility and those who are managed and have responsibility taken from them. This is a division more important than the division between the rich and poor.[2]

Certainly the modern industrial worker has improved his material standard of living at the cost of becoming more and more dependent on larger and larger groups. Not only his dignity but also his security has suffered. And so he reaches out for new "skyhooks"—for something to believe in, for something that will give meaning to his job.

**Disillusionment with science.** A second trend which seems to bear some relation to our urgent need for a faith grows out of our disillusionment with science. As a result of the rapid advance of science, the curtains of ignorance and superstition have been pulled wide on all fronts of human curiosity and knowledge. Many of the bonds of our intellectual enslavement have been broken. Reason and scientific method were called on to witness to the truth, the whole truth, and nothing but the truth. We were freed from the past—its traditions, beliefs, philosophies, its mores, morals, and religion. Science became our religion, and reason replaced emotion.

However, even before the atom bomb there was a growing realization that science did not represent the whole truth, that with all its pretensions it could be dead wrong, and, finally and particularly, that without proper moral safeguards the truth did not necessarily make men free. Atomic fission intensified the fear and insecurity of every one of us who contemplated the possibility of the concentration of power in the hands of men without morals. We want science to be in the hands of men who not only recognize their responsibility to man-made ethical standards (which are easily perverted) but have dedicated themselves to the eternal and absolute standards of God. Thus, while the evidence of material science has been welcomed, our own personal experiences will not permit us to believe that life is merely a whirl of atoms without meaning, purpose, beauty, or destiny.

**Trend toward bigness.** A third factor contributing to our insecurity is the trend toward bigness and the resulting loss of individuality. This is the day of bigger and bigger business—in every aspect of life. The small is being swallowed by the big, and the big by the bigger. This applies to business, to unions, to churches, to education, to research and invention, to newspapers, to our practice of the professions, to government, and to nations. Everything is getting bigger except the individual, and he is getting smaller and more insignificant and more dependent on larger social units. Whether we like it or not, this is becoming an administrative society, a planned and controlled society, with ever-increasing concentration of power. This is the day of collectivism and public-opinion polls. It is the day when the individual must be *adjusted to the group*—when he must above all else be sensitive to the feelings and attitudes of others, must get an idea of how others expect him to act, and then react to this.

This is the insecure world which David Riesman has described so well in his book, *The Lonely Crowd*.[3] He pictures man as being no longer "tradition directed" as was primitive man, nor as in Colonial days is he "inner directed" as if by the gyroscope of his own ideals, but today he is "outer directed" as if by radar. He must constantly keep his antenna tuned to the attitudes and reactions of others to him. The shift has been from morals to morale and from self-reliance to dependence on one's peer group. However, the members of one's peer group are each responding to each other. Obviously these shifting sands of public opinion offer no stable values around which life can be consistently integrated and made meaningful. The high-water mark of adjustment in such a society is that the individual be socially accepted and above all else that he appear to be *sincere*.

This is certainly not a favorable environment for the development of steadfast character. It is essentially a neurotic and schizophrenic environment which breeds insecurity.

This socially dependent society also offers an ideal market for the wares of the "huckster," the propagandist, and the demagogue. Lacking a religious interpretation of the divine nature of man, these merchants in mass reaction have sought the least common denominator in human nature and have beamed the movies and newspapers at the ten-year mental level. One wonders if this approach to people does not make them feel that they have been sold short and that they are capable of much better than is expected of them. Has this demoralizing exposure of the cheapness of our values not intensified our search for something better to believe in?

On top of all these disturbing socioeconomic trends came the war. This certainly was materialism, science, and humanism carried to the logical conclusion. The war made us question our values and our direction. It left us less cocksure that we were right, and more fearful of ourselves as well as of others. It made us fearful of the power which we had gained, and led us to search our soul to determine whether we had the moral strength to assume the leadership role that had been given to us. We have been humbled in our efforts to play god and are about ready to give the job back. Note, however, that this is not a characteristic reaction to war. Typically wars have been followed by a noticeable deterioration of moral standards, of traditional values, and of social institutions.

Perhaps none of these rationalizations for our return to religion is entirely valid. I suspect that the search for some kind of overarching integrative principle or idea is the expression of a normal human need. Certainly history would indicate that man's need for a god is eternal even though it may be more keenly sensed in times of adversity. A religion gives a point of philosophical orientation around which life's experiences can be organized and digested. Without the equivalent, a personality cannot be whole and healthy. Short-term goals which need to be shifted with the changing tide do not serve the same integrative function as do the "skyhooks" which are fastened to eternal values. I do not personally regard the current religious revival as a cultural hangover, nor as a regression. Being a mystic I prefer instead to view the need for such a faith as the spark of the Creator in us to drive us on to achieve His will and our own divine destiny.

### Why Monday through Friday?

If we may grant for the moment that modern man *is* searching for deeper meanings in life, we may then ask: What has this to do with industry? If he needs "skyhooks," let him get them in church, or work out his own salvation. The business leaders of the past insisted that "business is business" and that it had little bearing on the individual's private life and philosophy.

There are several reasons why "skyhooks" must be a primary concern of the business administrator:

For the individual the job is the center of life, and its values must be in harmony with the rest of life if he is to be a whole and healthy personality.

This is an industrial society, and its values tend to become those of the entire culture.

The public is insisting that business leaders are in fact responsible for the general social welfare — that the manager's responsibilities go far beyond those of running the business. They have delegated this responsibility to the business executive whether he wishes to play this role or not.

Even if the administrator insists on a narrow definition of his function as merely the production of goods and services as efficiently as possible, it is nevertheless essential that he take these intangibles into account, since they are the real secrets of motivating an organization.

Besides all this the administrator needs a better set of "skyhooks" himself if he is to carry his ever-increasing load of responsibility without cracking up. The fact that so many administrators are taking time to rationalize, defend, and justify the private enterprise system is an outward indication of this need for more significant meanings.

### Anything Wrong with Capitalism?

We may ask, then: What specifically is wrong with our capitalistic system of private enterprise? What is wrong with production or with trying to improve our present standard of living? What is wrong with a profit, or with private ownership of capital, or with competition? Is this not the true American way of life?

Nothing is necessarily wrong with these values. There are certainly worse motives than the profit motive. A refugee from communism is reported to have observed: "What a delight to be in the United States, where things are produced and sold with such a nice clean motive as making a profit."

I am not an economist, and it is beyond the scope of this article to attempt a revision of our economic theory. I am tempted, however, to make a couple of observations about these traditional economic concepts:

1. That while the values represented by them are not necessarily wrong, they are certainly pretty thin and do not challenge the best in people.

2. That many of the classical economic assumptions are outmoded and are no longer adequate descriptions of the actual operation of our present-day economy.

For example, the concept of economic man as being motivated by self-interest not only is outmoded by the best current facts of the social sciences, but also fails to appeal to the true nobility of spirit of which we are capable.

The concept of the free and competitive market is a far cry from the highly controlled and regulated economy in which business must operate today. General Motors does not appear to want to put Chrysler out of business, and apparently the union also decided to take the heat off Chrysler rather than to press its economic advantage to the logical conclusion. The assumption that everyone is out to destroy his competitors does not explain the sharing of technology through trade associations and journals. No, we also have tremendous capacity for co-operation when challenged by larger visions. We are daily denying the Darwinian notion of the "survival of the fittest"—which, incidentally, William Graham Sumner, one of the nineteenth-century apologists for our economic system, used for justifying unbridled self-interest and competition.

Certainly the traditional concept of private ownership of capital does not quite correspond to the realities of today's control of large blocks of capital by insurance companies and trusteed funds.

The notion of individual security through the accumulation of savings has largely given way to the collectivist means of group insurance, company annuities, and Social Security.

The concept that all profits belong to the stockholders is no longer enthusiastically supported by either the government or the unions, since both are claiming an increasing cut.

And so, while we may argue that the system of private enterprise is self-regulatory and therefore offers maximum individual freedom, the simple, cold fact is that it is in ever-increasing degree a managed or controlled economy—partly at the insistence of the voters, but largely as the result of the inevitable economic pressures and the trend toward bigness.[4]

Regardless of the rightness or wrongness of these changes in our system of enterprise, the changes have been considerable, and I doubt that classical economic theory can be used as an adequate rationale of its virtues. I am therefore not particularly optimistic about the efficacy of the current campaign to have businessmen "save the private enterprise system and the American way of life" by engaging in wholesale economic education, much of which is based on outmoded concepts.

Much as economic theory needs revision, I fear that this is not likely to cure our ills. Nor do I believe that profit-sharing or any other device for increasing the workers' cut (desirable as these efforts may be) will give us what we really want. It is, rather, another type of sharing that is needed, a sharing of more worthy objectives, a sharing of the management function, and a sharing of mutual respect and Christian working relationships.

**Goals and purposes.** What is wrong is more a matter of goals and purposes—of our assumptions about what we are trying to do and how we can dignify and improve ourselves in the doing. There is nothing wrong with production, but we should ask ourselves: *Production for what?* Do we use people for production or production for people? How can production be justified if it destroys personality and human values both in the process of its manufacture and by its end use? Clarence B. Randall of Inland Steel, in his book, *A Creed for Free Enterprise*, says:

> We have come to worship production as an end in itself, which of course it is not. It is precisely there that the honest critic of our way of life makes his attack and finds us vulnerable. Surely there must be for each person some ultimate value, some purpose, some mode of self-expression that makes the experience we call life richer and deeper.[5]

So far, so good, Mr. Randall. But now notice how he visualizes industry making its contribution to this worthy objective:

> To produce more and more with less and less effort is merely treading water unless we *thereby release time and energy for the cultivation of the mind and the spirit* and for the achievement of those ends for which Providence placed us on this earth.[6]

Here is the same old dichotomy—work faster and more efficiently so that you can finish your day of drudgery and cultivate your soul on your own time. In fact he says: "A horse with a very evil disposition can nevertheless pull the farmer's plow." No, I am afraid the job *is* the life. *This* is what must be made meaningful. We cannot assume that the end of production justifies the means. What happens to people in the course of producing may be far more important than the end product. Materialism is not a satisfactory "skyhook." People are capable of better and want to do better. (Incidentally, I have the impression that Mr. Randall's practices line up very well with my own point of view even if his words do not.)

Perhaps we should ask: What is the really important difference between Russian communism and our system? Both worship production and are determined to produce more efficiently, and do. Both worship science. Both have tremendously improved the standard of living of their people. Both share the wealth. Both develop considerable loyalties for their system. (In a mere 40 years since Lenin started the communist revolution a third of the world's people have come to accept its allegiance.) True, in Russia capital is controlled by the state, while here it is theoretically controlled by individuals, although in actual practice, through absentee ownership, it is controlled to a considerable extent by central planning agencies and bureaus, both public and private.

No, the real difference is in the philosophy about people and how they may be used as means to ends. It is a difference in the assumptions made about the origin of rights—whether the individual is endowed with rights by his Creator and yields these only voluntarily to civil authority designated by him, or whether rights originate in force and in the will of the government. Is God a myth, or is He the final and absolute judge to whom we are ultimately responsible? Are all standards of conduct merely man-made and relative, or absolute and eternal? Is man a meaningless happenstance of protoplasm, or is he a divine creation with a purpose, with potential for improvement, and with a special destiny in the overall scheme of things? These are some of the differences—or at least I hope that they still are. And what a difference these intangible, perhaps mythical "skyhooks" make. They are nevertheless the most real and worthwhile and enduring things in the world. The absence of these values permitted the Nazis to "process" people through the gas chambers in order to recover the gold in their teeth.

### The Administrator Contributes

This, then, is part of our general cultural heritage and is passed on to us in many ways. However, it really comes to life in people—in their attitudes, aspirations, and behaviors. And in a managerial society this brings us back to the quality of the individual administrator. He interprets or crystallizes the values and objectives for his group. He sets the climate within which these values either *do* or *do not* become working realities. He must define the goals and purposes of his group in larger and more meaningful perspective. He integrates the smaller, selfish goals of individuals into larger, more social and spiritual, objectives for the group. He provides the vision without which the people perish. Conflicts are resolved by relating the immediate to the long-range and more enduring values. In fact, we might say this *integrative function* is the core of the administrator's contribution.

The good ones have the mental equipment to understand the business and set sound long-term objectives, but the best ones have in addition the philosophical and character values which help them to relate the overall goals of the enterprise to eternal values. This is precisely the point at which deep-seated religious convictions can serve an integrative function, since they represent the most long-range of all possible goals.[7] Most really great leaders in all fields of human endeavor have been peculiarly sensitive to their historic role in human destiny. Their responsibility and loyalty are to some distant vision which gives calm perspective to the hot issues of the day.

This function of the administrator goes far beyond being a likable personality, or applying correct principles of organization, or being skillful in the so-called techniques of human relations. I am convinced that the difficulties which so many executives have with supervisory relationships cannot be remedied by cultivation of the so-called human relations skills. These difficulties spring, rather, from one's conception of his function or role as a boss, his notion about the origin and nature of his authority over others, the assumptions he makes about people and their worth, and his view of what he and his people are trying to accomplish together. To illustrate:

If, for example, my personal goal is to get ahead in terms of money, position, and power; and if I assume that to achieve this I must best my competitors; that the way to do this is to establish a good production record; that my employees are means to this end; that they are replaceable production units which must be skillfully manipulated; that this can be done by appealing to the lowest form of immediate selfish interest; that the greatest threat to me is that my employees may not fully recognize my authority or accept my leadership—if these are my values, then I am headed for trouble—all supervisory techniques notwithstanding.

I wish I could be quite so positive in painting the picture of the right values and approaches to management. I suspect there are many, many different right answers. No doubt each company or enterprise will have to define its own long-term purposes and develop its own philosophy in terms of its history, traditions, and its real function in our economy. I am also certain that no one philosophy would be equally useful to all managers. The character of an organization is, to a large extent, set by the top man or the top group, and it is inevitable that this be the reflection of the philosophy of these individuals. No one of us can operate with another's philosophy. I have also observed that in most enterprises the basic faith or spirit of the organization is a rather nebulous or undefined something which nevertheless has very profound meaning to the employees.

**A successful executive.** Recognizing then the futility of advocating any one pattern of values, it occurs to me that it might, however, be suggestive or helpful if I told you something of the philosophy of one extremely successful executive whom I have pumped a good deal on this subject (for he is more inclined to live his values than to talk about them).

As near as I can piece it together, he believes that this world was not an accident but was created by God and that His laws regulate and control the universe and that we are ultimately *responsible to Him.* Man, as God's supreme creation, is in turn endowed with creative ability. Each individual represents a unique combination of talents and potentials. In addition, man is the only animal endowed with freedom of choice and with a high capacity for making value judgments. With these gifts (of heredity and cultural environment) goes an obligation to give the best possible accounting of one's stewardship in terms of maximum self-development and useful service to one's fellows in the hope that one may live a rich life and be a credit to his Creator.

This executive also assumes that each individual possesses certain God-given rights of self-direction which only *the individual* can voluntarily delegate to others in authority over him, and that this is usually done in the interest of achieving some mutual cooperative good. The executive therefore assumes that his *own* authority as boss over others must be exercised with due regard for the attendant obligations to his employees and to the stockholders who have temporarily and voluntarily yielded their rights in the interest of this common undertaking. (Notice that he does not view his authority as originating with or derived from his immediate superior.) This delegated authority must, of course, be used to advance the common good rather than primarily to achieve the selfish ambitions of the leader at the expense of the led.

He further assumes that the voluntary association of employees in industry is for the purpose of increasing the creativity and productivity of all members of the group and thus of bringing about increased benefits to all who may share in the ultimate use of these goods and services. What is equally important, however, is that in the course of this industrial operation each individual should have an opportunity to develop the maximum potential of his skills and that the working relationships should not destroy the individual's ability to achieve his greatest maturity and richness of experience. As supervisor he must set the working conditions and atmosphere which will make it possible for his employees to achieve this dual objective of increasing productivity and maximizing self-development.

These goals can best be achieved by giving employees maximum opportunity to exercise their capacity for decision making and judgment within their assigned area of responsibility. The supervisor is then primarily a coach who must instruct, discipline, and motivate all the members of the group, making it possible for each to exercise his special talent in order to maximize the total team contribution. Profits are regarded as a measure of the group's progress toward these goals, and a loss represents not only an improper but even an immoral use of the talents of the group.

There is nothing "soft" about his operation. He sets high quality standards and welcomes stiff competition as an additional challenge to his group. He therefore expects and gets complete cooperation and dedication on the part of everyone. Incidentally, he views the activity of working together in this manner with others as being one of life's most rewarding experiences. He holds that this way of life is something which we have not yet fully learned, but that its achievement is part of our divine destiny. He is firmly convinced that such conscientious efforts *will* be rewarded with success. He manages with a light touch that releases creativity, yet with complete confidence in the outcome.

This is probably a poor attempt at verbalizing the basic philosophy which this man lives so easily and naturally. I hope, however, that it has revealed something of his conception of his role or function as an executive, and his view of what he and his organization are trying to do together. With this account of his values I am sure that you would have no difficulty completing the description of his administrative practices and operating results. They flow naturally from his underlying faith, without benefit of intensive training in the principles and art of administration.

As you would suspect, people like to work for him — or with him. He attracts good talent (which is one of the real secrets of success). Those with shoddy values, selfish ambitions, or character defects do not survive — the organization is self-pruning. Those who remain develop rapidly because they learn to accept responsibility. He not only advocates but practices decentralization and delegation. His employees will admit that they have made mistakes, but usually add with a grin that they try not to make the same one twice. People respond to his leadership because he has faith in them and expects the best in them rather than the worst. He speaks well of the members of his organization, and they appear to be proud of each other and of their record of performance. He takes a keen interest in developing measurements of performance and in bettering previous records or competitive standards. He feels that no one has a right to "louse up a job" — a point on which he feels the stockholders and the Lord are in complete agreement.

While he does not talk much about "employee communications" or stress formal programs of this type, his practice is to spend a large proportion of his time in the field with his operating people rather than in his office. He is "people oriented," and he does a particularly good job of listening. The union committee members have confidence in his fairness, yet do a workmanlike job of bargaining. In administering salaries he seems to be concerned about helping the individual to improve his contribution so that a pay increase can be justified.

In his general behavior he moves without haste or hysteria. He is typically well organized, relaxed, and confident, even under trying circumstances. There is a high degree of consistency in his behavior and in the quality of his decisions because his basic values do not shift. Since he does not operate by expediency, others can depend on him; and this consistency makes for efficiency in the discharge of delegated responsibility. Those operating problems which do come to him for decision seem to move easily and quickly to a conclusion. His long-term values naturally express themselves in well-defined policies, and it is against this frame of reference that the decisions of the moment easily fall into proper perspective.

In policy-level discussions his contributions have a natural quality of objectivity because "self-concern" does not confuse. Others take him at face value because his motives are not suspect. When differences or conflicts do arise, his approach is not that of compromise; rather, he attempts to integrate the partisan views around mutually acceptable longer-range goals. The issues of the moment then seem to dissolve in a discussion of the best means to the achievement of the objective. I have no doubt that he also has some serious problems, but I have tried to give a faithful account of the impression which he creates. There is a *sense of special significance* about his operation which is shared by his associates.

### This Is the Key

It is precisely this "sense of special significance" which is the key to leadership. We all know that there are many different ways of running a successful operation. I am certainly not recommending any particular set of administrative practices — although admittedly some are better than others. Nor am I suggesting that his set of values should be adopted by others, or for that matter could be. What I am saying is that a man's real values have a subtle but inevitable way of being communicated, and they affect the significance of everything he does.

These are the vague intangibles — the "skyhooks" — which are difficult to verbalize but easy to sense and tremendously potent in their influence. They provide a different, invisible, fundamental structure into which the experiences of every day are absorbed and given meaning. They are frequently unverbalized, and in many organizations they defy definition. Yet they are the most real things in the world.

The late Jacob D. Cox, Jr., formerly president of Cleveland Twist Drill Company, told a story that illustrates my point:

> Jimmy Green was a new union committee member who stopped in to see Mr. Cox after contract negotiations had been concluded. Jimmy said that every other place he had worked, he had always gone home grouchy; he never wanted to play with the children or take his wife to the movies. And then he said, "But since I have been working here, all that has changed. Now when I come home, the children run to meet me and we have a grand romp together. It is a wonderful difference and I don't know why, but I thought you would like to know."[8]

As Mr. Cox observed, there must be a lot of Jimmy Greens in the world who want an opportunity to take part freely in a cooperative effort that has a moral purpose.

### *APPENDIX*

It's time I level with HBR readers about how "Skyhooks" came about. In a very real sense, I did not write it. It came as a stream of consciousness — but only after I had worked very hard for several weeks at putting my ideas together. I wrote the paper mainly to clear my own thinking, and to try it out for criticism on the Cleveland Philosophical Club. After much reading and thinking, I got absolutely nowhere. In desperation I was about to abandon the idea and write on a different subject. Deep inside my consciousness I said in effect to my silent partner within, "Look, if you want me to do this, you better help."

About 2 a.m. that morning the ideas flowed in a continuous stream, and I put them down in shorthand notes as fast as I could.

The word "Skyhooks" for the title came in the heat of a discussion with a group of business executives attending the Institute of Humanistic Studies at Aspen, Colorado. As we debated the limits of the rational and scientific approach to life, it occurred to me that science appears rational on the surface, but at its very foundation typically lies a purely intuitive, non-rational assumption made by some scientist. He just hooked himself on a "piece of sky out there" and hung on. It was a complete leap of faith that led him.

In my studies of exceptional executives I had found a mystery not easily explainable by rational elements. These men, too, were hanging on skyhooks of their own—hidden and secret missions which went way beyond their corporate business objectives. Sometimes the mission was a "nutsy" one. Often it had long roots back in the executive's childhood and was emotional, intuitive, beyond rationality, selfless—but it stuck. For example, it might be like John F. Kennedy's determination to become President; reportedly he was doing it for his older brother, who had the ambition to be President but never made it because he was a war casualty.

Or perhaps the mission was like that of the president of one of our largest corporations. When he was 12 years old, his father died. He promised his mother he would help her work the farm in the hills so that his eight younger brothers could go through school. This is what he continued to do all of his life—helping other young men to make something of themselves. He was a great developer of managers.

I could fill a book with such examples. Many great executives I have known have something deep inside that supports them; something they trust when the going gets tough; something ultimate; something personal; something beyond reason—in short, a deep-rooted skyhook which brings them calm and confidence when they stand alone.

There is another interesting aspect to this question. In our rational, analytical, and highly successful Western culture, we have come to place great value on the material gains which represent the end results of our achievements. This is what our kids are complaining about: that we have gone overboard on material values and made a culture of *things*. But the *results* of our strivings are dead works; the life is in the *process* of achieving, in the leap of faith. David was great not when he slew Goliath, but when he decided to try.

So it seems to me that the skyhooks mystique is also characterized by a commitment to value the *process*, the working relationships with others, the spiritual bonds growing out of the faith in the God-potential deep within another person, and the basis of genuine community. The rest is the means, not the end.

In 1955, when my article was published, the generation gap had not been invented, and Marshall McLuhan had not alerted us to the fact that "the medium is the message." Yet a quick look backward reveals the considerable impact of youth and "McLuhanism" on our history and our future. The "McCarthy Kids" have ousted a President and his party, halted the military domination of our foreign policy, radically changed our educational and religious institutions, revised industry's approach to management recruiting, and made the Peace Corps type of job competitive with the "goodies" offered by business. Generalizing about the medium having greater impact than the message, they have pointed out that our values are dictated by our social systems—especially the technological, political, and managerial systems. More important than the things we create in industry, they say, is the *way* we create them—the kind of community we establish in our working together.

Without debating the merits of "pot" versus liquor, or anarchy versus order, I believe their emphasis on social process is introducing a new dimension into our corporate life and values.

"Skyhooks" was written for myself and not for publication. For a while I refused to give anybody a copy, but under pressure I duplicated a small number of copies for my friends, and they wanted copies for their friends. When the Editor of HBR got his copy and asked, "How about publishing it?" I answered, "Only if you take it as it is; I don't want to revise it." I see little need for revising it now—except perhaps the reference to the increase in membership in the institutional church. The search for ultimate values and meanings is keener than in 1955, but it is apparently no longer satisfied merely by church affiliation.

### NOTES

1. New York: W.W. Norton, 1954.
2. John Kord Lagemann, "Job Enlargement Boosts Production," *Nation's Business*, December 1954, p. 36.
3. New Haven: Yale University Press, 1950.
4. See John Kenneth Galbraith, *American Capitalism* (Boston: Houghton Mifflin, 1952).
5. Boston: Little, Brown, 1952, p. 16.
6. Ibid.
7. For further elaboration, see Gordon W. Allport, *The Individual and His Religion* (New York: Macmillan, 1953).
8. *Material Human Progress* (Cleveland: Cleveland Twist Drill Company, 1954), p. 104.

# 6

# Ethical Managers Make Their Own Rules

### SIR ADRIAN CADBURY

In 1900 Queen Victoria sent a decorative tin with a bar of chocolate inside to all of her soldiers who were serving in South Africa. These tins still turn up today, often complete with their contents, a tribute to the collecting instinct. At the time, the order faced my grandfather with an ethical dilemma. He owned and ran the second-largest chocolate company in Britain, so he was trying harder and the order meant additional work for the factory. Yet he was deeply and publicly opposed to the Anglo-Boer War. He resolved the dilemma by accepting the order, but carrying it out at cost. He therefore made no profit out of what he saw as an unjust war, his employees benefited from the additional work, the soldiers received their royal present, and I am still sent the tins.

My grandfather was able to resolve the conflict between the decision best for his business and his personal code of ethics because he and his family owned the firm which bore their name. Certainly his dilemma would have been more acute if he had had to take into account the interests of outside shareholders, many of whom would no doubt have been in favor both of the war and of profiting from it. But even so, not all my grandfather's ethical dilemmas could be as straight-forwardly resolved.

So strongly did my grandfather feel about the South African War that he acquired and financed the only British newspaper which opposed it. He was also against gambling, however, and so he tried to run the paper without any references to horse racing. The effect on the newspaper's circulation was such that he had to choose between his ethical beliefs. He decided, in the end, that it was more important that the paper's voice be heard as widely as possible than that gambling should thereby receive some mild encouragement. The decision was doubtless a relief to those working on the paper and to its readers.

The way my grandfather settled these two clashes of principle brings out some practical points about ethics and business decisions. In the first place, the possibility that ethical and commercial considerations will conflict has always faced those who run companies. It is not a new problem. The difference now is that a more widespread and critical interest is being taken in our decisions and in the ethical judgments which lie behind them.

Secondly, as the newspaper example demonstrates, ethical signposts do not always point in the same direction. My grandfather had to choose between opposing a war and condoning gambling. The rule that it is best to tell the truth often runs up against the rule that we should not hurt people's feelings unnecessarily. There is no simple, universal formula for solving ethical problems. We have to choose from our own codes of conduct whichever rules are appropriate to the case in hand; the outcome of those choices makes us who we are.

Lastly, while it is hard enough to resolve dilemmas when our personal rules of conduct conflict, the real difficulties arise when we have to make decisions which affect the interests of others. We can work out what weighting to give to our own rules through trial and error. But business decisions require us to do the same for others by allocating weights to all the conflicting interests which may be involved. Frequently, for example, we must balance the interests of employees against those of shareholders. But even that sounds more straightforward than it really is, because there may well be differing views among the shareholders, and the interests of past, present, and future employees are unlikely to be identical.

Eliminating ethical considerations from business decisions would simplify the management task, and Milton Friedman has urged something of the kind in arguing that the interaction between business and society should be left to the political process. "Few trends could so thoroughly undermine the very foundation of our free society," he writes in *Capitalism and Freedom*," as the acceptance by corporate officials of a social responsibility other than to make as much money for their shareholders as possible."

But the simplicity of this approach is deceptive. Business is part of the social system and we cannot isolate the economic elements of major decisions from their social consequences. So there are no simple rules. Those who make business decisions have to assess the economic and social consequences of their actions as best as they can and come to their conclusions on limited information and in a limited time.

As will already be apparent, I use the word ethics to mean the guidelines or rules of conduct by which we aim to live. It is, of course, foolhardy to write about ethics at all, because you lay yourself open to the charge of taking up a position of moral superiority, of failing to practice what you preach, or both. I am not in a position to preach nor am I promoting a specific code of conduct. I believe, however, that it is useful to all of us who are responsible for business decisions to acknowledge the part which ethics plays in those decisions and to encourage discussion of how best to combine commercial and ethical judgments. Most business decisions involve some degree of ethical judgment; few can be taken solely on the basis of arithmetic.

While we refer to a company as having a set of standards, that is a convenient shorthand. The people who make up the company are responsible for its conduct and it is their collective actions which determine the company's standards. The ethical standards of a company are judged by its actions, not by pious statements of intent put out in its name. This does not mean that those who head companies should not set down what they believe their companies stand for—hard though that is to do. The character of a company is a matter of importance to those in it, to those who do business with it, and to those who are considering joining it.

What matters most, however, is where we stand as individual managers and how we behave when faced with decisions which require us to combine ethical and commercial judgments. In approaching such decisions, I believe it is helpful to go through two steps. The first is to determine, as precisely as we can, what our personal rules of conduct are. This does not mean drawing up a list of virtuous notions, which will probably end up as a watered-down version of the Scriptures without their literary merit. It does mean looking back at decisions we have made and working out from there what our rules actually are. The aim is to avoid confusing ourselves and everyone else by declaring one set of principles and acting on another. Our ethics are expressed in our actions, which is why they are usually clearer to others than to ourselves.

Once we know where we stand personally we can move on to the second step, which is to think through who else will be affected by the decision and how we should weight their interest in it. Some interests will be represented by well-organized groups; others will have no one to put their case. If a factory manager is negotiating a wage claim with employee representatives, their remit is to look after the interests of those who are already employed. Yet the effect of the wage settlement on the factory's costs may well determine whether new employees are likely to be taken on. So the manager cannot ignore the interest of potential employees in the outcome of the negotiation, even though that interest is not represented at the bargaining table.

The rise of organized interest groups makes it doubly important that managers consider the arguments of everyone with a legitimate interest in a decision's outcome. Interest groups seek publicity to promote their causes and they have the advantage of being single-minded: they are against building an airport on a certain site, for example, but take no responsibility for finding a better alternative. This narrow focus gives pressure groups a debating advantage against managements, which cannot evade the responsibility for taking decisions in the same way.

In *The Hard Problems of Management*, Mark Pastin has perceptively referred to this phenomenon as the ethical superiority of the uninvolved, and there is a good deal of it about. Pressure groups are skilled at seizing the high moral ground and arguing that our judgment as managers is at best biased and at worst influenced solely by private gain because we have a direct commercial interest in the outcome of our decisions. But as managers we are also responsible for arriving at business decisions which take account of all the interests concerned; the uninvolved are not.

At times the campaign to persuade companies to divest themselves of their South African subsidiaries has exemplified this kind of ethical high-handedness. Apartheid is abhorrent politically, socially, and morally. Those who argue that they can exert some influence on the direction of change by staying put believe this as sincerely as those who favor divestment. Yet many anti-apartheid campaigners reject the proposition that both sides have the same end in view. From their perspective it is self-evident that the only ethical course of action is for companies to wash their hands of the problems of South Africa by selling out.

Managers cannot be so self-assured. In deciding what weight to give to the arguments for and against divestment, we must consider who has what at stake in the outcome of the decision. The employees of a South African subsidiary have the most direct stake, as the decision affects their future; they are also the group whose voice is least likely to be heard outside South Africa. The shareholders have at stake any loss on divestment, against which must be balanced any gain in the value of their shares through severing the South African connection. The divestment lobby is the one group for whom the decision is costless either way.

What is clear even from this limited analysis is that there is no general answer to the question of whether companies should sell their South African subsidiaries or not. Pressure to reduce complicated issues to straightforward alternatives, one of which is right and the other wrong, is a regrettable sign of the times. But boards are rarely presented with two clearly opposed alternatives. Companies faced with the same issues will therefore properly come to different conclusions and their decisions may alter over time.

A less contentious divestment decision faced my own company when we decided to sell our foods division. Because the division was mainly a U.K. business with regional brands, it did not fit the company's strategy, which called for concentrating resources behind our confectionery and soft drinks brands internationally. But it was an attractive business in its own right and the decision to sell prompted both a management bid and external offers.

Employees working in the division strongly supported the management bid and made their views felt. In this instance, they were the best organized interest group and they had more information available to them to back their case than any of the other parties involved. What they had at stake was also very clear.

From the shareholders' point of view, the premium over asset value offered by the various bidders was a key aspect of the decision. They also had an interest in seeing the deal completed without regulatory delays and without diverting too much management attention from the ongoing business. In addition, the way in which the successful bidder would guard the brand name had to be considered, since the division would take with it products carrying the parent company's name.

In weighing the advantages and disadvantages of the various offers, the board considered all the groups, consumers among them, who would be affected by the sale. But our main task was to reconcile the interests of the employees and of the shareholders. (The more, of course, we can encourage employees to become shareholders, the closer together the interests of these two stakeholders will be brought.) The division's management upped its bid in the face of outside competition, and after due deliberation we decided to sell to the management team, believing that this choice best balanced the diverse interests at stake.

Companies whose activities are international face an additional complication in taking their decisions. They aim to work to the same standards of business conduct wherever they are and to behave as good corporate citizens of the countries in which they trade. But the two aims are not always compatible: promotion on merit may be the rule of the company and promotion by seniority the custom of the country. In addition, while the financial arithmetic on which companies base their decisions is generally accepted, what is considered ethical varies among cultures.

If what would be considered corruption in the company's home territory is an accepted business practice elsewhere, how are local managers expected to act? Companies could do business only in countries in which they feel ethically at home, provided always that their shareholders take the same view. But this approach could prove unduly restrictive, and there is also a certain arrogance in dismissing foreign codes of conduct without considering why they may be different. If companies find, for example, that they have to pay customs officers in another country just to do their job, it may be that the state is simply transferring its responsibilities to the private sector as an alternative to using taxation less efficiently to the same end.

Nevertheless, this example brings us to one of the most common ethical issues companies face — how far to go in buying business? What payments are legitimate for companies to make to win orders and, the reverse side of that coin, when do gifts to employees become bribes? I use two rules of thumb to test whether a payment is acceptable from the company's point of view: Is the payment on the face of the invoice? Would it embarrass the recipient to have the gift mentioned in the company newspaper?

The first test ensures that all payments, however unusual they may seem, are recorded and go through the books. The second is aimed at distinguishing bribes from gifts, a definition which depends on the size of the gift and the influence it is likely to have on the recipient. The value of a case of whiskey to me would be limited, because I only take it as medicine. We know ourselves whether a gift is acceptable or not and we know that others will know if they are aware of the nature of the gift.

As for payment on the face of the invoice, I have found it a useful general rule precisely because codes of conduct do vary round the world. It has legitimized some otherwise unlikely company payments, to the police in one country, for example, and to the official planning authorities in another, but all went through the books and were audited. Listing a payment on the face of the invoice may not be a sufficient ethical test, but it is a necessary one; payments outside the company's system are corrupt and corrupting.

The logic behind these rules of thumb is that openness and ethics go together and that actions are unethical if they will not stand scrutiny. Openness in arriving at decisions reflects the same logic. It gives those with an interest in a particular decision the chance to make their views known and opens to argument the basis on which the decision is finally taken. This in turn enables the decision makers to learn from experience and to improve their powers of judgment.

Openness is also, I believe, the best way to disarm outside suspicion of companies' motives and actions. Disclosure is not a panacea for improving the relations between business and society, but the willingness to operate an open system is the foundation of those relations. Business needs to be open to the views of society and open in return about its own activities; this is essential for the establishment of trust.

For the same reasons, as managers we need to be candid when making decisions about other people. Dr. Johnson reminds us that when it comes to lapidary inscriptions, "no man is upon oath." But what should be disclosed in references, in fairness to those looking for work and to those who are considering employing them?

The simplest rule would seem to be that we should write the kind of reference we would wish to read. Yet "do as you would be done by" says nothing about ethics. The actions which result from applying it could be ethical or unethical, depending on the standards of the initiator. The rule could be adapted to help managers determine their ethical standards, however, by reframing it as a question: If you did business with yourself, how ethical would you think you were?

Anonymous letters accusing an employee of doing something discreditable create another context in which candor is the wisest course. Such letters cannot by definition be answered, but they convey a message to those who receive them, however warped or unfair the message may be. I normally destroy these letters, but tell the person concerned what has been said. This conveys the disregard I attach to nameless allegation, but preserves the rule of openness. From a practical point of view, it serves as a warning if there is anything in the allegations; from an ethical point of view, the degree to which my judgment of the person may now be prejudiced is known between us.

The last aspect of ethics in business decisions I want to discuss concerns our responsibility for the level of employment; what can or should companies do about the provision of jobs? This issue is of immediate concern to European managers because unemployment is higher in Europe than it is in the United States and the net number of new jobs created has been much lower. It comes to the fore whenever companies face decisions which require a trade-off between increasing efficiency and reducing numbers employed.

If you believe, as I do, that the primary purpose of a company is to satisfy the needs of its customers and to do so profitably, the creation of jobs cannot be the company's goal as well. Satisfying customers requires companies to compete in the marketplace, and so we cannot opt out of introducing new technology, for example, to preserve jobs. To do so would be to deny consumers the benefits of progress, to short-change the shareholders, and in the longer run to put the jobs of everyone in the company at risk. What destroys jobs certainly and permanently is the failure to be competitive.

Experience says that the introduction of new technology creates more jobs than it eliminates, in ways which cannot be forecast. It may do so, however, only after a time lag, and those displaced may not, through lack of skills, be able to take advantage of the new opportunities when they arise. Nevertheless, the company's prime responsibility to everyone who has a stake in it is to retain its competitive edge, even if this means a loss of jobs in the short run.

Where companies do have a social responsibility, however, is in how we manage that situation, how we smooth the path of technological change. Companies are responsible for the timing of such changes and we are in a position to involve those who will be affected by the way in which those changes are introduced. We also have a vital resource in our capacity to provide training, so that continuing employees can take advantage of change and those who may lose their jobs can more readily find new ones.

In the United Kingdom, an organization called Business in the Community has been established to encourage the formation of new enterprises. Companies have backed it with cash and with secondments. The secondment of able managers to worthwhile institutions is a particularly effective expression of concern, because the ability to manage is such a scarce resource. Through Business in the Community we can create jobs collectively, even if we cannot do so individually, and it is clearly in our interest to improve the economic and social climate in this way.

Throughout, I have been writing about the responsibilities of those who head companies and my emphasis has been on taking decisions, because that is what directors and managers are appointed to do. What concerns me is that too often the public pressures which are put on companies in the name of ethics encourage their boards to put off decisions or to wash their hands of problems. There may well be commercial reasons for those choices, but there are rarely ethical ones. The ethical bases on which decisions are arrived at will vary among companies, but shelving those decisions is likely to be the least ethical course.

The company which takes drastic action in order to survive is more likely to be criticized publicly than the one which fails to grasp the nettle and gradually but inexorably declines. There is always a temptation to postpone difficult decisions, but it is not in society's interests that hard choices should be evaded because of public clamor or the possibility of legal action. Companies need to be encouraged to take the decisions which face them; the responsibility for providing that encouragement rests with society as a whole.

Society sets the ethical framework within which those who run companies have to work out their own codes of conduct. Responsibility for decisions, therefore, runs both ways. Business has to take account of its responsibilities to society in coming to its decisions, but society has to accept its responsibilities for setting the standards against which those decisions are made.

# 7

# Storytellers' Ethics

## ROBERT COLES

At one moment in *The Great Gatsby* the narrator, Nick Carraway, looking for his host, wanders into Gatsby's enormous, oak-paneled, Gothic library. There he encounters a drunk and excited man who gestures toward the bookshelves and says, "They're real. . . . Absolutely real—have pages and everything. I thought they'd be a nice durable cardboard. Matter of fact, they're absolutely real. . . . It's a triumph. What thoroughness! What realism! Knew when to stop, too—didn't cut the pages."

At one level, of course, Fitzgerald is exploring the shallow ostentation that can accompany wealth. But Gatsby's unread books also ask us to reflect on all the wisdom they might have offered the enormously (and mysteriously) successful entrepreneur, all the moral energy, the personal and ethical reflection they might have prompted in him had he opened them.

In the late 1930s and 1940s, another American writer was struggling hard with his own moral issues. William Carlos Williams, the New Jersey poet and physician, worked among the poor in cities such as Paterson and so was not always well paid—indeed, had a number of patients who couldn't or didn't pay him at all. At what point should he abandon them—see only the well-to-do, the well educated, many of whom were all too willing to buy his time because he was by then a well-known writer? How was he to come to terms with the social and cultural distance between himself and those mostly immigrant, working-class families whose homes he kept visiting as an old-fashioned general practitioner? Not rarely he found himself annoyed, perplexed, irritated, angry, as he tried to do an earnest doctor's job, yet felt himself misunderstood or ignored or provoked. Why bother at all?

To answer such questions, he wrote a series of stories, published in 1937 under the title *Life Along the Passaic River*—a tough look, really, at the ethical questions a medical practice prompts. Each of the stories is relatively short and quite powerfully provocative. Again and again the doctor has to confront not only his patients' blind spots or moments of selfishness or insensitivity, but also his own egoism and self-importance, his narrowness and imperiousness. The doctor engages in a kind of Augustinian self-scrutiny—offering the reader through fiction a chance to do likewise: look candidly inward and see what he or she finds.

Williams the writer had a far-reaching grasp: he wrote poems, of course, and the short stories I have just mentioned; but he also had a strong interest in

America's political and economic history. He never forgot that Paterson was where Alexander Hamilton founded the first American manufacturing enterprise; nor did he lack interest in his own wife's family.

His father-in-law, Paul Herman, had been a poor immigrant from Germany in 1890s Manhattan. Soon enough he would become a skilled printer and, eventually, a rich entrepreneur, a man who owned his own business and lived exceedingly well. So even as Williams tried to evoke in stories the moral dilemmas doctors keep confronting (or ignoring willfully), he kept his writing eyes on his own world, on the comfortable town of Rutherford—a contrast, indeed, during the 1930s with Paterson—including the fortunes of his in-laws. In 1937, the same year *Life Along the Passaic River* was published, he saw *White Mule* come to print, a substantial novel that was destined to be the first part of the trilogy that includes *In the Money* and *The Buildup*.

Much of what Paul Herman did along the road to business success is chronicled in the trilogy: once an associate of Samuel Gompers, he crossed picket lines, arranged the financing necessary to compete with his old bosses, and in general proved himself to be a smart, knowing, and enterprising businessman. But these books offer something more than a social history of one family's rise. Williams bears down on the private side of things—the manner in which someone gets to think about life and people (including members of his or her own family) as the deals are cut, the bargains struck, the decisions made. These three novels, in essence, cast a close look at the ethical trials and temptations that a competitive industrial order always puts in the way of those who want to become its forceful protagonists.

I came to know Dr. Williams as an undergraduate; I wrote my thesis on the first two books of his major poem "Paterson," a lyrical examination of an important part of America's history, the old factory towns in the Northeast. He was intent in that poem on reminding his readers (and himself) of the distance that all too often separates theory from practice, ideas from conduct. "Smart isn't necessarily good," he once observed. Even in the realm of ethical reflection that tension holds: one can do brilliantly in a course on ethics and not necessarily carry such knowledge into the world of action.

Hitler had at his side, early on, all sorts of intelligent, well-educated people, including, alas, philosophers and psychoanalysts, not to mention religious leaders. Williams kept mentioning such terrible ironies to us (in his writing, in conversations) because, after all, he had been witness to them during the 1930s and 1940s in a personal way. He was a friend of Ezra Pound, whose aesthetic genius, vast store of knowledge, cultivated sensibility, and enormous gifts as a poet did not spare him from becoming a rabid, hate-filled propagandist for Mussolini and Hitler. "His life forced me to think about moral reflection in a new way," Williams once said.

In response to such a dilemma he did not take up programmatic moral analysis (what we should do under X, Y, or Z circumstances) but rather, through story telling, tried to reach the mind, the heart, the soul of his readers—"to affect them deeply," he once put it, "to excite their moral imagination in such a way that they sweat and tremble, toss and turn." He wanted not only the effort of intelligent consideration but also a "moral immersion"—a degree of empathy perhaps—that connects a reader's intellect with his or her personal life.

By moral imagination he meant an emotional as well as an intellectual response:

Those stories [about doctors] and the Stecher books [the trilogy] are aimed at the conscience, my own and anyone else's who reads them. The last thing I want for them is someone's clever interpretation of them, someone's egotistical delight in figuring them out, someone's enjoyment of them as "interesting." I'm out to unnerve people—get them worried about what they might be doing, or not doing. Oh—not to hector them and point a finger at them, no; but if I can get people wondering about how they're doing in life, or how they might be doing in life—whether they're doing good or doing bad, and how much of each!—then I'll have done something myself. And if I've listened to myself, and my words have made a difference in my own way of living—well, that's the test, right? If you don't get nudged into practicing what you preach, or what you read—then you're at a moral standstill, I suspect.

Vintage Williams—blunt talk, the shrewdness about the mind's capacity for self-deception, the essential modesty, the capacity for self-criticism, the lack of (even antagonism toward) academic pretentiousness, and not least, the knack with words and phrases: "moral imagination," "moral standstill." I remember, while in medical school, asking him how some of us going into one or another profession might do the kind of reading that would get our moral imagination going—help us break out of whatever particular moral standstill threatened us. He had no easy or pat answers, of course; but he had faith in story telling: "Hell, from the Bible onward, a parable, a tale, a story well told creeps into your chest, turns your stomach, makes your eyes widen up, your ears, too. It's not only the brain we're after!" Again, vintage Williams—the doctor's inquiry called into service by a writer who wanted to reach people in such a way that his words made a difference in their lives.

His words sure made a difference in my life; they got me thinking, got me ultimately to try medicine, got me also to work with children, as he did: to train in pediatrics and child psychiatry. Eventually, I ended up working with young people themselves caught in various moral struggles (school desegregation, the civil rights movement), and later, I was offered a chance to teach college students and medical students.

But what to teach? Williams's own fiction, of course, for reasons already mentioned: the "doctor stories," glimpses of doctors struggling with irritation, boredom, self-importance, prejudice, and yes, their own vulnerabilities, their moments of irrationality; and *White Mule*, which has a way of getting readers to look at their own family histories—whence they've come, socially and economically, and where they'd like to go, and at what, if any, moral cost.

But Williams is not the only twentieth-century American writer who has taken on such issues. Walker Percy, also a physician, has given us *The Moviegoer*, in which a 29-year-old stockbroker named Binx Bolling takes a sharp, searching look at the world around him, at himself as well.

"Life in Gentilly is very peaceful," Binx tells us early on. "I manage a small branch office of my uncle's brokerage firm. I am a model tenant and a model citizen and take pleasure in doing all that is expected of me. My wallet is full of identity cards, library cards, credit cards. Last year I purchased a flat olive-drab strong box, very smooth and heavily built with double walls for fire protection, in which I placed my birth certificate, college diploma, honorable discharge, G.I.

insurance, a few stock certificates and my inheritance." By then, of course, we are sorting out in our own minds what all those identity cards mean — how we become what we are, and where, as a consequence, we are headed.

Dr. Percy is a wonderfully comic writer, with a keen sense of how so many of us stumble or plow our way through life — forgetting all too often to ask what really matters — what (after all is said and done) we value and hope to leave behind us as our contribution to the world. His novel uses gentle humor, and sometimes social satire, in the service of philosophical reflection. The doctor in him knows that sickness and the threat of death (in others, in ourselves) often prompt us to stop and wonder where we're headed; and so he works such themes into his story, and in so doing gets the rest of us not only to laugh with him, and with Binx, but also to consider our present direction, its pluses and minuses.

Another Southern novelist of distinction, Flannery O'Connor, has contributed a masterpiece to this century's moral fiction in "The Displaced Person." On one level, the story is an account of a landowner's struggles with her workers: her dissatisfaction with one of them, her decision to replace him with another. "Mrs. McIntyre sighed with pleasure," O'Connor writes. " 'At last,' she said, 'I've got somebody I can depend on. For years I've been fooling with sorry people. Sorry people. Poor white trash and niggers,' she muttered."

Yet the author is really taking up the much broader subject of moral purpose — the motives that prompt our actions, whether they be business decisions or personal ones. Like Dr. Percy, Flannery O'Connor has a penetrating sense of humor and a suggestive way with words and images. A story ostensibly about the impact of a "displaced person" (come to our South from Europe after the Second World War) on a seemingly complacent small-town business (farm) turns into something else — a comment on how "displaced" some of our values can on close inspection turn out to be.

I mention all of this because it provides a necessary background to how I arrived at the Harvard Business School in the spring of 1985 to teach a seminar titled "The Business World: Moral and Social Inquiry Through Fiction." By then I had become a bit of an old hand at pushing novels and short stories and occasional poems on Harvard College students and Harvard Medical School students. I'd also ventured elsewhere in the university — to the Graduate School of Education, the law school, and the Kennedy School of Government.

One day in a law school class a student put this question to me: "Why not cross the river and teach at the business school?" The young man was in a joint program at the two schools and was himself grappling with plenty of personal and professional questions — how to combine two kinds of education, where to do so, and with what long-range goals in mind. He had a strong interest in international law, international business — and Third World social problems: a sure recipe for anguish as one gets ready to start out in life!

I was stymied for a while by his question. What would I teach? Who would be interested in studying what I'd teach, if I could muster the kind of reading list I was used to handing out to students — lists of paperback novels or collections of short stories? Where would such a class be headed — the drifts of its explanations and the thrusts of its objectives? My wife, a high school English teacher (and the daughter of a Harvard Business School graduate), gave a lot of thought to those questions, and together we came up with a reading list and with a sequence for the use of the books.

We decided to start with F. Scott Fitzgerald's *The Great Gatsby*, an American classic, which many of the students, I would learn, had read in college but which they now read with different eyes: the story of a parvenu of sorts, but also the story of others, well established in the world of Wall Street—their 1920s moral sensibility tested by an ambitious, aspiring, lavishly hospitable outsider. We followed with Fitzgerald's *The Last Tycoon*, an effort, never fully completed, to evoke the world of Hollywood—and the struggles there between artistic and commercial forces. Fitzgerald was intent on depicting a major industry in transformation—becoming consolidated and integrated into other aspects of the economy (banking, advertising).

Both books offer a provocative inquiry into the lives of successful and powerful people—and as well, an author's mix of personal responses to such individuals: curiosity, admiration, even awe, but also apprehension, ironic amusement, and, occasionally, decided disapproval. Since both novels were turned into movies, we were able to use them as well, and examine the way two morally energetic stories were turned into screenplays, into films.

We moved from Fitzgerald to Flannery O'Connor's gem, "The Displaced Person" and to the film made of that story. When a businesswoman (a landowner) decides to replace an inefficient worker, she sets in motion all sorts of psychological, ethical, and religious events. O'Connor was a Biblical moralist, and her interest is to examine, in microcosm, such enduring aspects of humanity as greed, selfishness, and hate. Such qualities of mind and heart are found in all sorts of people, she suspects. Her story is not meant to embody a confrontation between an employer and her onetime employee, or her new one, but rather an analysis of what people do—with themselves, with one another once certain decisions (in this case, a business one) are made.

We moved on to Saul Bellow's novel *Seize the Day*, with its struggling, beleaguered commodities broker whose efforts to come to terms with his wife, his father, and, indeed, life in general are chronicled with a gifted writer's wry, sardonic shrewdness. There is an antic, loony quality to this novel, and for a while I hesitated to use it; but my wife reminded me of the everyday life of commodity speculators—*their* presumable struggles to find sanity, or at least stability and success, amid so much noise, if not wildly fluctuating frenzy. We kept the novel on the reading list, used it—and the students took to it eagerly.

Next came *The Moviegoer*, the novel by Walker Percy, which I described briefly before. As the stockbroker Binx Bolling tries to figure out how he should live his life, the reader is offered a wonderfully humorous and slyly observant examination of the upper middle class in mid-twentieth-century America. Percy also works over certain themes the European existentialist philosophers and theologians and storytellers have found congenial. Binx's alternation between an aloof interest in self-fulfillment and moments of intense moral self-scrutiny mirrors some of the swings of attitude and behavior many of us note in ourselves.

With *The Moviegoer* I hand out copies of a Percy essay "The Man on the Train"—an essay in moral philosophy, really, but rendered humorously, in the story of a suburban commuter who comes into Manhattan day after day by train and sees so very little on his way. This "fog," this blindness that descends on so many of us so commonly—the way we turn off or tune out at certain moments—is a central preoccupation of Percy: we get lost, as it were, to ourselves, and for reasons he wants to examine. His writing is at once droll and spirited, occasionally melancholy, always instructive—a tonic when we are worried about the ruts into which we have fallen, the automatons we have become.

The next writer, John Cheever, continues an examination, through stories, of the privileged lives some of us live. His territory is not Percy's South but Connecticut's Fairfield County and Manhattan's Upper East Side—the apartment houses that line Fifth Avenue and Park Avenue. Like Percy's, his approach is gentle, affectionate, but not without moments of rueful and somber contemplation. Some of his characters have conquered the world, yet drink too much or seem strangely isolated or withdrawn—their marriages not by any means as successful as their careers, and their children rather hurt or ailing. Cheever's affection for these men and women is obvious—as is Percy's; still, the two novelists wonder (as we all do at moments in our lives) what we lose as we gain: the personal vulnerabilities that come upon us as we live our fast-paced and demanding and productive lives.

The last spell of the course was given over to the astonishing trilogy by William Carlos Williams, mentioned earlier: *White Mule*, *In the Money*, and *The Buildup*. The novels evoke the moral and psychological challenges faced by those who fight to leave the ranks of the working poor to take on the risks and opportunities of the entrepreneur. The point of reading them, of reading all this fiction, is to stir a group of men and women (students and teacher alike) to take stock of themselves: what they believe in, what they want out of life, how they want to live that life. Fiction can be infectiously engaging, can prompt us to sift and sort, to consider ups and downs, desirable possibilities and potentially hurtful impasses or dead-end streets. The point, ultimately, is to stir the moral imagination—to encourage us as readers to look inward as we keep moving through our days and ways.

It is true that there are important and valuable alternatives to this mode of moral inquiry—the case history, for instance. In medicine and business, morally challenging incidents are constantly taking place—decisions about whether (as a doctor) one ought to pull a plug, an intravenous needle, a stomach tube, or (as a businessperson) make this kind of arrangement, embark on that direction. No wonder then that ethics courses devoted to cases are an increasingly familiar presence in many of our medical and business schools.

Still, ethical inquiry can have another, broader dimension to it, can be directed not only at one or another occupational choice but also at the kind of life being lived by one or another doctor, lawyer, businessperson, teacher, architect. Novels and short stories lend themselves especially well to this kind of reflection. They need not become the basis for didactic insistence—the urging of a social or cultural or political agenda. Nor are they meant to be diagnostic or prescriptive. What they do is nudge us to connect our lives to the lives of the various characters in their various stories—to immerse ourselves in a world with plenty of moral drama at work.

Talking about his trilogy, William Carlos Williams said:

You won't find answers in those novels, but you'll find lots of questions asked—by indirection. How do you balance your business life and your home life? How do you resist the temptation to become callous and selfish? How do you hold to moral and religious values in the face of all sorts of challenges at work? What happens to people, emotionally and spiritually, when they compromise with certain important principles—start down the road of rationalizations and self-justifications? The slope is gradual—sometimes imperceptible—but real. I try to survey the slope carefully—to bring the reader up close, so close that his empathy puts him in the shoes of the characters. You hope when he closes the book his own character is influenced!

That last comment is especially interesting—the impact of characters in a story on the character of the reader. It reminds me of the important distinction Emerson made in 1837 in his essay "The American Scholar": "Character is higher than intellect." Novels don't supply the intellect its prized formulations, but rather, suggest various moral, social, and psychological possibilities—stimulate the mind's capacity to wonder, to dream, to put itself in all sorts of situations, and to be shaped by such imaginative experiences. Novels help us shape a general attitude toward living a life—encourage us to think about what we want and at what personal or professional cost. Such a mode of moral inquiry complements the other kind, in which specific situations are analyzed and choices of action discussed.

Efforts to look inward morally with the help of storytellers can run into trouble. The teacher can become self-righteous or a scold—can use the various books assigned as thinly disguised instruments of polemical assertion or condemnation. Tone is all-important—as students themselves quickly appreciate. Do you really want to pour rain on a parade—use F. Scott Fitzgerald's ironies or John Cheever's gentle satire as severe and provocative challenges, to the point that students become antagonistic and feel themselves and their future work arraigned, condemned? The point in a course is not only the students' attitudes—the effort to encourage moral introspection of a personal and heartfelt kind—but the teacher's attitudes: his or her willingness to come clean, so to speak, about what a course intends.

I have seen plenty of arrogance and selfishness in the supposedly gentler, more "humanistic" professions—snobbishness or self-importance and meanness or hardness of spirit in doctors, in the clergy, in educators, in the so-called arts, and certainly, among us in my own branch of medicine, psychoanalytic psychiatry. Years of personal analysis, of education, of postgraduate supervision have not prevented many of us from becoming dogmatic, smug, and fiercely antagonistic to those who happen to disagree with us.

I try to keep such thoughts in mind when I ask future corporate leaders or financiers to take a sharp and candid look, or a smiling and wry one, at certain moral pitfalls. The labor leader, the political reformer, the egalitarian theorist, the medical healer, the minister or priest, the college teacher, even the moral philosopher or wise novelist are in the end all flawed human beings, no less in jeopardy as they go about their lives than those out there in the marketplace.

I found it important, in this last regard, to share with my students a few stories of my own, never mind urge on them the stories of a Flannery O'Connor, a Walker Percy—stories of physician-healers or civil rights activists I'd come to know whose moral struggles were no less serious than any conveyed in the books we read. Nor is the point ingratiation. I simply want to take these novelists on their own merits and not fix them to someone else's political, social, or moral agenda.

I was enormously impressed with the diversity of the business school students I taught: with their moral earnestness, with their willingness to work long and hard at the reading assigned, both in and out of class. Their papers were singularly affecting: in a page or two they connected their experiences to those of the characters in this or that novel. Our class became progressively more relaxed and intimate. We drank beer toward the end. We had a dinner. Months after the course was over and the students had left for the world of business, I received letters with ideas for further reading, and, yes, repeated suggestions that the class have a reunion. Individual readers became members of a particular, inquiring community whose bonds still hold at this writing, almost a year later.

Meanwhile, I hope to keep teaching the course—adding this time around Tolstoy's powerful story "Master and Man," in which a Russian winter storm envelops a businessman and his servant: a morally suggestive drama of great intensity. My hunch is that the men and women who took the course last year will keep doing their own reading of the kind we all did together—or so it seems, given their letters to me with thoughts for the course in future years. After all, these books are available in paperback, some with good introductions. As one student put it to me (he's now on Wall Street by day, Oyster Bay by night), "Reading these novels can become a habit, a habit of being." He was referring to a phrase Flannery O'Connor once used that became the title for a collection of her letters, assembled by Sally Fitzgerald, her biographer.

It was nice, I thought, hearing an existentialist description given to the idea of staying in touch with novels and short stories over the course of one's life. The existentialists emphasize the finite individuality of each of us, our private and personal struggles to comprehend this confused and confusing world; and they emphasize the aloneness each of us experiences, our lonely search for meaning. Hence the appropriateness of that former student's phrase as he tried to let me know that fiction as a moral source can work not only in a class at Harvard Business School but also in an individual's continuing life: again, "a habit of being" acquired.

I had intended that the previous paragraph be the last one, but as I was editing my own words a letter arrived that I believe deserves partial quotation:

> All my friends are talking about Ivan Boesky. They want to know what made him tick. I want to know, too. But yesterday, as we talked, I realized that I did know—as much, probably, as anyone ever will know. I'd read *The Great Gatsby*, and suddenly, as I sat there, in a Wall Street restaurant, Jay Gatsby came to my mind, and our long discussions of what Gatsby is meant to tell us about ourselves. I told my buddies: go get *The Great Gatsby*, read it, think about it, and then we can talk some more about Boesky, and some others we read about in the papers, too.

The letter followed with a renewed invitation for a class reunion in New York City—and as I put it down I realized that such a correspondence, and the classroom course that prompted it, amounted to an answer to that perennial question teachers hear put to them: What is the purpose of your course? The point of those weekly meetings in Morgan Hall was to help us contemplate the likes of an Ivan Boesky—the significance of his ilk for all of us; but the main point was to help us look inward morally, focus sharply on our own values and standards as we get on with our jobs, not to mention our lives.

# PART
## TWO

# The Corporation as Moral Environment

## Introduction

The nine articles in Part II, miscellaneous in origin and emphasis, all bear on the influence of the corporation upon the ethics of the individual. I have ordered them according to their views of the corporation. First is the concept of the corporation as an economic agent with no special ethical obligation, that is, to the extent feasible an amoral environment. The Friedman model, according to which the only social responsibility of the corporation is to make profits within the limits of the law and the rules of the game, leaves moral outcome to the invisible hand of the competitive market and the definition of ethical custom to the rationalizations of those playing the game. On the other hand, a broader definition of the corporation with responsibilities and influential relationships to customers, employees, communities, and shareholders is implicit as the dominant theme of the last four articles. But in either case, the corporation as a culture influences or determines the ethical behavior of the morally movable individuals we looked at in Part I.

"Note on the Corporation as a Moral Environment," by Kenneth E. Goodpaster, which has not appeared in the *Harvard Business Review*, is an item from the Harvard Business School course called "Ethical Aspects of Business Policy." It was designed to be useful in the analysis of cases. It is included here so that readers may apply it to their own organizations and responsibilities. To observe, describe, and evaluate a corporation as a moral environment is a useful undertaking even for a follower of Friedman, for these days the pursuit of profit attended by loosened ethical custom can be abruptly interrupted by a subpoena from the SEC, a delegation with handcuffs from the prosecuting attorney, or suspension by the Department of Defense. For those interested in managing or sharing in the direction of a company in such a way as to permit expression of ethical doubts in troublesome situations, to maintain or even elevate moral judgment, and to ensure clean pursuit of economic goals, this paper should prove helpful.

In what some have considered an outrageous tour de force, Albert Z. Carr asks with no hint of tongue in cheek whether bluffing is ethical. His allegiance to Friedman carries him closer to the line between right and wrong than the master probably ever intended, and frankly describes ethical custom in business as defensible deception. His view of business as a game, like poker, in which no one expects truth to be the language of conversation, must still be reckoned with. It becomes quite clear to what ethical level consensus has lowered the rules. That business as practiced by corporations has developed a special ethics may indeed be suggested by companies in which citizens, allegedly upright in private life, have bribed procurement officials, purchased senatorial favors through noticeably large contributions, adulterated baby food, concealed adverse side effects of pharmaceuticals, approved deceptive advertising copy, sold inside information, or within companies misled superiors, rigged financial reports, or taken credit belonging to others.

The assertion that the standards of right and wrong in business differ from the prevailing traditions of morality in our society, however contested by business leaders, is still widely believed by the public. Such a presumption by individuals confronting moral questions would obviously be most helpful to those on the brink of rationalization before an unethical choice. A hint of sardonic intent is discernible in Carr's statement that "a sudden submission to Christian ethics by businessmen would bring about the greatest economic upheaval in history."

The uproar provoked by this article is the subject of Timothy Blodgett's summary of reader response at the time of first publication. Mr. Carr, in reaction to the objections raised, says that his article plainly indicates that "sound long-range business strategy and ethical considerations are usually served by the same policy." I must confess I missed that wholesome message and find it a late arrival to the discussion.

The article "Is the Ethics of Business Changing?" by Steven N. Brenner and Earl A. Molander repeats in 1976 an inquiry first made in 1961. The *HBR* readers who responded to a questionnaire have accepted the concept of corporate responsibility as "a legitimate and achievable goal for business" in greater numbers than fifteen years earlier. Only 28 percent endorsed the traditional Friedman position. Whether ethical standards in business had improved was a subject of much disagreement. Most respondents favored the development of ethical codes in companies but felt that codes alone would not improve business conduct. The author of the original survey concluded from the data and other signs of the times that business behavior had become more ethical, but that the "expectations of a better educated and ethically sensitized public have risen more rapidly than the behavior." The phenomenon of rising expectations has had much to do with the discovery, publication, and punishment of recent unethical or illegal behavior that would have been ordinary practice in Albert Carr's business world. This article, like the others here from the past, indicates once again that concern for ethics has a long history, both in corporate practice and at the *Harvard Business Review*. The significance of that longtime concern may seem minor in the glare of the high-wattage spotlight wielded at present by newly concerned moralists unentangled in the root problem of combining ethical behavior with economic achievement.

A more profound inquiry into the relation of ethical behavior to the proper function of the corporation is embodied in Douglas S. Sherwin's "The Ethical Roots of the Business System." His definition of ethical behavior is derived from his view of the corporation as exclusively the economic agent of society. To fully realize the potential of economic performance (which rather than profit, he says, is the purpose of a business), managers must realize that "employees, as well as shareholders, and customers must derive benefits commensurate with their performance." Managers' values govern how a business is run. "If in any of the businesses' operations, managers do not realize potential economic performance, either the values of the leadership are not congruent with society's values (that economic performance is the good desired from business) or the leadership is failing to extend its own value system throughout the organization." When business behavior wanders from the values that "connect with the purpose and nature of business" — that is, economic performance — it is unethical.

Sherwin, less simplistic than Friedman, acknowledges that for success three constituencies must be addressed, and he is aware that life inside the corporation can disrupt the free play of even the economic values he confines himself to. He notes, for example, how management-by-objective and return-on-investment criteria can lead managers astray. If such programs are administered so that long-term performance is prejudiced, then (as Carr suggests) they are unethical. Social action falls outside the economic sphere that "society and public policy have assigned to the business system" and also becomes unethical. The reader may question again how clear is society's mandate (now a complex medley of demands for equal opportunity, comparable worth, clean air and water, product safety, and the like) that the corporation concentrate exclusively on economic performance. Who speaks for society?

Unlike Kenneth Goodpaster and John B. Matthews, authors of "Can a Corporation Have a Conscience?" Sherwin says no. Fortunately, the corporation is not a real person, for real persons have values that go beyond the values that connect with the assigned role for private business. Real persons' consciences — variable, open-ended, and inimical to society's aims — would not produce behavior society can depend upon.

Goodpaster and Matthews espouse the thesis that just as persons are moral when they approach decisions carefully and rationally and are concerned about the effect of the decision on others, so "rationality" and "respect" can become characteristic of the corporation. Corporations that "monitor their employment practices and the effects of their production processes and products on the environment and human health" show the rationality and respect that morally responsible individuals do. People organized as a group can act as a unit. When they do, under the direction of established policy, they can be thought of as exhibiting character. Where Sherwin sees attention to the needs of employees, customers, and shareholders as essential to optimal economic performance, Goodpaster and Matthews add a moral justification for treating all those affected by corporate decisions not merely as means and resources but also as ends in themselves.

A close reading of these two articles sheds light on the separation of corporate and personal ethics that is dramatized in the Carr and Learned essays. The separation is perpetuated by different definitions of what society expects of corporations. A pluralistic society does not speak with one voice. Each person has a choice, then, of which voice to attend to, once the literal demands of the law and administrative regulation are satisfied. That choice is surely influenced, one way or another, by the conscience of the persons making it. Readers checking on their own position will find the summary of arguments for and against the assumption by a corporation of moral responsibility comprehensive and illuminating. The outcome has everything to do with the nature of the corporation as an environment that shapes behavior.

The last three articles in this part make important statements about real life inside our companies. Policy that concentrates on economic outcomes without regard to the effects of competition on motivation or without concern for how individuals perceive their own interest has unfortunate consequences never intended by naive policy makers. Robert Jackall brings the perspective of a sociologist to his close observation of two large companies and overview of others. To the extent that his data are representative (selection of the article by a diverse panel of practitioner-judges as the best of the year suggests that they may be), the connection between success and hard work embodied by the Protestant ethic has been eroded by the bureaucracy of formal organization. The administrative hierarchies, standardized work procedures, regularized timetables, uniform policies, and centralized control characteristic of modern production and distribution systems have had a devastating effect. The subordinate owing fealty to his immediate boss suppresses his opinions; all subordinates share an overriding deference to the chief executive officer. Success is no longer objectively determined; it becomes a political achievement, marked by such social definitions of performance as dress, style, reputation as a team player, and relation to a powerful mentor. Managers thus are distracted from sheer performance by the perceived capriciousness of organizational life.

The bureaucratic ethic, as here illustrated perhaps unwittingly by unethical management, is a deadly force. It ties moral choices to personal fates. It substitutes for standards of morality internal rules and social context as the "principal moral gauges for action." "Men and women in bureaucracies turn to each other for moral cues for behavior and come to fashion specific situational moralities for specific significant people in their worlds."

Before you shrug off these corrosive observations about morality gone astray as being unrepresentative, consider price fixing almost anywhere, but for the moment in the folding-carton industry. Jeffrey Sonnenfeld and Paul R. Lawrence in "Why Do Companies Succumb to Price Fixing?" spell out quite crisply the industry and company characteristics that led to flagrant price fixing and the obvious steps that have since been taken to prevent it. That forty-seven executives in twenty-two companies were fined, put on probation, or jailed, and that incalculable damage was done to company morale and reputation should command the attention of anybody wondering what might be going on in his or her organization and how one might detect an illegal and unethical way of life. Jackall knows how to explain it, more usefully than Carr, but cannot be expected to know how to change it. Sonnenfeld and Lawrence directly confront the problem of changing corporate culture. The harder problem is to recognize its character when one is caught up in it and the rationalizations that sustain it.

Bowen H. McCoy knew at the time what his moral problem was—whether to abandon his ambition and that of his group to scale a mountain pass before the sun melted the steps cut in the ice or to carry a nearly naked holy man in the opposite direction to a village far below. His and his group's decision to press on lead him to examine the reasoning that made abandonment of the sadhu defensible and to conclude that it was wrong. He realizes that like many people every day in many companies he had walked through a classic moral dilemma without seeing it or thinking through the consequences. His analysis of the failure of his group to recognize what he now sees was its obligation is extended to the corporation. He concludes that those who would remain moral persons in large organizations must have corporate support or be lost. Without the help of a corporate tradition that encourages openness of inquiry and freedom to operate from a reasoned set of personal values, the need for both individuality and corporate success cannot be met. To change the values of a company or of any group to permit pursuit of the moral alternative is a challenge to management that many economists would reject as irrelevant. The corporate executive, however, is beginning to think it necessary.

The corporation, or any cooperative group to which one belongs, is a powerful constraint on the moral autonomy of any manager confronted with the conflict of corporate economic values and concerns for one's own well-being and that of his or her family. To advance the ethical performance of the present-day corporation, these papers suggest, it is essential to be aware of the inevitable tendencies of bureaucracy, of the fragility of personal rectitude against the attractions of rationalization, reputation, and advancement, and of the alternatives for constructive action possible for those who have become aware of what is happening around them. We are preparing for the courses of action suggested by the articles in Part III.

# 1

# Note on the Corporation as a Moral Environment

KENNETH E. GOODPASTER

Ethics does not treat of the world. Ethics must be a condition of the world, like logic.

— Ludwig Wittgenstein[1]

General managers are like ecologists who anticipate and monitor the effects of corporate policy on environments both inside and outside the corporation. One way of understanding the corporation is to divide its transactions into two types that are central to the functions of the general manager and ethically important in their own right.[2] First, the corporation acts as a moral agent when its policies and actions affect outside constituencies, including the welfare of society as a whole. Second, when policies affect inside constituencies, the corporation can be viewed as a moral environment, and should therefore be managed with a view to the freedom and well-being of its members.

This note focuses on how policy formulation and implementation can affect the moral environment of an organization. More specifically, it examines the corporation's obligations and responsibilities regarding not only the rights and welfare of its employees but also its influence on their moral character.

We begin by looking at management of the work environment from a historical perspective. The next section maps the areas in which policies can influence the corporation as a moral environment. In the following two sections we discuss the particular responsibilities of the corporation in these areas. Finally, the last section offers some analytical questions for evaluating cases.

## Historical Overview

The Industrial Revolution effected three important changes in the activity of work. First, mechanization diminished the need for skilled labor. Second, the size of production required standardized procedures and precluded close personal interaction between owners and workers. And third, industrialization required people not only to work outside of their homes, but sometimes to relocate from rural communities into urban areas. These changes dramatically affected social relations and moral values. People, cut off from traditional communities, also lost control of their work under the new organization of labor — making "alienation" the disease of modernity.

Karl Marx said that alienation resulted from private ownership of the means of production and the advent of wage labor. Both placed the capitalist in an advantageous position vis-à-vis labor. According to Marx, capitalist exploitation came in the form of surplus labor value. The need for profits required workers to produce far beyond what was necessary for the owner to break even and pay their wages. Therefore, Marx claimed, employees never received the full value of their labor. Indeed, he said, the value of a worker's labor decreased as his or her production increased when wages remained constant.[3] This caused one of the essential tensions of work under capitalism and held the seeds of an unhealthy moral environment because the capitalist regularly needed to find means for increasing productivity from a sometimes recalcitrant work force. The result of this, according to Marx, was that workers were not treated like persons but like instruments of production.[4]

For Marx then, the problem with capitalism was not so much a matter of unfair wages or inhuman working conditions, as the fact that the capitalist would always have to extract more than the necessary production from workers.[5] A recent study of labor-management relations in a midwestern company dramatized this issue.[6] While profit-sharing and quality-of-work life programs improved the welfare of employees, these measures did not quiet the debate over what constituted a full workday. Management sought the maximum productivity possible per day, while labor wanted to work only as long as it took to reach a set amount of production.

A later theory, scientific management, conceived of work in terms of objective, causal relationships between human and mechanical parts. In *The Principles of Scientific Management*, Frederick Winslow Taylor expressed the belief that most workers tended to work too slowly, making any system based on a worker's initiative inefficient.[7] Because Taylor considered human individuality cumbersome, he shaped a standardized work system that made employees replaceable, like the parts of a machine. He divided the work process into thinking and acting — managers did the former while workers did the latter. This eliminated work done by rule of thumb or learned through the apprenticeship system. Management selected and trained workers, and all tasks were standardized. Under Taylor's system, labor required little skill and was, therefore, cheap.

Enormously successful, scientific management was used to organize all kinds of work from government bureaucracies to hospitals. Fueled by wage incentives and controlled by strict discipline, this system did not depend on promises, obligations, duties, rights, and responsibilities. Efficiency became the primary value in a workplace that had come to be regarded as an amoral arena for wages and profit.

This belief that productivity could be improved by rearranging physical variables was reflected in research conducted at Western Electric's Hawthorne Works in 1924. Scientists studying the relationship between the intensity of light in a workroom and employee productivity were surprised to find that productivity increased when the lights were turned up *and* when they were turned down. While they concluded that light had very little to do with worker output, they decided that other uncontrolled variables probably did.

Looking for another set of physical variables, Harvard University researchers Fritz Roethlisberger, W. Lloyd Warner, and Professor Elton Mayo redefined the Hawthorne research into a study of the physical factors involved in fatigue and monotony.[8] During the five years of this research, productivity in the study group remained higher than in other areas of the operation. Further research at the Hawthorne facility demonstrated that physical changes did not account for productivity as much as the complex social dynamics of the experimental group and their interactions with management.[9]

The Hawthorne studies suggested that worker groups had their own values, norms of behavior, and informal communication systems—all with their own underlying logic. In contrast to Taylor's mechanistic approach to management, the "systems" approach developed. This approach viewed employees as members of a social system and attempted to understand how they were motivated within this context.[10] Its foundations lie in a social rather than a physical understanding of productivity.

Highlighting the need for empathetic managers who understood and cared about the social needs of employees, the Hawthorne studies also suggested that employee participation could reduce resistance to change.[11] Yet critics claimed the studies presented an inadequate view of society, smoothed over inherent conflicts of interest, and assumed a pro-management bias in order to manipulate labor. They wondered whether psychological manipulation was replacing physical manipulation.[12]

The writings of Marx and Taylor along with the debate over the Hawthorne studies underscore the moral challenge to management. How does a manager secure cooperation from employees without manipulation or coercion? How does a corporation balance its economic interests with the interests of its employees? A company's answers to these questions determine the nature of its moral environment.

## Mapping the Territory

As a moral environment, the modern American corporation consists of a complicated web of interactions. Individual values of corporate leaders, managers, and employees interweave with organizational values, policies, and practices. The well-being of the corporation as a whole depends on both the technical and the moral excellence of its employees. By technical excellence, we mean the skills necessary for a particular job, whereas moral excellence refers both to how employees are treated and to traits that are encouraged such as honesty, fairness, compassion, loyalty, and so forth. Technical excellence without moral excellence can lead to serious problems (e.g., a government contractor may be brilliant at solving problems, but have fraudulent billing practices). On the other hand, moral excellence without technical excellence can lead to bankruptcy or business failure.[13]

Managing the corporate *moral* environment, then, includes two broad areas of responsibility. First, management is responsible for the freedom and well-being of employees or quality work life. Second, corporate policies and practices exert influence on employees' moral character. For example, programs like employee assistance or company day-care centers directly impact the welfare of workers, while corporate codes of ethics often aim in part at improving the moral character of people within the corporation. Some policies affect both aspects of the moral environment—i.e., worker participation programs may not only enrich daily work experience, but may also cultivate certain virtues in employees.

The matrix below relates these two areas of responsibility to the general management tasks of policy formulation and implementation. The axis lines in this diagram are broken because these areas are not, and should not be, rigidly separated. They also imply that the diagram is a tool for organizing one's thoughts—not inhibiting or constraining them.

|  | Work Life Quality Considerations | Influence on Moral Character |
|---|---|---|
| Policy Formulation | 1 | 3 |
| Policy Implementation | 2 | 4 |

The matrix can be used to analyze the intentional and unintentional effects that a policy might have in particular cases. Some policies that appear morally neutral on the surface can change considerably when implemented. A management incentive program at the H.J. Heinz Company illustrates this point.[14] Heinz intended to reward effective managers, but the system encouraged misrepresentation of income to protect bonuses. While formulated to serve the welfare of the company and its managers (quadrant 1), the system had an unanticipated impact on the employees' ethical code (quadrant 3). The implemented policy essentially fulfilled its goals (quadrant 2)—profit increased and managers got bonuses. Yet the implementation produced the undesirable effect of encouraging dishonesty (quadrant 4) by not emphasizing and enforcing the use of appropriate means for achieving corporate goals.

Other policies might attempt to influence both areas of the moral environment but fail because of inattention to implementation. Policies concerning sexual harassment may have this result if they aim only at overt wrongs. Hence, sneers, jokes, and whispers may go unchecked. This undermines the policy's intention by giving the illusion of protection without actually providing it. The same thing holds true with virtually any provision of a corporate code of ethics. Some companies think that by simply putting such a code on paper, they have met their moral obligations to employees and others involved. However, ethical codes that are never practiced can lead to either cynicism or complacency or both.

Management policies that negatively affect any of these four matrix areas will injure the moral health of the corporation. Although some policies appear morally neutral, many actually result in ethical problems which, if left unchecked, can lead to legal problems or increased government regulation. For example, companies that fail to consider employee safety may have to answer to the Occupational Safety and Health Administration (OSHA). Those that violate employee rights may hear from the Equal Employment Opportunity Commission (EEOC), whereas companies that break promises and contracts may be brought before the National Labor Relations Board (NLRB). While avoiding such external sanctions is not the primary purpose of morally motivated corporate policies, it does offer significant secondary motivation for managers who need it.

## Work Life Quality Considerations

As illustrated earlier, modern managers take the first step toward viewing the corporation as a moral environment when they cease to regard employees as mere tools for achieving corporate goals and begin to view them from a social perspective. The next step involves recognizing the value and dignity of each employee. By taking this step, the corporation assumes a moral viewpoint, which entails certain duties and obligations. The following list indicates the kinds of moral obligations that the corporation has in this domain:[15]

Avoiding direct harm to employees
Respecting employee rights
Communicating honestly
Keeping promises and labor contracts
Obeying laws and complying with government regulations
Helping employees in need
Treating employees fairly

When we consider the corporation as a moral environment, these moral guidelines, while essential, are not entirely sufficient. Their application must be guided by a larger vision of the community's well-being—one that accounts for both the welfare of the community as a whole and the welfare of the people in it.

As to the welfare of those within the corporation, management should supply the necessary physical and psychological conditions for employees to have a decent work life. This usually requires a safe work environment and reasonable working conditions. Lunch rooms and athletic facilities can improve the work experience, while programs like flex-time and company day-care centers make work more compatible with family arrangements. Beyond this, some companies have added innovations such as quality circles, participatory management, profit sharing, and job enrichment. Many companies also provide means for dealing with personal problems through employee assistance programs.

Some argue that these innovations are nothing but frills, i.e., why not pay employees a dollar an hour more rather than giving them cloth napkins in the lunchroom? Others contend that the corporation providing all of these things will begin to resemble a welfare state. Still others warn that an overly paternalistic management could eventually bankrupt the business. As labor leader Samuel Gompers once said, "The worst crime against the working people is a company which fails to make a profit." The corporation as a moral environment must tend to its own success for the sake of its employees.

Yet, how does one determine the parameters of a corporation's moral responsibility to the welfare of its people? How does the obligation to provide for the health and safety of its employees differ from a corporation's responsibility to provide athletic facilities? The boundaries of corporate responsibility for employee welfare have changed over time. What once seemed a frill might become a necessity and vice versa. For example, most corporations consider health care a basic responsibility but do not at present view day care that way.

But these innovations and benefits, all containing some notion of how to improve people's work lives, are not enough. A company must also concern itself with individual rights. Attorney David Ewing believes that many companies in the United States violate the civil liberties of employees — particularly freedom of speech, privacy, and conscience because these freedoms seem to interfere with the efficient operation of business.[16] Sometimes civil liberties do conflict with corporate goals. For example, employees should not exercise their right to freedom of speech by giving competitors important financial information. However, corporations cannot justify restricting freedom of speech in areas that do not affect the welfare of the business. In one case, a Texas oil company employee was asked to resign after writing an article for *Look* magazine about the Kennedy assassination.[17] Did the company have a right to ask the employee to refrain from publicly expressing his opinions? Cases like this one led law professor Clyde Summers to argue that not only must employers guarantee individual rights, they should also implement fair procedures for protecting employees from unjust dismissal.[18]

Some believe that too much attention to employee rights will adversely affect employees and the corporation. One could argue, for example, that too much emphasis on entitlements and legal protections for employees detracts from responsibility to perform well on the job, causing laziness, insubordination, or shoddy workmanship. Another argument against excessive emphasis on employee rights is that it would, in effect, deny owners and employers some of *their* legitimate rights. Obviously, the rights and interests of both parties need to be balanced.

But suppose a corporation adopted a moral point of view, provided a satisfying work life, respected individuals' rights, and protected them from unjust dismissal. Would this exhaust its responsibilities to its employees? The American work ethic connects hard work with the moral worth of the individual. Many of our beliefs about merit and fairness are linked to the notion of "doing a good job." Most of us believe people have a moral obligation to do their best and consider it unfair when an incompetent person gets paid the same as someone who works with care and skill. The values that underlie corporate policy generally rest on the things needed to make the corporation prosper. So providing reasonable working conditions and incentives for employee excellence is a responsibility that the corporation has both to itself and to its people.

A well-run corporation from both moral and business viewpoints fulfills its responsibility to the well-being and rights of its employees by providing them with the things necessary to have a good work life. However, *having* a good work life differs from *leading* a good work life. Institutions in our society can provide the conditions necessary for people to have a good life. But the moral character of a person determines whether he or she will lead a good life.

### Influence on Moral Character

In the fourth century B.C., Aristotle realized that one could not discuss the nature of a morally good person without discussing the social conditions necessary for developing and sustaining such people. In other words, personal morality required certain institutional or organizational arrangements. According to Aristotle, the just city-state provided the conditions necessary for citizens to become morally good, and these good citizens would in turn create and perpetuate a good society.[19]

Like Aristotle's city-state, the corporation should, for the sake of itself and its stakeholders, be a place that fosters and sustains morally good people. This involves two responsibilities: making sure that neither the formulation nor the implementation of a policy undermines the ethical beliefs of employees, and communicating in word and deed the ethical standards of the corporation. Both of these require that the corporation respect the dignity and moral autonomy of each employee.

What we generally mean by morality is a set of values and principles that are practiced with some consistency. A person may, in some respects, behave differently at work than at home and still remain autonomous. However, it is not as easy for people to change their beliefs and intuitions about what is right or wrong. Employees are placed under tremendous stress when required to do something that they think is ethically wrong. The choice may be between doing what is morally right (i.e., "blowing the whistle") and losing one's job, or "keeping one's mouth shut" and losing self-respect. Consultant Albert Z. Carr suggests that the psychological stress from the conflict between personal ethics and business practices can be resolved by thinking of business as a game.[20] Whether Carr's suggestion would work is questionable. Business, unlike poker, lies in the real world — not in the fictitious domain of play. A person who feels that he or she can lie or cheat in good conscience at work is likely to be able to do so in other contexts as well.

Conflicting policy goals, unethical practices, poor leadership, and sloppy controls can all have a bad effect on the moral character of employees. In the Heinz case, a code of ethics conflicted with an efficient means for attaining corporate goals. Account juggling became an accepted practice that was either sanctioned by leaders or went undetected by them. Many of the managers had probably come to believe over the years that juggling the books was the "sensible thing to do." Nobody seemed to be hurt and the company showed steady growth. This kind of rationale and the general consensus on the use of the practice contributed to its spread over seven years.

In a more recent case of check kiting at E.F. Hutton, a similar dynamic may have been at work. Some blamed the practice of deliberately and strategically overdrawing company checking accounts on poor leadership. When leaders do not clearly articulate standards of behavior, the assumption can spread that what is not explicitly prohibited is permitted. Obviously it is impossible for a corporation to articulate all of its prohibitions. But when a potentially unethical practice emerges, management needs to promptly identify it as such and clarify its policy on the matter. This is difficult to do without appropriate controls and decisive leadership.

Doing the morally right thing in an organizational context is sometimes difficult. Because of their desire to be accepted, employees are subject to peer group pressures. This, in addition to the desire to succeed, makes them susceptible to certain temptations. Good leaders can provide positive role models for the kind of character traits that "make sense" and are rewarded in a company. The promotion of competent people of dubious moral character can lead to cynicism and/or moral deterioration on the part of those willing to lower their ethical standards to get ahead.

Focusing on the character traits that are nurtured in corporations, psychoanalyst Michael Maccoby observed that some of the executives he studied were saddened when they realized that the very qualities that made them successful at work had led them to fail in their personal lives. Maccoby pointed out that business needs to take a long-range look at the effect that it has on its employees:

> The larger society, of which business is only a sub-system, depends for its greatness not only on the head, but on the heart — the qualities of courage, compassion, generosity, and idealism. If the most dynamic sector of society continues to select out these qualities, where will we find future leaders who possess the moral strength to know right from wrong and the courage to act on those convictions?[21]

So beyond the corporation's responsibility to avoid policies and practices that undermine the moral values of its employees, there is also a more positive duty or obligation to foster individual growth and development. Certain kinds of controls, such as those that keep employees from engaging in unethical practices and those that nip wrongdoing in the bud, can prevent harm. But this does not mean that the corporation should be run like a totalitarian state. On the contrary, in order to fulfill its duty to foster personal development, the corporation must respect and encourage initiative and creativity among all employees. This requires giving them freedom and flexibility.

Morality not only requires consistency but the freedom of choice for a person to become truly responsible for his or her actions. The more input employees have into the work process, the more responsibility they have for the success and failure of a project. By respecting employee know-how, keeping lines of communication open, instilling a sense of community and pride in workmanship, a corporation can make work more meaningful and set the stage for personal growth.

A corporation also needs to have a set of goals or ideals that goes beyond profit making. For example, the Borg-Warner Corporation drew up a statement of ethical and humanistic beliefs as a means of unifying its diversified holdings under one vision.[22] Such statements can be an effective means for articulating the ideals of a company in relation to all of its stakeholders. If these values are reflected in corporate policies, business practices, and leadership, they can have a positive influence on the pride, loyalty, and self-esteem of employees.

Matsushita, a Japanese electronics company, also has a set of guiding principles that it calls "spiritual" values. These values are specifically intended to balance efficiency with countervailing human values and provide both labor and management with a way of linking their spiritual lives to their productive lives. Matsushita's values are: national service through industry, fairness, harmony and cooperation, struggle for betterment, courtesy and humility, adjustment and assimilation, and gratitude.[23] For this company, emphasis on such character traits is intended to help people make some sense out of the moral dilemmas that arise between the individual, his or her work, and society.

American companies might produce a somewhat different list of virtues because of different priorities. For example, Americans might list initiative rather than humility, not because they do not think that humility is a good thing, but because initiative is a trait that American culture has traditionally valued and reinforced. Hence, one way that the values of a corporation come to "make sense" is when they reflect traditional social values.

However, a corporation may also have a responsibility to confront on ethical grounds the mores of a society. American corporations operating under the Sullivan Principles in South Africa offer one such example. Basic human rights to freedom and due process, along with the principles of moral common sense, are universal moral requirements. These should not be violated by the corporation even if they are acceptable in the country in which it operates.

Perhaps the most important way in which the moral environment of a corporation can be measured is in terms of employee morale. This is easily illustrated by the fact that it is one of the first things affected by corporate scandals and poor management.[24] The term "morale" is commonly used to mean happiness or enthusiasm. Webster's dictionary defines it as: "the moral or mental condition as regards courage, zeal, confidence, discipline, enthusiasm, and willingness to endure hardship." Philosophers throughout the ages have argued that the road to a happy life is best traveled by leading a morally good life—that morale is intimately connected to morality. As Harvard professor Fritz Roethlisberger once observed: "Morale is something that nobody thinks about until it's gone."

## Some Questions for Case Analysis

The following analytical questions can help to describe and evaluate a corporation as a moral environment. Although they are divided into the two general areas of our discussion, some of the questions overlap.

*Considerations Regarding Work Life Quality*

1. Do policies and practices fairly balance the interests of the corporation and its employees?

2. Do managers attempt to manipulate employees?

3. Are the incentive systems fair? Do they place equal emphasis on using the correct means for achieving corporate goals?

4. How does the corporation understand its moral obligations to employees? In terms of benefits and costs, rights, or duties?

5. Is there concern for employees' physical and mental health? How does the corporation demonstrate this concern? Are there opportunities for learning and/or job enrichment?

6. Are individual rights and civil liberties protected? Does the corporation obey the letter and the spirit of the law? Does it keep promises and contracts? Does it enforce its own rules? Are the hiring and firing procedures fair?

*Considerations Regarding Influence on Moral Character*

1. Are managers genuine—do they mean what they say? Do they practice their moral beliefs?

2. Do corporate policies and practices in any way undermine the moral integrity of employees?

3. Are employees encouraged to be forthright? Are they given access to top management? Does the corporation treat its employees as intelligent individuals capable of doing more than just following orders?

4. What kinds of behavior "make sense" in this organization? What kinds of people make it to the top? What moral traits and dispositions are reinforced?

Perhaps the most important questions one must ask when looking at the corporation as a moral environment are: Does the corporation, as an institution, have a clear sense of its moral standards? Are the policies and practices of a corporation consistent with its espoused moral beliefs?

The corporation is inextricably connected to the wider social, political, and physical environment. Harboring its own system of logic and set of dispositions, it exerts a tremendous influence on its stakeholders' lives. For this reason it is essential that business leaders increase both their understanding and their commitment to managing the corporation as a moral environment.

### NOTES

1. Quoted in W.H. Auden, *A Certain World: A Commonplace Book* (New York: Viking, 1970).
2. "Some Avenues for Ethical Analysis in General Management" (HBS Case Services #9-383-007).
3. Karl Marx, *Capital*, vol. I (Moscow: Progress Publishers, 1978), p. 173.
4. Karl Marx, "1844 Manuscripts," *Karl Marx: Selected Writings*, David McLellan, ed. (Oxford: Oxford University Press, 1977), p. 78.
5. Ibid., p. 85. Marx says that raising wages "would only mean a better payment of slaves and would not give human meaning and worth to either the worker or his labor."
6. "Building Trust at Warner Gear" (HBS Case Services #0-386-011).
7. Frederick Winslow Taylor, *The Principles of Scientific Management* (New York: W.W. Norton, 1967), p. 19.
8. See Elton Mayo, *The Human Problems of Industrial Civilization* (New York: Macmillan, 1933).
9. See Fritz Roethlisberger and W.J. Dickson, *Management and the Worker* (Cambridge: Harvard University Press, 1939).
10. See L.W. Porter, E.E. Lawler, and J.R. Hackman, *Behavior in Organizations* (New York: McGraw-Hill, 1975).
11. Jeffrey Sonnenfeld, "Shedding Light on the Hawthorne Studies," *Journal of Occupational Behavior*, vol. 6, 1985, pp. 111–130.
12. Ibid., p.115.
13. It is interesting to note that the Greek word for virtue (*areté*) refers to both moral and technical excellence. The Greek ideal of a good person entailed not only moral excellence but the ability to perform one's function with skill (*techné*) and knowledge (*epistemé*). In these terms, the corporation as a moral environment requires not only good people, but people who work well.
14. "H.J. Heinz Company, The Administration of Policy" (HBS Case Services #9-382-034).

15. Adapted from "Some Avenues for Ethical Analysis in General Management" (HBS Case Services #9-383-007).
16. David Ewing, "Civil Liberties in the Corporation," *New York State Bar Journal* (April 1978), pp. 188–191; 223–229.
17. "The Individual and the Corporation" (HBS Case Services #9-368-018).
18. Clyde Summers, "Protecting All Employees Against Unjust Dismissal," *Harvard Business Review*, January–February 1980, pp. 132–139.
19. Aristotle, *The Nicomachean Ethics*, tr. by Martin Ostwald (Indianapolis: Bobbs-Merrill, 1975), book 10 (1179a 33).
20. Albert Z. Carr, "Is Business Bluffing Ethical?" *Harvard Business Review*, January–February 1968, pp. 143–153.
21. Michael Maccoby, *The Gamesman* (New York: Simon and Schuster, 1976), p. 32.
22. "The Beliefs of Borg-Warner" (HBS Case Services #9-383-091).
23. Richard Pascale and Anthony Athos, *The Art of Japanese Management* (New York: Warner Books, 1981), p. 75.
24. See, "When Scandal Haunts the Corridors," The *New York Times*, July 7, 1985, section 3, p. 1.

# 2

# Is Business Bluffing Ethical?

## ALBERT Z. CARR

A respected businessman with whom I discussed the theme of this article remarked with some heat, "You mean to say you're going to encourage men to bluff? Why, bluffing is nothing more than a form of lying! You're advising them to lie!"

I agreed that the basis of private morality is a respect for truth and that the closer a businessman comes to the truth, the more he deserves respect. At the same time, I suggested that most bluffing in business might be regarded simply as game strategy — much like bluffing in poker, which does not reflect on the morality of the bluffer.

I quoted Henry Taylor, the British statesman who pointed out that "falsehood ceases to be falsehood when it is understood on all sides that the truth is not expected to be spoken" — an exact description of bluffing in poker, diplomacy, and business. I cited the analogy of the criminal court, where the criminal is not expected to tell the truth when he pleads "not guilty." Everyone from the judge down takes it for granted that the job of the defendant's attorney is to get his client off, not to reveal the truth; and this is considered ethical practice. I mentioned Representative Omar Burleson, the Democrat from Texas, who was quoted as saying, in regard to the ethics of Congress, "Ethics is a barrel of worms"[1] — a pungent summing up of the problem of deciding who is ethical in politics.

I reminded my friend that millions of businessmen feel constrained every day to say *yes* to their bosses when they secretly believe *no* and that this is generally accepted as permissible strategy when the alternative might be the loss of a job. The essential point, I said, is that the ethics of business are game ethics, different from the ethics of religion.

He remained unconvinced. Referring to the company of which he is president, he declared:

> Maybe that's good enough for some businessmen, but I can tell you that we pride ourselves on our ethics. In 30 years not one customer has ever questioned my word or asked to check our figures. We're loyal to our customers and fair to our suppliers. I regard my handshake on a deal as a contract. I've never entered into price-fixing schemes with my competitors. I've never allowed my salesmen to spread injurious rumors about other companies. Our union contract is the best in our industry. And, if I do say so myself, our ethical standards are of the highest!

He really was saying, without realizing it, that he was living up to the ethical standards of the business game — which are a far cry from those of private life. Like a gentlemanly poker player, he did not play in cahoots with others at the table, try to smear their reputations, or hold back chips he owed them.

But this same fine man, at that very time, was allowing one of his products to be advertised in a way that made it sound a great deal better than it actually was. Another item in his product line was notorious among dealers for its "built-in obsolescence." He was holding back from the market a much-improved product because he did not want it to interfere with sales of the inferior item it would have replaced. He had joined with certain of his competitors in hiring a lobbyist to push a state legislature, by methods that he preferred not to know too much about, into amending a bill then being enacted.

In his view these things had nothing to do with ethics; they were merely normal business practice. He himself undoubtedly avoided outright falsehoods — never lied in so many words. But the entire organization that he ruled was deeply involved in numerous strategies of deception.

## Pressure to Deceive

Most executives from time to time are almost compelled, in the interests of their companies or themselves, to practice some form of deception when negotiating with customers, dealers, labor unions, government officials, or even other departments of their companies. By conscious misstatements, concealment of pertinent facts, or exaggeration — in short, by bluffing — they seek to persuade others to agree with them. I think it is fair to say that if the individual executive refuses to bluff from time to time — if he feels obligated to tell the truth, the whole truth, and nothing but the truth — he is ignoring opportunities permitted under the rules and is at a heavy disadvantage in his business dealings.

But here and there a businessman is unable to reconcile himself to the bluff in which he plays a part. His conscience, perhaps spurred by religious idealism, troubles him. He feels guilty; he may develop an ulcer or a nervous tic. Before any executive can make profitable use of the strategy of the bluff, he needs to make sure that in bluffing he will not lose self-respect or become emotionally disturbed. If he is to reconcile personal integrity and high standards of honesty with the practical requirements of business, he must feel that his bluffs are ethically justified. The justification rests on the fact that business, as practiced by individuals as well as by corporations, has the impersonal character of a game—a game that demands both special strategy and an understanding of its special ethics.

The game is played at all levels of corporate life, from the highest to the lowest. At the very instant that a man decides to enter business, he may be forced into a game situation, as is shown by the recent experience of a Cornell honor graduate who applied for a job with a large company.

This applicant was given a psychological test which included the statement, "Of the following magazines, check any that you have read either regularly or from time to time, and double-check those which interest you most. *Reader's Digest, Time, Fortune, Saturday Evening Post, The New Republic, Life, Look, Ramparts, Newsweek, Business Week, U.S. News & World Report, The Nation, Playboy, Esquire, Harper's, Sports Illustrated.*"

His tastes in reading were broad, and at one time or another he had read almost all of these magazines. He was a subscriber to *The New Republic*, an enthusiast for *Ramparts*, and an avid student of the pictures in *Playboy*. He was not sure whether his interest in *Playboy* would be held against him, but he had a shrewd suspicion that if he confessed to an interest in *Ramparts* and *The New Republic*, he would be thought a liberal, a radical, or at least an intellectual, and his chances of getting the job, which he needed, would greatly diminish. He therefore checked five of the more conservative magazines. Apparently it was a sound decision, for he got the job.

He had made a game player's decision, consistent with business ethics.

A similar case is that of a magazine space salesman who, owing to a merger, suddenly found himself out of a job.

This man was 58, and, in spite of a good record, his chance of getting a job elsewhere in a business where youth is favored in hiring practice was not good. He was a vigorous, healthy man, and only a considerable amount of gray in his hair suggested his age. Before beginning his job search he touched up his hair with a black dye to confine the gray to his temples. He knew that the truth about his age might well come out in time, but he calculated that he could deal with that situation when it arose. He and his wife decided that he could easily pass for 45, and he so stated his age on his résumé.

This was a lie; yet within the accepted rules of the business game, no moral culpability attaches to it.

## The Poker Analogy

We can learn a good deal about the nature of business by comparing it with poker. While both have a large element of chance, in the long run the winner is the man who plays with steady skill. In both games ultimate victory requires intimate knowledge of the rules, insight into the psychology of the other players, a bold front, a considerable amount of self-discipline, and the ability to respond swiftly and effectively to opportunities provided by chance.

No one expects poker to be played on the ethical principles preached in churches. In poker it is right and proper to bluff a friend out of the rewards of being dealt a good hand. A player feels no more than a slight twinge of sympathy, if that, when—with nothing better than a single ace in his hand—he strips a heavy loser, who holds a pair, of the rest of his chips. It was up to the other fellow to protect himself. In the words of an excellent poker player, former President Harry Truman, "If you can't stand the heat, stay out of the kitchen." If one shows mercy to a loser in poker, it is a personal gesture, divorced from the rules of the game.

Poker has its special ethics, and here I am not referring to rules against cheating. The man who keeps an ace up his sleeve or who marks the cards is more than unethical; he is a crook, and can be punished as such—kicked out of the game or, in the Old West, shot.

In contrast to the cheat, the unethical poker player is one who, while abiding by the letter of the rules, finds ways to put the other players at an unfair disadvantage. Perhaps he unnerves them with loud talk. Or he tries to get them drunk. Or he plays in cahoots with someone else at the table. Ethical poker players frown on such tactics.

Poker's own brand of ethics is different from the ethical ideals of civilized human relationships. The game calls for distrust of the other fellow. It ignores the claim of friendship. Cunning deception and concealment of one's strength and intentions, not kindness and open-heartedness, are vital in poker. No one thinks any the worse of poker on that account. And no one should think any the worse of the game of business because its standards of right and wrong differ from the prevailing traditions of morality in our society.

## Discard the Golden Rule

This view of business is especially worrisome to people without much business experience. A minister of my acquaintance once protested that business cannot possibly function in our society unless it is based on the Judeo-Christian system of ethics. He told me:

> I know some businessmen have supplied call girls to customers, but there are always a few rotten apples in every barrel. That doesn't mean the rest of the fruit isn't sound. Surely the vast majority of businessmen are ethical. I myself am acquainted with many who adhere to strict codes of ethics based fundamentally on religious teachings. They contribute to good causes. They participate in community activities. They cooperate with other companies to improve working conditions in their industries. Certainly they are not indifferent to ethics.

That most businessmen are not indifferent to ethics in their private lives, everyone will agree. My point is that in their office lives they cease to be private citizens; they become game players who must be guided by a somewhat different set of ethical standards.

The point was forcefully made to me by a Midwestern executive who has given a good deal of thought to the question:

So long as a businessman complies with the laws of the land and avoids telling malicious lies, he's ethical. If the law as written gives a man a wide-open chance to make a killing, he'd be a fool not to take advantage of it. If he doesn't, somebody else will. There's no obligation on him to stop and consider who is going to get hurt. If the law says he can do it, that's all the justification he needs. There's nothing unethical about that. It's just plain business sense.

This executive (call him Robbins) took the stand that even industrial espionage, which is frowned on by some businessmen, ought not to be considered unethical. He recalled a recent meeting of the National Industrial Conference Board where an authority on marketing made a speech in which he deplored the employment of spies by business organizations. More and more companies, he pointed out, find it cheaper to penetrate the secrets of competitors with concealed cameras and microphones or by bribing employees than to set up costly research and design departments of their own. A whole branch of the electronics industry has grown up with this trend, he continued, providing equipment to make industrial espionage easier.

Disturbing? The marketing expert found it so. But when it came to a remedy, he could only appeal to "respect for the golden rule." Robbins thought this a confession of defeat, believing that the golden rule, for all its value as an ideal for society, is simply not feasible as a guide for business. A good part of the time the businessman is trying to do unto others as he hopes others will *not* do unto him.[2] Robbins continued:

Espionage of one kind or another has become so common in business that it's like taking a drink during Prohibition — it's not considered sinful. And we don't even have Prohibition where espionage is concerned; the law is very tolerant in this area. There's no more shame for a business that uses secret agents than there is for a nation. Bear in mind that there already is at least one large corporation — you can buy its stock over the counter — that makes millions by providing counterespionage service to industrial firms. Espionage in business is not an ethical problem; it's an established technique of business competition.

### "We Don't Make the Laws"

Wherever we turn in business, we can perceive the sharp distinction between its ethical standards and those of the churches. Newspapers abound with sensational stories growing out of this distinction.

We read one day that Senator Philip A. Hart of Michigan has attacked food processors for deceptive packaging of numerous products.[3]

The next day there is a Congressional to-do over Ralph Nader's book, *Unsafe At Any Speed*, which demonstrates that automobile companies for years have neglected the safety of car-owning families.[4]

Then another Senator, Lee Metcalf of Montana, and journalist Vic Reinemer show in their book, *Overcharge*, the methods by which utility companies elude regulating government bodies to extract unduly large payments from users of electricity.[5]

These are merely dramatic instances of a prevailing condition; there is hardly a major industry at which a similar attack could not be aimed. Critics of business regard such behavior as unethical, but the companies concerned know that they are merely playing the business game.

Among the most respected of our business institutions are the insurance companies. A group of insurance executives meeting recently in New England was startled when their guest speaker, social critic Daniel Patrick Moynihan, roundly berated them for "unethical" practices. They had been guilty, Moynihan alleged, of using outdated actuarial tables to obtain unfairly high premiums. They habitually delayed the hearings of lawsuits against them in order to tire out the plaintiffs and win cheap settlements. In their employment policies they used ingenious devices to discriminate against certain minority groups.[6]

It was difficult for the audience to deny the validity of these charges. But these men were business game players. Their reaction to Moynihan's attack was much the same as that of the automobile manufacturers to Nader, of the utilities to Senator Metcalf, and of the food processors to Senator Hart. If the laws governing their businesses change, or if public opinion becomes clamorous, they will make the necessary adjustments. But morally they have in their view done nothing wrong. As long as they comply with the letter of the law, they are within their rights to operate their businesses as they see fit.

The small business is in the same position as the great corporation in this respect. For example:

In 1967 a key manufacturer was accused of providing master keys for automobiles to mail-order customers, although it was obvious that some of the purchasers might be automobile thieves. His defense was plain and straightforward. If there was nothing in the law to prevent him from selling his keys to anyone who ordered them, it was not up to him to inquire as to his customers' motives. Why was it any worse, he insisted, for him to sell car keys by mail, than for mail-order houses to sell guns that might be used for murder? Until the law was changed, the key manufacturer could regard himself as being just as ethical as any other businessman by the rules of the business game.[7]

Violations of the ethical ideals of society are common in business, but they are not necessarily violations of business principles. Each year the Federal Trade Commission orders hundreds of companies, many of them of the first magnitude, to "cease and desist" from practices which, judged by ordinary standards, are of questionable morality but which are stoutly defended by the companies concerned.

In one case, a firm manufacturing a well-known mouthwash was accused of using a cheap form of alcohol possibly deleterious to health. The company's chief executive, after testifying in Washington, made this comment privately:

We broke no law. We're in a highly competitive industry. If we're going to stay in business, we have to look for profit wherever the law permits. We don't make the laws. We obey them. Then why do we have to put up with this "holier than thou" talk about ethics? It's sheer hypocrisy. We're not in business to promote ethics. Look at the cigarette companies, for God's sake! If the ethics aren't embodied in the laws by the men who made them, you can't expect businessmen to fill the lack. Why, a sudden submission to Christian ethics by businessmen would bring about the greatest economic upheaval in history!

It may be noted that the government failed to prove its case against him.

### Cast Illusions Aside

Talk about ethics by businessmen is often a thin decorative coating over the hard realities of the game.

Once I listened to a speech by a young executive who pointed to a new industry code as proof that his company and its competitors were deeply aware of their responsibilities to society. It was a code of ethics, he said. The industry was going to police itself, to dissuade constituent companies from wrongdoing. His eyes shone with conviction and enthusiasm.

The same day there was a meeting in a hotel room where the industry's top executives met with the "czar" who was to administer the new code, a man of high repute. No one who was present could doubt their common attitude. In their eyes the code was designed primarily to forestall a move by the federal government to impose stern restrictions on the industry. They felt that the code would hamper them a good deal less than new federal laws would. It was, in other words, conceived as a protection for the industry, not for the public.

The young executive accepted the surface explanation of the code; these leaders, all experienced game players, did not deceive themselves for a moment about its purpose.

The illusion that business can afford to be guided by ethics as conceived in private life is often fostered by speeches and articles containing such phrases as, "It pays to be ethical," or, "Sound ethics is good business." Actually this is not an ethical position at all; it is a self-serving calculation in disguise. The speaker is really saying that in the long run a company can make more money if it does not antagonize competitors, suppliers, employees, and customers by squeezing them too hard. He is saying that oversharp policies reduce ultimate gains. That is true, but it has nothing to do with ethics. The underlying attitude is much like that in the familiar story of the shopkeeper who finds an extra $20 bill in the cash register, debates with himself the ethical problem—should he tell his partner?—and finally decides to share the money because the gesture will give him an edge over the s.o.b. the next time they quarrel.

I think it is fair to sum up the prevailing attitude of businessmen on ethics as follows:

We live in what is probably the most competitive of the world's civilized societies. Our customs encourage a high degree of aggression in the individual's striving for success. Business is our main area of competition, and it has been ritualized into a game of strategy. The basic rules of the game have been set by the government, which attempts to detect and punish business frauds. But as long as a company does not transgress the rules of the game set by law, it has the legal right to shape its strategy without reference to anything but its profits. If it takes a long-term view of its profits, it will preserve amicable relations, so far as possible, with those with whom it deals. A wise businessman will not seek advantage to the point where he generates dangerous hostility among employees, competitors, customers, government, or the public at large. But decisions in this area are, in the final test, decisions of strategy, not of ethics.

## The Individual and the Game

An individual within a company often finds it difficult to adjust to the requirements of the business game. He tries to preserve his private ethical standards in situations that call for game strategy. When he is obliged to carry out company policies that challenge his conception of himself as an ethical man, he suffers.

It disturbs him when he is ordered, for instance, to deny a raise to a man who deserves it, to fire an employee of long standing, to prepare advertising that he believes to be misleading, to conceal facts that he feels customers are entitled to know, to cheapen the quality of materials used in the manufacture of an established product, to sell as new a product that he knows to be rebuilt, to exaggerate the curative powers of a medicinal preparation, or to coerce dealers.

There are some fortunate executives who, by the nature of their work and circumstances, never have to face problems of this kind. But in one form or another the ethical dilemma is felt sooner or later by most businessmen. Possibly the dilemma is most painful not when the company forces the action on the executive but when he originates it himself—that is, when he has taken or is contemplating a step which is in his own interest but which runs counter to his early moral conditioning. To illustrate:

The manager of an export department, eager to show rising sales, is pressed by a big customer to provide invoices which, while containing no overt falsehood that would violate a U.S. law, are so worded that the customer may be able to evade certain taxes in his homeland.

A company president finds that an aging executive, within a few years of retirement and his pension, is not as productive as formerly. Should he be kept on?

The produce manager of a supermarket debates with himself whether to get rid of a lot of half-rotten tomatoes by including one, with its good side exposed, in every tomato six-pack.

An accountant discovers that he has taken an improper deduction on his company's tax return and fears the consequences if he calls the matter to the president's attention, though he himself has done nothing illegal. Perhaps if he says nothing, no one will notice the error.

A chief executive officer is asked by his directors to comment on a rumor that he owns stock in another company with which he has placed large orders. He could deny it, for the stock is in the name of his son-in-law and he has earlier formally instructed his son-in-law to sell the holding.

Temptations of this kind constantly arise in business. If an executive allows himself to be torn between a decision based on business considerations and one based on his private ethical code, he exposes himself to a grave psychological strain.

This is not to say that sound business strategy necessarily runs counter to ethical ideals. They may frequently coincide; and when they do, everyone is gratified. But the major tests of every move in business, as in all games of strategy, are legality and profit. A man who intends to be a winner in the business game must have a game player's attitude.

The business strategist's decisions must be as impersonal as those of a surgeon performing an operation—concentrating on objective and technique, and subordinating personal feelings. If the chief executive admits that his son-in-law owns the stock, it is because he stands to lose more if the fact comes out later than if he states it boldly and at once. If the supermarket manager orders the rotten tomatoes to be discarded, he does so to avoid an increase in consumer complaints and a loss of goodwill. The company president decides not to fire the elderly executive in the belief that the negative reaction of other employees would in the long run cost the company more than it would lose in keeping him and paying his pension.

All sensible businessmen prefer to be truthful, but they seldom feel inclined to tell the *whole* truth. In the business game truth-telling usually has to be kept within narrow limits if trouble is to be avoided. The point was neatly made a long time ago (in 1888) by one of John D. Rockefeller's associates, Paul Babcock, to Standard Oil Company executives who were about to testify before a government investigating committee: "Parry every question with answers which, while perfectly truthful, are evasive of *bottom* facts."[8] This was, is, and probably always will be regarded as wise and permissible business strategy.

### For Office Use Only

An executive's family life can easily be dislocated if he fails to make a sharp distinction between the ethical systems of the home and the office—or if his wife does not grasp that distinction. Many a businessman who has remarked to his wife, "I had to let Jones go today" or "I had to admit to the boss that Jim has been goofing off lately," has been met with an indignant protest. "How could you do a thing like that? You know Jones is over 50 and will have a lot of trouble getting another job." Or, "You did that to Jim? With his wife ill and all the worry she's been having with the kids?"

If the executive insists that he had no choice because the profits of the company and his own security were involved, he may see a certain cool and ominous reappraisal in his wife's eyes. Many wives are not prepared to accept the fact that business operates with a special code of ethics. An illuminating illustration of this comes from a Southern sales executive who related a conversation he had had with his wife at a time when a hotly contested political campaign was being waged in their state:

I made the mistake of telling her that I had had lunch with Colby, who gives me about half my business. Colby mentioned that his company had a stake in the election. Then he said, "By the way, I'm treasurer of the citizens' committee for Lang. I'm collecting contributions. Can I count on you for a hundred dollars?"

Well, there I was. I was opposed to Lang, but I knew Colby. If he withdrew his business I could be in a bad spot. So I just smiled and wrote out a check then and there. He thanked me, and we started to talk about his next order. Maybe he thought I shared his political views. If so, I wasn't going to lose any sleep over it.

I should have had sense enough not to tell Mary about it. She hit the ceiling. She said she was disappointed in me. She said I hadn't acted like a man, that I should have stood up to Colby.

I said, "Look, it was an either-or situation. I had to do it or risk losing the business."

She came back at me with, "I don't believe it. You could have been honest with him. You could have said that you didn't feel you ought to contribute to a campaign for a man you weren't going to vote for. I'm sure he would have understood."

I said, "Mary, you're a wonderful woman, but you're way off the track. Do you know what would have happened if I had said that? Colby would have smiled and said, 'Oh, I didn't realize. Forget it.' But in his eyes from that moment I would be an oddball, maybe a bit of a radical. He would have listened to me talk about his order and would have promised to give it consideration. After that I wouldn't hear from him for a week. Then I would telephone and learn from his secretary that he wasn't yet ready to place the order. And in about a month I would hear through the grapevine that he was giving his business to another company. A month after that I'd be out of a job."

She was silent for a while. Then she said, "Tom, something is wrong with business when a man is forced to choose between his family's security and his moral obligation to himself. It's easy for me to say you should have stood up to him—but if you had, you might have felt you were betraying me and the kids. I'm sorry that you did it, Tom, but I can't blame you. Something is wrong with business!"

This wife saw the problem in terms of moral obligation as conceived in private life; her husband saw it as a matter of game strategy. As a player in a weak position, he felt that he could not afford to indulge an ethical sentiment that might have cost him his seat at the table.

### Playing To Win

Some men might challenge the Colbys of business—might accept serious setbacks to their business careers rather than risk a feeling of moral cowardice. They merit our respect—but as private individuals, not businessmen. When the skillful player of the business game is compelled to submit to unfair pressure, he does not castigate himself for moral weakness. Instead, he strives to put himself into a strong position where he can defend himself against such pressures in the future without loss.

If a man plans to take a seat in the business game, he owes it to himself to master the principles by which the game is played, including its special ethical outlook. He can then hardly fail to recognize that an occasional bluff may well be justified in terms of the game's ethics and warranted in terms of economic necessity. Once he clears his mind on this point, he is in a good position to match his strategy against that of the other players. He can then determine objectively whether a bluff in a given situation has a good chance of succeeding and can decide when and how to bluff, without a feeling of ethical transgression.

To be a winner, a man must play to win. This does not mean that he must be ruthless, cruel, harsh, or treacherous. On the contrary, the better his reputation for integrity, honesty, and decency, the better his chances of victory will be in the long run. But from time to time every businessman, like every poker player, is offered a choice between certain loss or bluffing within the legal rules of the game. If he is not resigned to losing, if he wants to rise in his company and industry, then in such a crisis he will bluff—and bluff hard.

Every now and then one meets a successful businessman who has conveniently forgotten the small or large deceptions that he practiced on his way to fortune. "God gave me my money," old John D. Rockefeller once piously told a Sunday school class. It would be a rare tycoon in our time who would risk the horse laugh with which such a remark would be greeted.

In the last third of the twentieth century even children are aware that if a man has become prosperous in business, he has sometimes departed from the strict truth in order to overcome obstacles or has practiced the more subtle deceptions of the half-truth or the misleading omission. Whatever the form of the bluff, it is an integral part of the game, and the executive who does not master its techniques is not likely to accumulate much money or power.

### NOTES

1. The *New York Times*, March 9, 1967.
2. See Bruce D. Henderson, "Brinkmanship in Business," HBR March–April 1967, p. 49.
3. The *New York Times*, November 21, 1966.
4. New York: Grossman, 1965.
5. New York: David McKay, 1967.
6. The *New York Times*, January 17, 1967.
7. Cited by Ralph Nader in "Business Crime," *The New Republic*, July 1, 1967, p. 7.
8. Babcock in a memorandum to Rockefeller (Rockefeller Archives).

## 3

# Showdown on "Business Bluffing"

## TIMOTHY B. BLODGETT

### Foreword

Few articles that HBR has published have aroused a response as great and as vociferous as Albert Z. Carr's "Is Business Bluffing Ethical?" (January–February 1968). Mr. Carr contended that business's ethical standards differ from society's and that, in business, deception is accepted and indeed necessary if one is to succeed. He likened this "game strategy" of the businessman to the poker player's bluffing. Quoting liberally from letters, Mr. Blodgett, Associate Editor of HBR, reports readers' reactions. Mr. Carr responds (be sure to read his last paragraph).

"This article presents a very realistic and accurate account of the standards used in business decisions, at least for those companies and individuals who are subject to competitive pressures and therefore feel that they must take every legally permissible advantage in order to survive and grow."

"Fortunately, Mr. Carr's view does not appear to be the prevailing view, except, perhaps, along the few remaining frontiers of civilization, such as the upper Amazon."

These two quotations—the first from a letter written by Rawson L. Wood, Chairman of the Board of Arwood Corporation, Rockleigh, New Jersey, and the second from a letter by Leon P. Chemlen, who is on the marketing staff of Dynamics Research Corporation, Stoneham, Massachusetts — distill the contrasting reactions of HBR readers to Mr. Carr's article.

Of the many readers who responded, more than twice as many are critical of the article as are favorable to it. Many others seem uncertain or are noncommittal about Mr. Carr's position, devoting themselves mainly to discussion of the state of business ethics today.

The tone of the letters ranges from enthusiastic to shocked. Interestingly, a couple of the most favorable letters have come from persons in the advertising business, an endeavor not noted for understatement about the virtues and powers of goods being marketed.

A few correspondents question HBR's motives in publishing the article. One indignant writer gives this title to a lengthy dissertation: "Is the Article on Business Bluffing Ethical?" Another even questions the existence of "A.Z. Carr" and suggests that the Editors may have been playing an early April Fool's joke.

But most readers have been as serious and thoughtful in answering Mr. Carr as he was in presenting his view of the way things are.

### "No Medals for Honesty"

Was Mr. Carr "telling it like it is" (in the current expression)? One reader who thinks so is Richard O. Lundquist, an underwriter in Washington, D.C., with The Equitable Life Assurance Society of the United States. He cites this case:

"A young manager was upset because his boss had told a prospective salesman, 'The minimum income a new man earned with us last year was $8,900.' That was about $2,000 from the truth. When the senior manager was questioned about this, he answered, 'Well, that's not important. We are just trying to attract him into the business.' "

Mr. Lundquist mentions two similar examples and then concludes:

"What is universal about these examples is that these managers, each functioning on a different corporate level, are concerned with one thing — *getting the job done*. Most companies give numerous awards for achievement and accomplishment, for sales, for growth, for longevity and loyalty; but there are no medals in the business world for honesty, compassion, or truthfulness."

A person in church affairs discourses in similar vein, but offers a different motive for such behavior. Morton O. Nace, Jr., Executive Director of the Episcopal Churchmen of the Diocese of Chicago, mentions a series of vocational seminars sponsored by his organization. He describes in this way some comments of more than 1,000 persons who have participated in them:

"The vocational seminars have shown that *self-preservation* and *self-indulgence* are the real motivations behind the decisions that businessmen and women make — rather than their conscience! Our evidence clearly supports the premise of Mr. Carr that it is a 'special game of business ethics' that governs the lives of most, if not all, businessmen. Salesmen have said, 'The important thing for me is to make my sales quota, and not whether I should tell the whole truth about a product.' Engineers have said, 'What can I do if my company's main concern is for greater profit instead of using the best materials and design?' Office workers have said, 'Why shouldn't I steal a little from the company? They owe me more than I make now anyhow!' And realtors have said, 'If I show my listing to a Negro, I'll be out of business. I'm not about to do that.' "

Another reader takes particular note of Mr. Carr's discussion of conflicts between personal ethical standards and "game strategy" in business. Bob L. Plunkett, Accounting and Office Manager of Tic Toc Markets, Inc., Costa Mesa, California, confides:

"When I first started telling my wife some of the decisions that I was making, she just couldn't understand how I could be so unsympathetic at the office and so kind at home. My answer to her has always been that we are playing a game just as I used to play football; some make the team and some don't. I have to see that the best players are on the team. It is unfortunate that it poses a problem for those that do not make the team, but that is the breaks of the game."

From abroad comes a comment indicating that the ethical problem, if it exists as such, cannot be characterized as American only. Kees Lievense, a consultant on organization and planning in Amsterveen, Holland, writes:

"The author is trying to express things which live at the verge of our consciousness and is bringing them into the open. He is definitely clarifying our position. Certainly most revealing! And dangerous? Certainly most dangerous as well, as all revelations are, and at the same time greatly liberating! I don't think I am going to read the article again; I don't like shivering. However, I am afraid it will have done its work of unraveling liberation, which, after all, you always try to resist as long as you can."

### A Matter of "Mutual Trust"

Many readers have given careful thought to refutation of Mr. Carr's contention that deception is an integral part of the business "game." I shall try to present their views fairly by quoting representative selections from letters.

Some readers take particular exception to Mr. Carr's claim that deception succeeds:

"All of us in business know that 'playing the game' yields only short-term rewards. We'll admit our faults, but we'll not endorse them as part of our philosophy. To do so would bring the house of business down on itself." (John Valiant, New Product Manager, William H. Rorer, Inc., Fort Washington, Pennsylvania)

"My own experience in dealing with hundreds of companies has led me to believe that sharp dealing or the slightest prevarication on the part of a businessman usually results in informal excommunication to the back alleys of the business world or to obscurity." (Mark Rollinson, President, Greater Washington Industrial Investments, Inc., Washington, D.C.)

"I think a better strategy in business is to work hard, be honest, and be smarter than anyone else." (L.D. Barre, Vice President-Marketing, RTE Corporation, Waukesha, Wisconsin)

Warren R. Howard, Technical Director of Wall Industries, Inc., Beverly, New Jersey, wonders where such practices would lead us:

"Should a quality control engineer falsify a certified test report simply because he knows that his customer will not test a particular lot of material, and because he has slipped such 'out-of-spec' material through in the past? Should a manager shade the facts in his application for funds from top management in order to make his ROI forecast meet management's minimum requirements? Just where can we draw the limits when dishonesty is adopted as a game strategy? Is it proper to insist on strict integrity and honesty? Does it actually harm the mental and ethical life of the executive to tell the truth as a matter of rule?"

Mr. Carr cited as an accurate description of "bluffing" in business and poker this utterance of a British statesman: "Falsehood ceases to be falsehood when it is understood on all sides that the truth is not expected to be spoken." This has moved Alan B. Potter, Vice President of the Dye Division (Dorval, Quebec) of Ciba Company Limited, to comment:

"But it is not at all the case that businessmen do not expect the truth to be spoken. On the contrary, almost all day-to-day business is conducted verbally or on the basis of nonlegal documents. The economic system would collapse without mutual trust on a practically universal scale among business executives.

"Mr. Carr apparently assumes that 'not telling the whole truth' is synonymous with 'telling a lie.' Businessmen know that it would be ridiculous to expect anything more than a straight answer to a straight question. Moreover, it is perfectly acceptable to withhold the truth by saying, 'I am sorry, I am not willing to discuss that subject.' There are many reasons of self-interest or discretion which would justify a refusal to answer any question, and businessmen do not expect that those reasons need be given."

Another recurrent theme in the letters is an insistence that business's ethics cannot be separated from those of society. Typical is the response of J. Douglas McConnell, Marketing Economist at Stanford Research Institute and Lecturer at San Francisco State College:

"Mr. Carr's argument would be sound if business functioned in a vacuum. Because business is an integral part of society, however, it will always be judged by societal criteria.

"It is inevitable that the ethics of business and those of society will always have a considerable degree of commonality. For one thing, business as a group is large and powerful in our society, and many of its values are accepted by society at large. Business's goal is to function at a profit, and to a considerable extent making money is also a value of society.

"Another point of commonality is that most people are members of several groups. The business executive is likely to be a veteran, a member of a school or college board, a member of a local church, or a committeeman for the Community Chest; and he and his family are also consumers. The norms of these other groups carry over to his business life to a greater or lesser extent.

"We live in a highly complex world, with diverse pressures and interests, where simple answers seldom fit simple questions such as 'Is business bluffing ethical?' Business's principal role is that of the wealth-generating group in society—and its ethics will always reflect this. However, the other groups in society—such as education, health services, religion, the military, government, and the consumer—will occasionally be in conflict with these ethics, and there will be (as there is now) pressure to bring business ethics more into conformity with those of society."

Harry R. Wrage, Manager of the MEDINET Application Operation of the General Electric Company (Watertown, Massachusetts), takes up the question of responsibility:

"Business is not a closed society, free to operate by special rules as long as all the players understand them. Nor does business want this status. The responsible businessman recognizes a great responsibility to nonplayers in Mr. Carr's 'game'—to employees and suppliers, to customers, and to the general public. It is this responsibility, and the challenge it presents, that makes the career of the executive one of the most exciting and rewarding of our society. If we do not all meet all of these responsibilities all of the time, that is understandable; but this is not evidence of the existence of, or a need for, special and looser ethical standards for the business community."

A distaff view of the businessman's ethic comes from the wife of one, Mrs. Philip D. Ryan of Wyckoff, New Jersey:

"Plainly, the true meaning of a man's job escapes Mr. Carr. A man's work is not a card game; it is the sum of his self-expression, his life's effort, his mark upon the world, his pride. Men who peddle useless products of poor quality, buy their business at the cost of their integrity, and cherish a sense of worth which is merely a sense of net worth had best stick to card games and send their wives out to work. Men who think ethics are a 'sentiment,' that the law is the only path to honor, that 'there's no obligation on [them] to stop and consider who is going to get hurt'—such men may gain the world (though I doubt it), but plainly they have lost their souls."

One of Mr. Carr's anecdotes particularly struck a chord and has produced some interesting comments. It concerns the Cornell honor graduate who applied for a job and was confronted with a list of magazines running the gamut from *The Reader's Digest* to *Ramparts*. Mr. Chemlen, whom I quoted at the beginning of this article, excuses the young man's deception in reporting his reading tastes:

"This is merely one of the more amusing and illogical aspects of the organizational dialectic and has precious little to do with ethics or poker. It is more akin to coming in out of the rain. Just as no one faults the matador for sidestepping the headlong thrust of his adversary, no one may fault the Cornell honor graduate for parrying the charge of the clumsy buffalo of bureaucracy."

But Mr. Potter, whom I also quoted earlier, sees grave implications in this anecdote:

"There is no evidence that the candidate would not have been given the job if he had answered truthfully. On the contrary, if the company included *Playboy* magazine in the list, it almost certainly meant it would appreciate truthfulness. In modern business we are desperately searching for intelligent liberals, radicals, and intellectuals.

"This story is the most unpleasant example of all. It clearly shows how business can become corrupted when it is thought, erroneously, to reward corruption. What are we to think of this young man? How can he elevate business standards, believing as he does that he needed to lie before he could even be recruited?"

Several readers object to Mr. Carr's poker analogy on the ground that it oversimplifies the process of decision making and the nature of personal relationships in business. One of these correspondents is Henry Johnson, President of The Johnson Wire Works Limited of Montreal. After acknowledging that "there is a substantial element of truth" in likening business to a game in which "duplicity" is an accepted practice, he goes on:

"But the fact is that the businessman is engaged in many games at the same time, with vastly differing rules. At one end of the spectrum, he may be engaged in a labor negotiation where the rules are well known and the protestations of either side are never seriously regarded. At the other pole, the businessman is dealing with an individual employee or customer. These people are not playing games. Anything but straightforward dealing should indeed cause the businessman some guilty insomnia.

"In between lie the ethical question marks, and I do not think we can avoid them as easily as Mr. Carr implies, simply by reason of the fact that we are 'in the office.' Each matter that arises poses its own question: 'How much games-manship, if any, can I use here?'

"But it is surely the function of what we call conscience to extend the area where truth is used, and to 'play games' only on recognized playing fields."

Implicit or stated in many letters is the idea that Mr. Carr *approved* of what he called "game strategy" (a notion to which he vigorously objects, as pointed out in his comments. The stricture of F.W. Henrici, Systems Analyst for Schering Corporation, Bloomfield, New Jersey, is typical:

"What really bothers me is Mr. Carr's attempt to give businessmen something with which to salve their consciences. Almost everyone knows that one doesn't reach a position of power in business, or even in the church, without a little hanky-panky. So be it. But if you lust for power, or money, or success, so that you are willing to put up with hanky-panky, then at least suffer those pangs of conscience. Know that other men scorn you in some small way for the things you condone.

"Mr. Carr doesn't make his case for hanky-panky, either. Business is not a game where lying is right and proper. His only justification is that you must do it because everybody else does. Using that philosophy, one can justify anything from slave trading to today's Mafia-type of business ethics. And the fact that there is no law against it doesn't make something right, either. Your conscience will tell you whether it is right or not."

Robert S. Hower, a salesman in York, Pennsylvania, for the National Gypsum Company, takes Mr. Carr to task with this reflection:

"My advice to Mr. Carr would be to read Aristotle again, and he will find that Aristotle was correct in his observation that much of our being is formed by personal, self-imposed discipline. If we permit ourselves to be weak in one area, it flows into our personality in other areas. Man cannot make excuses in one area by saying this is a game, and then become a strong, moral creature in other things—we just were not made that way."

**Abuse of freedom?** Many readers (often on the assumption that Mr. Carr is an advocate of the behavior he described) venture serious forebodings about our democratic and capitalist system if the attitude of the game player should prevail. "The shoddy results of the poker god are beginning to show around the world," is the way Arthur D. Margison expresses it.

Mr. Margison, who is President of a Don Mills, Ontario, engineering firm, A.D. Margison and Associates Limited, is worried about the state of business ethics, as represented by the "bluffing" strategy, at a time when " 'our way of life' is in competition with other systems."

Zeb V. Beck, Jr., Division Plant Manager in Charlotte, North Carolina, for the Southern Bell Telephone & Telegraph Company, conjures up the same specter:

"Of course there are conflicts that exist when our values oppose one another. However, the decisions we make on the basis of ethical values in these conflicts should far outweigh those based on 'profit,' social acceptability, or political ex-pediency. Unless they do, there is practically nothing to distinguish us from the materialistic value system of the Communists."

Dr. Carlos W. Moreno, an industrial engineer in Cincinnati, Ohio, also con-cerns himself on a broad canvas with the effects of the notion that "whatever is not forbidden by law is acceptable." He comments:

"One basis of a free society is reliance on self-restriction. We have seen all too often, and as expected, that abuse of freedom has resulted in its restriction and in a more regulated life.

"The conclusion that follows is that if many people do not practice self-control, the pressure of society at large will bring about the regulation of every meaningful action, such as business, to the point that future history books might describe the nineteenth and twentieth centuries as a period in which one section of humanity had a chance to live in freedom, but proved to be too undeveloped for it."

James B. Dickson of Dickson Associates, employee relations counselors in Neenah, Wisconsin, is more optimistic:

"In the long run, deception cannot compete against quality. Fortunately, we are beginning to see the emergence of business organizations which recognize that people have had their bellyful of shoddy merchandise. (And shoddy merchandise is the inevitable byproduct of a business that operates on the ethic of bluffing.)

"The analogy of business and the poker game would be excellent except for the fact that business ultimately must rely on the consuming public. The public may not be interested in joining the poker game when it finds it can get full value from a business enterprise that puts its time and effort into developing a product worthy of people."

**What can be done?** So if we have a problem—whether it can be defined in a broad frame of reference or only in the narrower one of business—what can we do about it? Graham R. Briggs, Executive Assistant to the First Vice President of Abex Corporation, New York City, offers this reflection:

"Business, like society, operates within a set of norms of acceptable behavior. A radical departure from these norms in either direction, toward idealism or toward complete immorality, spells trouble at least and ruin at worst. Moreover, it seems to me to be true that acceptable behavior in business includes much that would be unacceptable in one's personal life.

"However, Mr. Carr sidesteps the question of where an individual should draw the line between acceptable and immoral action. Every businessman is tempted to be just a little less moral than his competitors—not enough to be operating right outside the business 'moral code,' but enough to secure a competitive edge.

"Then how can the inevitable gradual decline of business morals to an eventual state of complete anarchy be prevented? The law is insufficient protection against this; it can cover only the most flagrant violations, it cannot change as quickly as circumstances nowadays require, and it is too easily circumvented by those who are quick-witted and prepared to take a risk.

"The only guard against a gradual decline in morals is the ideals of each businessman. All of us have (or if we do not, something is wrong with us) an ideal of how business should be conducted; how we would like to be able to behave, or, rather, how we wish we could rely on other businessmen to act. It is usually impossible to adhere to this ideal in practice, since we live in an imperfect world, but we should always have this ideal in mind, be prepared to make some sacrifices for its sake, and be conscious of what we are doing when we depart from it.

"Only in this way can we apply 'upward' pressure on business morality, which, if practiced by a sufficient number of businessmen, will tend over time to raise the level of business values closer to the ideal. Most of us would like to be able to trust our fellow businessmen more than we can now. I see no other way of ever achieving this result."

John M. Vivian, a Philadelphia management consultant, considers the "frankly amoral business ethic" in terms of what he views as a decline in business's economic and political power:

"Mr. Carr suggests that the pursuit of profit is restrained only by the 'letter of the law' and that business is justified in maintaining a morality which is a game, amoral or immoral, depending on your own personal ethic.

"If Mr. Carr is correct, aren't the liberals equally so when they claim that 'good business sense' is a root cause of the major ills of our time? To cite more dramatic cases than Mr. Carr used, since there are no specific laws against these activities: (1) The 'military-industrial establishment' is justified in actively fomenting 'limited' wars to produce profit; (2) slum landlords and shopkeepers are playing within the rules in charging our economically powerless Negro urban dwellers high prices for decaying tenements and shoddy merchandise; (3) the makers of thalidomide were fully justified in aggressively marketing their fetus-deforming product, without exhaustive pretesting, in countries which have lax controls.

"These suggestions are admittedly extreme, overstated, and, to some extent, unfair. I'm sure they offend Mr. Carr's personal values, but he must admit they are a logical extension of his interpretation of the business ethic. What troubles me is that statements such as these — not Mr. Carr's less inflammatory examples — are accepted as representative of the business ethic by much of the world's, and our own nation's, population. An increasingly powerful government, plus a better informed public opinion, simply will not be willing to accept the profit motive as justification for acts considered immoral or antisocial in personal (Judeo-Christian, if you must) ethical terms.

"I suggest that an increasing number of 'privately unethical,' but pragmatically acceptable, business practices will be exposed to public censure and control, and that if the present business ethic is not abandoned, private enterprise as we know it is doomed. The following reasons come to mind:

"1. The base of political power is broadening and shifting away from the business-oriented sectors of society. Youth, urban minorities, academic and government personnel, unionized workers — all nonbusiness or even antibusiness in attitude — are assuming political control of the nation.

"2. Economic power, once controlled by the industrial entrepreneurs, has passed to — and through — the hands of professional managers, and is rapidly being accumulated by the public sector and nonbusiness-oriented entities. The government, and to a lesser extent the huge philanthropic trusts and the union-influenced retirement funds, are amassing greater economic control, which will tend to be wielded in support of public opinion.

"3. The truly phenomenal growth of mass communications technology, culminating in the communications satellites, has exposed business foibles to instantaneous worldwide criticism. The name of one of our finest chemical manufacturers, for instance, has become synonymous with an unpopular war in some parts of the world because of a few student sit-ins over a small plant producing napalm. The insatiable appetite of the mass media for sensational material has made business muckraking a profitable and influential — but popularly an 'ethical' — pursuit; witness Ralph Nader's success in generating public indignation and helping direct government controls against several industries.

"4. Probably of most importance to business, wealth and power are no longer the exclusive reward of business. Government, universities, the arts, and other nonprofit enterprises increasingly offer opportunity for financial and personal success—without requiring employees to risk the ulcers that Mr. Carr attributes to the conflict between individual and business ethics. In the past, our best minds went into business; today, they are attracted to other pursuits, where they are not forced to compromise their individual moral values in pursuit of profits.

"My conclusion is that the business ethic has been its own undoing. The opportunity for individual and corporate success offered by the ethic has been so monumentally successful—has created such wealth in our nation—that society can now 'afford' to question its worth.

"Egalitarian influences in society have employed taxation directly and indirectly to remove the wealth from business control and distribute it throughout society. This wealth and the economic and political power that go with it are now being concentrated in the hands of nonbusiness or antibusiness forces not tolerating the business ethic.

"The growing rate of direct government controls over the practice and products of business is an indication of the future. As long as businessmen continue 'the game' and feel bound only by the letter of the law, an ethical society will continue to extend the law to coerce business into following generally accepted ethical values. And the better minds in the nation will increasingly be attracted by other pursuits.

"The ultimate result will be a bureaucratically overcontrolled and internally undertalented business community, 'creeping socialism' at a dead run, and the end of a dynamic free enterprise system."

I shall leave it to Mr. Wood, who opened this discussion, to close it:

"If business is to survive as an independent force in our society of free enterprise, it will have to accelerate its acceptance of social responsibilities. Because of the tremendous economic power of corporations in every industrial society, they cannot be allowed to use it without consideration of its effect on those outside the poker game.

"If the players in Mr. Carr's poker game shoot it out among themselves and thereby endanger the lives of the people living next door, someone is going to call the police and break up the game for good."

## Mr. Carr Comments:

I was especially struck by the high charge of emotion, ranging from fury to enthusiasm, in the letters received by HBR, as well as in a number of letters and even phone calls that have come directly to me. It may be significant that, of the *company heads* responding, a large majority ruefully agree that the state of business ethics portrayed in the article was accurate. The letters strongly suggest that the men who have "made it" are more willing to face the realities of the problem than are those farther down the ladder.

I have the distinct impression that many of HBR's more outraged respondents (one or two even burst into vituperative verse!) have not yet fully sensed the nature of the strategic questions confronting the men responsible for the profitability and growth of their companies.

Perhaps I can assuage some of the pain the article seems to have caused by listing below the main criticisms leveled against it, and appending a few comments of my own.

*"Business is too important to be regarded as a game."* This misses the point of the article, which is that—whether or not business ought to be regarded and conducted as a game—it *is* so regarded and conducted by many of its practitioners, including executives of great importance and high reputation. A businessman is certainly entitled to refuse to employ game strategy himself, but he may be at a severe disadvantage if he does not recognize that it is being used by others.

*"The comparison to poker is unfair and inaccurate."* Like all useful analogies, this one was intended to throw light on the subject, not to provide an exact parallel. The honorable poker player who, within the laws of the game, takes pleasure in outsmarting the other fellow has many a counterpart in the paneled offices of the corporate hierarchies. Again, it may be noted that there is no compulsion for any executive to mislead others, any more than there is for the poker player to bluff. The option is his; most players exercise it at one time or another.

*"The article condones unethical practices."* This complaint seems to me extraordinary. More than once, the article stresses the values of truth-telling and integrity in business, where, certainly, there are as many high-minded men as one will find in most walks of life. My point is that, given the prevailing ethical standards of business, an executive who accepts those standards and operates accordingly is guilty of nothing worse than conformity; he is merely playing the game according to the rules and the customs of society.

*"A man cannot separate the ethics of his business life from the ethics of his home life."* Over the long run, that is probably true. What happens is that, in too many instances, the ethical outlook of business comes to dominate in the home as well. Perhaps that accounts in part for the notorious instability of the middle-class home in our society, and the increasing revolt of the young against the corporate establishment. It may also explain why so many wives of businessmen have, like their husbands, been conscience-washed into undiscriminating acceptance of corporation policies.

*"The article is one-sided and extreme in its description of what goes on in business."* This I must deny. I regard the article as mild, objective, and, if anything, over-discreet. If it had incorporated all the facts in my files, it would have curled HBR readers' hair. And I am talking now not about violations of law, but of decisions within the realm of business ethics—the so-called "gray area," where complexity so often provides the executive with a rationalization for doing what serves his interests.

*"The article does not point out that if business fails to raise the moral level of its practices, it invites eventual reprisals from the public and the government."* This thought was not within the scope of the article, but I could not agree with it more. As the article plainly conveys, sound long-range business strategy and ethical considerations are usually served by the same policy.

# 4

# Is the Ethics of Business Changing?

STEVEN N. BRENNER AND EARL A. MOLANDER

What would you do if . . .

. . . the minister of a foreign nation where extraordinary payments to lubricate the decision-making machinery are common asks you for a $200,000 consulting fee? In return, he promises special assistance in obtaining a $100-million contract which would produce at least a $5-million profit for your company. The contract would probably go to a foreign competitor if your company did not win it.

. . . as the president of a company in a highly competitive industry, you learn that a competitor has made an important scientific discovery that will substantially reduce, but not eliminate, your profit for about a year? There is a possibility of hiring one of the competitor's employees who knows the details of the discovery.

. . . you learn that an executive earning $30,000 a year has been padding his expense account by about $1,500 a year?

These questions were posed as part of a lengthy questionnaire on business ethics and social responsibility completed by 1,227 *Harvard Business Review* readers—25% of the cross section of 5,000 U.S. readers polled (see *Exhibit I*).

Our study was prompted by the same concern that Raymond C. Baumhart had in 1961 when he conducted a similar study for HBR: the numerous comments on business ethics in the media contained little empirical evidence to indicate whether large numbers of business executives shared the attitudes, behavior, and experience of those whose supposedly unethical and illegal conduct was being represented (or denied) as typical of the business profession.[1]

In updating and expanding his study, we designed our survey around three main questions: Has business ethics changed since the early 1960s, and if so, how and why? Are codes the answer to the ethical challenges business people currently face? What is the relationship between ethical dilemmas and the dilemma of corporate social responsibility?

Here are some of the highlights of our study:

1. There is substantial disagreement among respondents as to whether ethical standards in business today have changed from what they were.

2. Respondents are somewhat more cynical about the ethical conduct of their peers than they were.

3. Most respondents favor ethical codes, although they strongly prefer general precept codes to specific practice codes.

4. The dilemmas respondents experience and the factors they feel have the greatest impact on business ethics suggest that ethical codes alone will not substantially improve business conduct.

## Exhibit I Profile of Respondents

|  | *1961 percentage* | *1976 percentage* |
|---|---|---|
| *Management position* | | |
| Top management—chairman of the board; board member; owner; partner; president; managing director | | 17% |
| Other top management—division or executive vice president; vice president; treasurer; secretary-treasurer; controller; secretary (to the corporation); general manager; general superintendent; editor, administrative director; dean and assistants thereto | 45% | 25 |
| (Total in 1961 is for first two categories.) | | |
| Upper middle management—functional department head (e.g., advertising, sales, promotion, production, purchasing, personnel, engineering, public relations, brand manager, and the like) | 27 | 13 |
| Lower middle management—assistant to functional department head; district manager; branch manager; section manager; and the like | 12 | 21 |
| Staff and nonmanagement personnel—all others employed in business | 9 | 13 |
| Professional —doctor; practicing lawyer; CPA; professor; consultant; military officer; government official; union official; clergy; and the like | 7 | 8 |
| Other or didn't answer | 0 | 3 |
| *Income group* | | |
| Under $20,000 | 57% | 15% |
| $20,000–29,999 | 23 | 28 |
| $30,000–39,999 | 8 | 24 |
| $40,000–49,999 | 4 | 10 |
| $50,000–74,999 | 4 | 13 |
| $75,000–99,999 | 2 | 5 |
| $100,000 and over | 2 | 4 |
| Didn't answer | 0 | 2 |
| *Company size by number of employees* | | |
| 1–99 | 22% | 19% |
| 100–999 | 29 | 25 |
| 1,000–9,999 | 26 | 23 |
| 10,000 and over | 23 | 25 |
| Didn't answer | 0 | 7 |
| *Formal education* | | |
| High school or less | 5% | 1% |

## Exhibit I Continued

| | | |
|---|---|---|
| Some college | 19 | 8 |
| Bachelor's degree | 36 | 30 |
| Graduate school | 40 | 60 |
| Didn't answer | 0 | 1 |
| *Functional area of most experience* | | |
| Accounting | * | 9% |
| Engineering | * | 10 |
| Finance | * | 15 |
| Marketing | * | 24 |
| Personnel or labor relations | * | 9 |
| Production | * | 9 |
| Public relations | * | 3 |
| Other | * | 18 |
| Didn't answer | * | 4 |
| *Age* | | |
| 29 or under | 6% | 13% |
| 30–39 | 28 | 37 |
| 40–49 | 35 | 26 |
| 50–59 | 23 | 19 |
| 60 and over | 8 | 5 |
| Didn't answer | 0 | 1 |
| *Sex* | | |
| Male | * | 94% |
| Female | * | 5 |
| Didn't answer | * | 1 |
| *Industry* | | |
| Manufacturing consumer goods | 16% | 13% |
| Manufacturing industrial goods | 25 | 22 |
| Engineering; research and development | 6 | 3 |
| Management consulting and business services | 6 | 8 |
| Banking; investment; insurance | 10 | 12 |
| Construction | 2 | 2 |
| Mining or extraction; oil | 2 | 3 |

## Exhibit I Continued

| | | |
|---|---|---|
| Retail or wholesale trade | 7 | 7 |
| Transportation; public utilities | 5 | 6 |
| Advertising; media; publishing | 4 | 3 |
| Consumer services | 3 | 4 |
| Other | 14 | 17 |
| Didn't answer | 0 | 2 |

*Not reported in 1961 study.
*Note:* Percentages calculated from 1,531 respondents in 1961 study and 1,227 respondents in 1976 study. Categories may not add up to 100 due to rounding errors.

5. Most respondents have overcome the traditional ideological barriers to the concept of social responsibility and have embraced its practice as a legitimate and achievable goal for business.

6. Most respondents rank their customers well ahead of shareholders and employees as the client group to whom they feel the greatest responsibility.

### Today versus 15 Years Ago

Like other professions, business is continually scrutinizing its behavior relative to its own standards and those of the society around it.

What do business executives see when they look at themselves? One thing we found was that they see their profession as less ethical than the professions of professors and doctors, but more ethical than those of government agency officials, lawyers, elected politicians, and union officials, in that order.

#### Common Dilemmas

Of course, the ethics of business includes not only the moral values and duties of the profession itself, but also the existing values and expectations of the larger society. Because ethical systems are created by fallible people, they generally have some inherent contradictions. Further, the values and ethics of various organizations differ from those of other sectors of society in which business people participate (such as the family, church, and political parties). For these reasons executives inevitably face some ethical dilemmas in their daily work.

To learn how chronic a problem such ethical dilemmas are in the contemporary business environment, we asked our respondents if they had ever experienced a conflict between what was expected of them as efficient, profit-conscious managers and what was expected of them as ethical persons. Four of every seven of those who responded (399 of 698) say they have experienced such conflicts, compared with three of four respondents in 1961 (603 of 796)—a substantial decrease of 19%.

One possible explanation for this decrease is that the internal pressures for profit and efficiency are not as great as they once were. Since we can find no evidence of such a change, two other possible explanations must be considered: ethical standards have declined from what they were or situations that once caused ethical discomfort have become accepted practice.

As *Exhibit II* shows, we did find that the *nature* of compromising circumstances has changed. Honesty in communication is a significantly greater problem in 1976 than it was in 1961. This includes honesty in advertising and in providing information to top management, clients, and government agencies. We found number manipulation to have become a particularly acute problem.

Dilemmas associated with firings and layoffs are significantly less of a problem in 1976. Either terminations and their related problems are becoming accepted as routine in today's business world, or they are being handled more equitably when they occur. Undoubtedly because of government prosecutions, price collusion is also far less of a problem.

We feel it particularly noteworthy that relations with superiors are the primary category of ethical conflict. Respondents frequently complained of superiors' pressure to support incorrect viewpoints, sign false documents, overlook supe-

## Exhibit II Conflicts between Company Interests and Personal Ethics

| | 1961 percentage | 1976 percentage |
|---|---|---|
| *In relations with:* | | |
| Superiors | * | 12.8% |
| Customers | * | 12.0 |
| Employees | * | 11.5 |
| Agents and customers | * | 9.5 |
| Competitors | * | 4.8 |
| Law; government; and society | * | 4.8 |
| Suppliers | * | 2.5 |
| Potential investors | * | 0.5 |
| Other and unspecified | * | 41.6 |
| *With regard to:* | | |
| Honesty in communication | 13.5% | 22.3% |
| Gifts; entertainment; and kickbacks | 8.9 | 12.3 |
| Fairness and discrimination | * | 7.0 |
| Miscellaneous law breaking | * | 5.8 |
| Honesty in executing contracts and agreements | * | 5.5 |
| Firings and layoffs | 16.2 | 4.8 |
| Price collusion and pricing practices | 12.5 | 2.3 |
| Other and unspecified | 48.8 | 40.1 |

*Not reported in 1961 study.

riors' wrongdoing, and do business with superiors' friends. Either superiors are expecting more than subordinates in 1976 or subordinates are less willing to do their bosses' bidding without questions, at least to themselves. Both possibilities suggest a weakening in the corporate authority structure and an attendant impact on ethical business conduct that deserves future study. The following examples demonstrate ethical dilemmas being faced in business today:

The vice president of a California industrial manufacturer "being forced as an officer to sign corporate documents which I knew were not in the best interest of minority stockholders."

A Missouri manager of manpower planning "employing marginally qualified minorities in order to meet Affirmative Action quotas."

A manager of product development from a computer company in Massachusetts "trying to act as though the product (computer software) would correspond to what the customer had been led by sales to expect, when, in fact, I knew it wouldn't."

A manager of corporate planning from California "acquiring a non-U.S. company with two sets of books used to evade income taxes—standard practice for that country. Do we (1) declare income and pay taxes, (2) take the "black money" out of the country (illegally), or (3) continue tax evasion?"

The president of a real estate property management firm in Washington "projecting cash flow without substantial evidence in order to obtain a higher loan than the project can realistically amortize."

A young Texas insurance manager "being asked to make policy changes that produced more premium for the company and commission for an agent but did not appear to be of advantage to the policyholder."

### Accepted Practices

Clearly, that ethical dilemmas do exist and are too often resolved in ways which leave executives dissatisfied seems to be a matter of substantial concern for today's business people. And too often unethical practices become a routine part of doing business. To determine just how routine, we asked: "In every industry there are some generally accepted business practices. In your industry, are there practices which you regard as unethical?"

If we eliminate those who say they "don't know," we see from *Exhibit III* that two-thirds of the responding executives in 1976 indicate that such practices exist, compared with nearly four-fifths who so responded in 1961.

Could this decrease be a sign of improvement in ethical *practices*? Perhaps, but it is also possible that such practices are now less visible than they once were. Even more disturbing is the possibility which we raised earlier—that ethical *standards* have, in fact, fallen in business so that practices once considered unethical are now not viewed as such. Further, these figures say nothing about the conduct that all agree is both unacceptable and unethical.

Nearly half (540) of all respondents and 84% of those indicating the existence of such practices were willing to tell us which practice or practices they would most like to see eliminated (see *Exhibit IV*). Both the changes and similarities in these "most unwanted" practices in the past 15 years are interesting.

As in 1961, the practice that most executives want to eliminate involves "gifts,

# Exhibit III Are There Industry Practices Which You Consider Unethical?

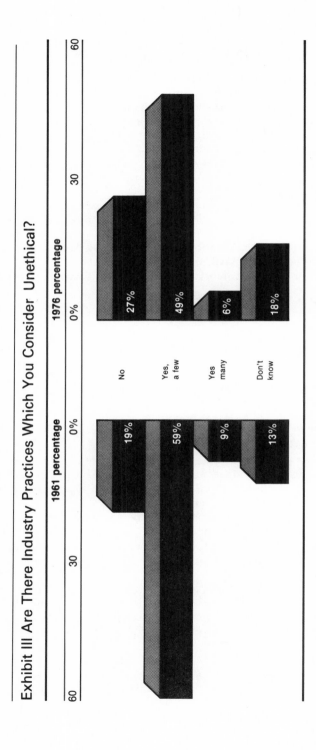

gratuities, bribes, and 'call girls.' " Typical examples given by the 144 respondents in this category are:

"Payoffs to a foreign government to secure contracts." [The vice president of an Oklahoma oil exploration company]

"Egg carton contracts with grocery chains can only be obtained by kickbacks —the egg packers do not have the freedom of choice in buying, thus stifling competition." [A young southern consumer goods executive vice president]

"Loans granted as favors to loan officers." [An Indiana bank vice president]

"Dealings with travel agencies that involve kickbacks, rebates, or other pseudonyms for 'bribes.' " [A Florida transportation industry executive]

Of the 80 respondents who mentioned practices which included cheating customers, unfair credit practices, or overselling, typical comments are:

"Substitution of materials without customer knowledge after the job has been awarded." [A young New York salesman]

"Misrepresenting the contents of products." [A Texas vice president of engineering]

"Scheduled delivery dates that are known to be inaccurate to get a contract." [A California director of engineering]

Both the sharp drop from 1961 to 1976 shown in *Exhibit IV* in concern over "price discrimination and unfair pricing" and "dishonest advertising" and the increase in concern over "unfairness to employees and prejudice in hiring" and "cheating customers" are probably attributable to government enforcement and higher legal standards, respectively.

### Economic Pressures

We have confirmed the continued existence both of ethical dilemmas inherent in everyday business and of generally accepted practices which individual managers feel are unethical. To observe the impact of such an environment on our respondents' ethical beliefs, we turned our attention to a number of issues of general ethical concern.

Simply returning our questionnaire reflected, we think, a general concern about business ethics among our respondents. Nevertheless, 65% of them feel that "society, not business, has the *chief* responsibility for inculcating its ethical standards into the educational and legal systems, and thus into business decision making."

Another important aspect of the debate over ethics focuses on whether any absolutes exist to strive for or whether ethics should be purely "situational" or "relative." Four out of five respondents agree that "business people should try to live up to an absolute moral standard rather than to the moral standard of their peer group."

Not only do executives believe in ethical absolutes; they also believe that "in the long run, sound ethics is good business." As in 1961, fewer than 2% of the respondents disagreed with this statement. Yet, in practice, many of these same executives see their associates losing sight of this standard. Again, as in 1961, close to half of our respondents agree that "the American business executive tends not to apply the great ethical laws immediately to work. He is preoccupied chiefly with gain."[2]

Our results suggest two explanations for this failure. First, despite its long-run value, ethical conduct apparently is not necessarily rewarded. Within the business organization, 50% of our respondents feel that one's superiors often do not want to know how results are obtained, as long as one achieves the desired outcome.

Second, competitive pressures from outside the organization push ethical consideration into the background. Of our executives, 43% feel that "competition today is stiffer than ever. As a result, many in business find themselves forced to resort to practices which are considered shady, but which appear necessary for survival."

### Societal Forces

In the period since Baumhart's study, American business has seen some significant changes. A sustained period of economic euphoria which began in 1961 has been replaced by recession, inflation, and resource scarcity. Charges of corporate irresponsibility relative to critical issues of the 1960s and 1970s (minority relations, consumerism, and the environment) combined with the recent disclosures of corporate wrongdoing at home and abroad have raised serious questions about the trend in business's ethical standards.

To determine if any such trend existed, we asked our HBR respondents: "How do you feel ethical standards in business today compare with ethical standards 15 years ago?"

The old French proverb, "The more things change, the more they stay the same," seems appropriate in describing the responses. Rather than reporting a clear-cut shift in either direction, our respondents split fairly evenly; 32% (388) feel standards are lower today, 41% (492) that they are about the same, and 27% (325) that they are higher.

But among those respondents who sense a more extreme change, a trend is identifiable with the 12% who believe ethical standards to be *considerably* lower outnumbering the 5% who believe them to be *considerably* higher by a 2.4-to-1 ratio.

We asked our respondents to describe "the single factor which has most influenced (or caused) the shift (you) observe in ethical standards." By splitting responses into two groups, those who see today's ethical standards as lower and those who see them as higher, it is possible to isolate which factors our respondents feel have influenced ethical standards in business.

The fact that 95% of the 713 respondents who see some shift in ethical standards provided further explanatory factors in brief sentences confirms our earlier assertion that ethics is an important personal concern to executives. The factors are listed in *Exhibit V.*

It is noteworthy that of the six major factors seen as causing *higher* standards, only two are subject to any significant measure of direct business influence and control — the education and professionalism of management and business's greater sense of awareness and responsiveness.

And of the six major factors seen as causing *lower* standards, only one is subject to such influence and control by business — pressure for profits in the organization.

Exhibit IV Unethical Practices Executives Want to Eliminate

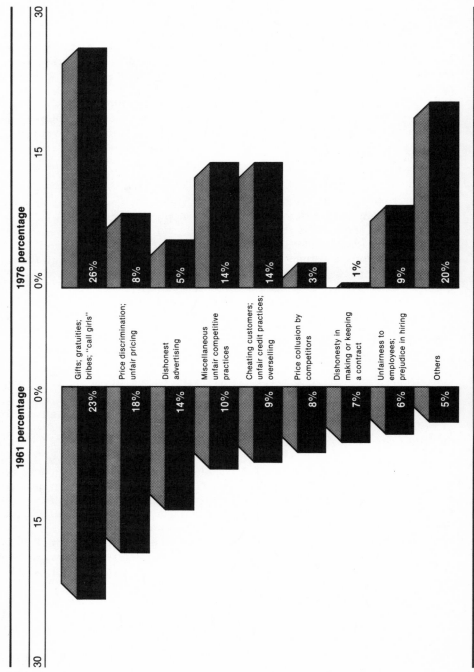

| | 1961 percentage | | 1976 percentage |
|---|---|---|---|

Gifts; gratuities; bribes; "call girls" — 23% (1961), 26% (1976)

Price discrimination; unfair pricing — 18% (1961), 8% (1976)

Dishonest advertising — 14% (1961), 5% (1976)

Miscellaneous unfair competitive practices — 10% (1961), 14% (1976)

Cheating customers; unfair credit practices; overselling — 9% (1961), 14% (1976)

Price collusion by competitors — 8% (1961), 3% (1976)

Dishonesty in making or keeping a contract — 7% (1961), 1% (1976)

Unfairness to employees; prejudice in hiring — 6% (1961), 9% (1976)

Others — 5% (1961), 20% (1976)

## Exhibit V Factors Influencing Ethical Standards

| | *Percentage of respondents listing factor* |
|---|---|
| *Factors causing higher standards* | |
| Public disclosure; publicity; media coverage; better communication | 31% |
| Increased public concern; public awareness, consciousness, and scrutiny; better informed public; societal pressures | 20 |
| Government regulation, legislation, and intervention; federal courts | 10 |
| Education of business managers; increase in manager professionalism and education | 9 |
| New social expectations for the role business is to play in society; young adults' attitudes; consumerism | 5 |
| Business's greater sense of social responsibility and greater awareness of the implications of its acts; business responsiveness; corporate policy changes; top management emphasis on ethical action | 5 |
| Other | 20 |
| *Factors causing lower standards* | |
| Society's standards are lower; social decay; more permissive society; materialism and hedonism have grown; loss of church and home influence; less quality, more quantity desires | 34% |
| Competition; pace of life; stress to succeed; current economic conditions; costs of doing business; more businesses compete for less | 13 |
| Political corruption; loss of confidence in government; Watergate; politics; political ethics and climate | 9 |
| People more aware of unethical acts; constant media coverage; TV; communications create atmosphere for crime | 9 |
| Greed; desire for gain; worship the dollar as measure of success; selfishness of the individual; lack of personal integrity and moral fiber | 8 |
| Pressure for profit from within the organization from superiors or from stockholders; corporate influences on managers; corporate policies | 7 |
| Other | 21 |

*Note:* Some respondents listed more than one factor, so there were 353 factors in all listed as causing higher standards and 411 in all listed as causing lower ones. Categories may not add up to 100 due to rounding errors.

Our respondents seem to be sending us three clearcut messages:

1. Public disclosure and concern over unethical business behavior are the most potent forces for improvement in ethical standards.

2. Hedonism, individual greed, and the general decay of social standards are the factors which most influence a decline in ethical standards.

3. The elements which influence shifts in ethical standards are ones over which they have little direct control.

### Growing Cynicism

The situation, then, is that today's executive often faces ethical dilemmas and observes generally accepted practices which he or she feels are unethical. At the same time he is more likely to attribute questionable conduct to his business colleagues than he is to himself.

In 1961, Baumhart found his respondents to be quite cynical when comparing their own ethical decisions with what they expected the "average" executive to do in the same circumstances. To measure cynicism, we presented four case situations in two different ways. We asked one half of our sample, "What would *you* do?" and the other half, "What would the *average* executive do?" (See *Exhibit VI.*)

The two groups' answers differ more than Baumhart's respondents'. In Case 1, current respondents report themselves as less willing to pad their own expense accounts and report others as more willing to do so than did respondents in 1961. This perception spread (between "I feel it is unacceptable" and "the average executive feels it is unacceptable") grew from 26% in 1961 to 36% in 1976.

In Case 2, while the spread is nearly the same (22% in 1961 versus 23% in 1976), the respondents indicate that both they and the average executive would be more inclined than 1961 respondents to hire a competitor's employee to get a technological secret.

The real magnitude of such cynicism is shown in Case 3's international situation where facilitative payments could help land a large contract: 42% of the respondents said they would refuse to pay a bribe no matter what the consequences, while only 9% felt that the average executive in the same situation would refuse to pay. Even more disturbing, seven-eighths of the respondents who report that the average executive would see such payments as unethical also feel that he would go ahead and pay them anyway! And more than one-third of the respondents who themselves see such payments as unethical admit a willingness to pay them to help cement the contract award. Apparently, economic values override ethical values.

Case 4 illustrates another aspect of cynicism. Here we presented a potential conflict of interest and asked half of our respondents what an inside director would do and half what an outside director would do. The results suggest that executives expect outside directors to be more likely than inside directors to find fault in this situation (64% versus 45%) and to be more overt in their opposition when they do (30% versus 16%).

Our respondents apparently are cynical not only when they compare their own motives and actions to those of others, but also when they consider how business people with different organizational perspectives handle identical situations. This makes sense; organizational loyalty tends to inhibit an employee's perception of an ethical dilemma and to constrain his actions when ethical dilemmas are recognized.

Could our results be simply a flaw in our sampling method or in our analysis? This possibility is unlikely. We split our sample at random into two equal groups. Demographically, our groups were virtually identical. So, too, were their responses to the other questions we asked. So the differences must indicate that while executives see themselves as being faced with ethical dilemmas and as handling them correctly, they are not so confident about their peers' reactions.

## Guideposts and Codes

What can be done to restore this confidence? And what can help reduce unethical acts?

We asked our respondents what factors they feel influence executives to make unethical decisions. As *Exhibit VII* shows, they believe that the behavior of one's superiors is the primary guidepost, with formal company policy a somewhat distant secondary influence.

In other words, when faced with ethical dilemmas, people first refer to their immediate organizational framework for guidance. If the unethical acts of others and the lack of formal company policy provide a rationale for unethical behavior, would a formal policy, that is, an ethical code, be beneficial? The current popularity of ethical codes would seem to suggest as much.

When we asked our respondents for their feelings about ethical codes for their industry, 25% said they favor no code at all. Of those who favor a code, 58% prefer one dealing with general precepts while only 17% prefer one delineating specific practices. Despite this lack of enthusiasm for specific codes, *Exhibit VIII* shows that the majority of respondents expect that such a code would help executives to (a) raise the ethical level of their industry, (b) define the limits of acceptable conduct, and (c) refuse unethical requests.

While respondents in 1976 are less certain of a code's efficacy than were their counterparts in 1961, these expectations support an argument many observers have made: the mere existence of a code, specific or general, can raise the ethical level of business behavior because it clarifies what is meant by ethical conduct. However, to an even greater extent than those in 1961, our respondents think a code is limited in its ability to change human conduct: 61% feel people would violate the code whenever they thought they could avoid detection and only 41% feel the code would reduce underhanded practices.

### Appropriate Enforcement

The single most negative response to our questions about a specific practice code concerns its enforceability: 89% of our respondents feel a specific practices code would *not* be easy to enforce. Anticipating this result since Baumhart's 1961 study had produced a similar response, we asked our respondents to identify an appropriate body for enforcing a code and the problems they foresaw in its enforcement.

In their choice of enforcement bodies, our respondents follow essentially the same pattern as Baumhart's did. Slightly more than a third favor self-enforcement at the company level, a third favor enforcement by a combined group of industry executives and members of the community, and slightly less than a third prefer enforcement at the industry level — either a trade association or a group of industry executives. Only 2.5% favor enforcement by a government agency.

Respondents foresee two major problems confronting all of these enforcement

# Exhibit VI I'm More Ethical than the Average Executive

Case 1 An executive earning $30,000 a year has been padding his expense account by about $1,500 a year.

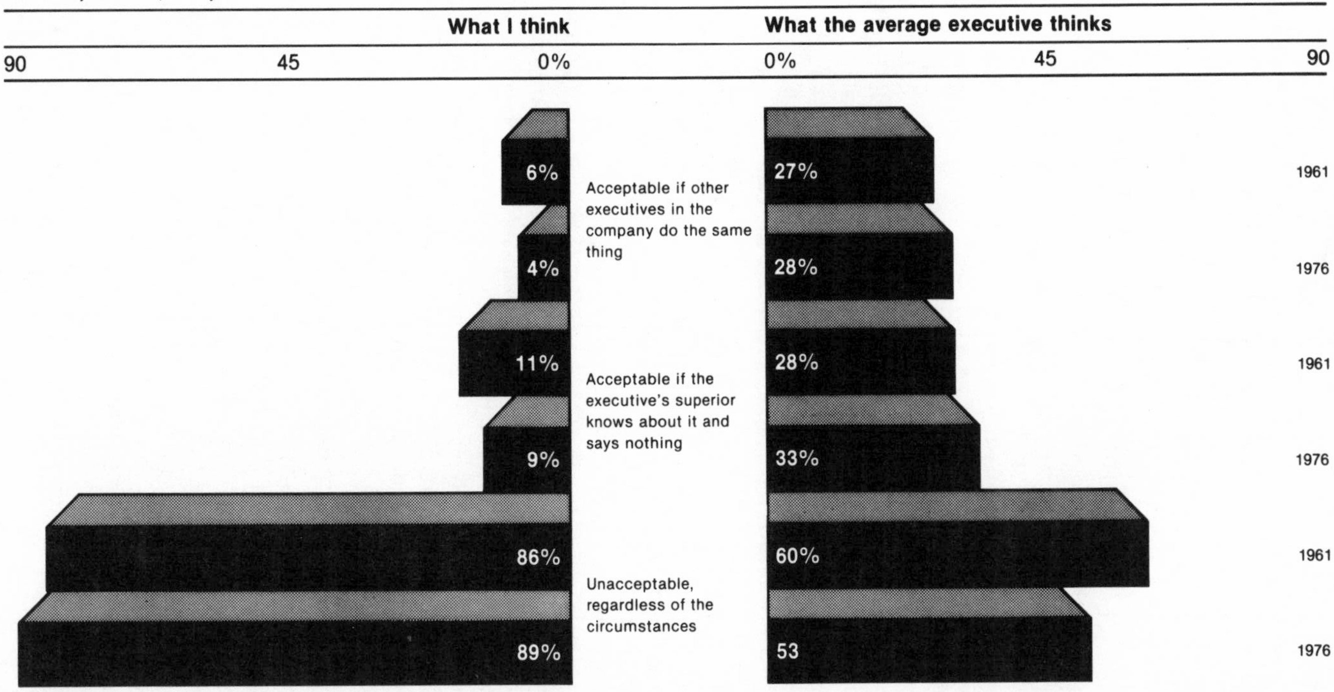

| | What I think | | | | What the average executive thinks | | |
|---|---|---|---|---|---|---|---|
| 90 | 45 | 0% | | | 0% | 45 | 90 |

Acceptable if other executives in the company do the same thing

6% / 4%  —  27% (1961) / 28% (1976)

Acceptable if the executive's superior knows about it and says nothing

11% / 9%  —  28% (1961) / 33% (1976)

Unacceptable, regardless of the circumstances

86% / 89%  —  60% (1961) / 53 (1976)

**Case 2** Imagine that you are the president of a company in a highly competitive industry. You learn that a competitor has made an important scientific discovery which will give him an advantage that will substantially reduce, but not eliminate the profits of your company for about a year. If there were some hope of hiring one of the competitor's employees who knew the details of the discovery, would you try to hire him?

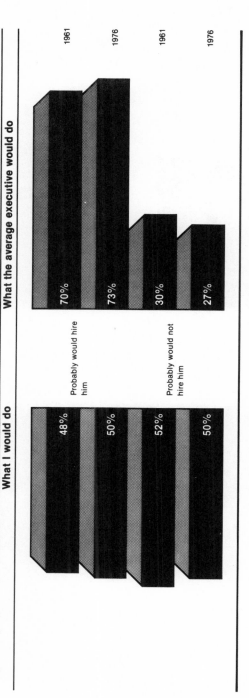

| | What I would do | What the average executive would do |
|---|---|---|
| Probably would hire him | 48% (1961) / 50% (1976) | 70% (1961) / 73% (1976) |
| Probably would not hire him | 52% (1961) / 50% (1976) | 30% (1961) / 27% (1976) |

# Exhibit VI

**Case 3** The minister of a foreign nation where extraordinary payments to lubricate the decision-making machinery are common asks you as a company marketing director for a $200,000 consulting fee. In return, he promises special assistance in obtaining a $100 million contract which should produce at least $5 million profit for your company. What would you do?

## What I would do

| 90 | 45 | 0% |

**Pay the fee,** feeling it was ethical in the moral climate of the foreign nation

36%

**Pay the fee,** feeling it was unethical but necessary to help ensure the sale

22%

**Refuse to pay,** even if the sale is thereby lost

42%

## What the average executive would do

| 0% | 45 | 90 |

45%

46%

9%

**Case 4\*** At a board meeting of High Fly Insurance Co. (HFI), a new board member learns that HFI is the "officially approved" insurer of the Private Pilots Benevolent Association (PPBA), which contains 200,000 members. On joining PPBA, members automatically subscribe to HFI's accident insurance for a premium included in the standard dues assessment. In return, HFI pays PPBA a fee tied to the volume of business PPBA members generate and gets use of the PPBA mailing list, which it uses to sell aircraft liability policies (its major source of revenues). PPBA's president sits on HFI's board of directors and the two companies are both located in the same office building.

What the average new director **who is a recently promoted HFI employee** would do in this situation

What the average new **outside** director would do in this situation

55% Would do nothing — 36%

29% Would privately and delicately raise the issue with the chairman of the board — 34%

13% Would express opposition in a director's meeting, but would go along with whatever position the board chose to take — 19%

3% Would express vigorous opposition and resign if corrective action is not undertaken — 11%

\*Not asked in 1961 study.

135

## Exhibit VII Factors Influencing Unethical Decisions

| | Rank | |
|---|---|---|
| | 1961 | 1976 |
| Behavior of superiors | 1.9 | 2.15 |
| Formal policy or lack thereof | 3.3 | 3.27 |
| Industry ethical climate | 2.6 | 3.34 |
| Behavior of one's equals in the company | 3.1 | 3.37 |
| Society's moral climate | * | 4.22 |
| One's personal financial needs | 4.1 | 4.46 |

*"Society's moral climate" was not asked in the 1961 study, which means that the rank cannot be compared numerically since 6 factors were used in 1976 and only 5 in 1961.
Note: The ranking is calculated on a scale of 1 (most influential) to 6 (least influential).

groups—getting information about violations and uniform and impartial enforcement. They feel that a third problem—lack of power and authority for enforcement—would be common to all groups except self-enforcement, which, understandably, they see as less of a problem. One young manager from Iowa hit on all three problems when he said, "You'll have problems with access to records, exceptions to the rules (and some may be legitimate), and punishment enforcement."

Our respondents feel that self-enforcement at the company level, the form of enforcement currently in widest use, has both substantial advantages and disadvantages compared with external enforcement.

Among the advantages they mentioned are:

1. Greater power and authority for those responsible for enforcement.
2. Easier access to information and detection of violations committed.
3. Easier interpretation when rules have been violated.
4. More natural definition of and execution of penalties to fit violations.

At the same time certain disadvantages exist:

1. Uniform and impartial enforcement.
2. Difficulty of securing the full-fledged commitment of the enforcers (top management).
3. Greater tendency to ignore or wink at the rules.
4. Greater difficulty in resolving profits-versus-ethics conflicts.
5. Continuous worry over actions of companies not covered by a code.

As a systems sales representative from California rather curtly put it, "Self-enforcement won't always work, because those who make 'em, break 'em."

The enforcement problems inherent in ethical codes led us to question their potential effectiveness. We reexamined the data concerning (1) the dilemmas our respondents have encountered (*Exhibit II*), (2) the practices they would most like to eliminate (*Exhibit IV*), and (3) the factors causing shifts in standards (*Exhibit V*), and we asked, "In which of these areas could ethical codes have an impact?"

In general, the responses suggest that codes can be most helpful in those areas where there is general agreement that certain unethical practices are widespread

# Exhibit VIII Consequences Expected from Industry-Specific Practice Codes

| | 1961 percentage | | | | | 1976 percentage | | | | |
|---|---|---|---|---|---|---|---|---|---|---|
| | Agree | Partly agree | Neutral | Partly disagree | Disagree | Agree | Partly agree | Neutral | Partly disagree | Disagree |
| Would raise the ethical level of the industry | 36% | 35% | 12% | 7% | 10% | 19% | 37% | 15% | 9% | 18% |
| Would help executives by defining clearly the limits of acceptable conduct | 48 | 33 | 7 | 5 | 7 | 29 | 38 | 11 | 9 | 12 |
| Managers would welcome as a useful aid when they wanted to refuse an unethical request impersonally | 59 | 28 | 5 | 4 | 4 | 45 | 34 | 8 | 6 | 6 |
| People would violate whenever they thought they could avoid detection | 13 | 44 | 8 | 20 | 15 | 22 | 39 | 11 | 19 | 9 |
| In situations of severe competition, would reduce the use of underhanded practices | 13 | 38 | 9 | 19 | 21 | 9 | 32 | 10 | 21 | 26 |
| Would be easy to enforce | 2 | 7 | 4 | 23 | 64 | 2 | 5 | 5 | 19 | 70 |

Note: Categories may not add up to 100 due to rounding errors.

and undesirable. Ethical codes do not, however, offer executives much hope for either controlling outside influences on business ethics or resolving fundamental ethical dilemmas. This is not to minimize the potential for codes to have an impact in narrow areas of concern. It is to emphasize that regardless of form they are no panacea for unethical business conduct.

## New View of Social Responsibility

The current revival of interest in business ethics coincides with a renewed focus on corporate social responsibility. To provide some insight into how our respondents see the relationship between "social responsibility" and "business ethics," we asked: Is social responsibility an *ethical* issue for the *individual business person*, or is it an issue that concerns the *role* the *corporation* should play in society?

The overwhelming response we got is that it is *both*—65% agree with the former statement and 83% with the latter.

But can it be both? The answer is, of course, yes. Whereas responsibility, for both the individual and the corporation, tends to be defined in the social arrangements and obligations which make up the structure of the society, ethics concerns the rules by which these responsibilities are carried out. As in numerous other settings, it is often difficult to separate the rules of the game from the game itself.

### Erroneous Caricature

One important finding of our study is the rejection of the traditional ideology that says business is a profit-bound institution. Only 28% of our respondents endorse the traditional dictum that "the social responsibility of business is to 'stick to business,' " most often associated with the writings of Milton Friedman.[3]

Further, only 23% agree that "social responsibility is good business only if it is also good public relations and/or preempts government interference." And 38% agree that "the social responsibility debate is the result of the attempt of liberal intellectuals to make a moral issue of business behavior."[4]

By contrast, 69% agree with George Lodge's observation that " 'profit' is really a somewhat ineffective measure of business's social effectiveness."[5]

Not only do those in our sample reject the traditional ideological barriers to corporate involvement in social responsibility, but they also reject the practical ones. Of our respondents, 77% disagree with the idea that "every business is in effect 'trapped' in the business system it helped create, and can do remarkably little about the social problems of our time."[6]

Have business executives abandoned their traditional profit orientation? Not necessarily. We still found strong support for long-term profit maximization among our executives. But these findings do indicate that the American business executive has incorporated a new view of his role and potential, and those of his company, into his profit concerns.

Those critics who continue to characterize the American business executive as a power-hungry, profit-bound individualist, indifferent to the needs of society, should be put on notice that they are now dealing with a straw man of their own making.

Before we go as far as to predict a revolution in corporate behavior, however, a word of caution is in order. First, the corporate organization still resists specific measures when trying to put social responsibility into practice. Of our respondents, 75% feel the rhetoric of social responsibility exceeds the reality in most corporations. And 58% agree that "the socially aware executive must show convincingly a net short-term or long-term economic advantage to the corporation in order to gain acceptance for any socially responsible measure he might propose."[7]

A second major barrier is uncertainty—uncertainty as to what "social responsibility" means. Almost half (46%) of our respondents agree with the assertion that "the meaning of social responsibility is so vague as to render it essentially unworkable as a guide to corporate policy and decisions."

This uncertainty as to meaning is further amplified by an uncertainty as to consequences. Our respondents were almost evenly split on two statements:

    1. Social responsibility invariably will mean *lower* corporate profits in the *short run*—41% agree, 16% are neutral, and 43% disagree.

    2. Social responsibility invariably will mean *higher* corporate profits in the *long run*—43% agree, 22% are neutral, and 36% disagree.

The nearly even split and the high number of neutral responses on these statements, together with the feeling of vagueness about the meaning of social responsibility, suggest that bringing social responsibility to the operating level is an objective which its advocates have yet to realize.

### Customer's Servant

    To further clarify our respondents' concept of social responsibility, we asked them to rank the various groups whose relations to the corporation define the corporation's place in the social system.

As *Exhibit IX* shows, the group to whom executives feel the greatest responsibility comes through clearly and unmistakably: *the customers*. Stockholders and employees are a clear second and third, and the interest of society at large and its elected governments—the "public interest"—appears to receive the least consideration.

This rather surprising result—the primacy of customer interest—suggests that we need to reexamine the thesis that the guiding principle of American business and the justification for its power is service to stockholders. We may be observing a return to the original capitalist doctrine of the customer as the client whom production is intended to serve and the replacement of the doctrine of "long-run profit maximization" with the "long-run customer satisfaction" doctrine.

The primacy of customer interests also raises some serious questions about any unethical conduct at the expense of customers which is rationalized on grounds of profit maximization. If the assertion of customer primacy is valid, it follows that business should also make ethical conduct in dealing with customers a first priority, a condition which our data suggest does not currently exist.

### Societal Obligations

    How do these attitudes affect policy and decision making on specific issues? We asked HBR readers to express the degree of responsibility they felt in each of nine areas along a scale of 1 (absolutely voluntary) to 5 (absolutely

## Exhibit IX Responsibility of Your Company to Various Groups

|  | Rank |
|---|---|
| Customers | 1.83 |
| Stockholders | 2.52 |
| Employees | 2.86 |
| Local community where company operates | 4.44 |
| Society in general | 4.97 |
| Suppliers | 5.10 |
| Government | 5.72 |

Note: The ranking is calculated on a scale of 1 (most responsibility) to 7 (least responsibility).

obligatory). The third-place standing of "maximizing long-run profits," shown in *Exhibit X*, confirms our observation that it is no longer perceived as the primary responsibility of today's executives.

But we were surprised to find two areas of general responsibility to *society* — "being an efficient user of energy and natural resources" and "assessing the potential environmental effects flowing from the company's technological advances" — are first and second. The strong feeling of obligation toward these areas, together with "using every means possible to maximize job content and satisfaction for the hourly worker," demonstrates the desire of the business person to define his responsibility in those areas which involve externalities directly associated with his operation, areas where he can see clearly the internalized benefits of his "socially responsible" actions, either in reduced costs or preempted government regulation.

By contrast, the strong voluntary rankings for the United Fund and hardcore hiring indicate that executives do not feel a significant obligation concerning social problems of a remedial or welfare nature whose benefits to the company are not readily apparent.

### Voluntary Measures

Perhaps not surprisingly, our respondents favor those measures for improving corporate social conduct that are both general in nature and leave room for voluntarism over those that involve compulsion and outside interference in corporate affairs. This result could be expected given our respondents' uncertainties about what social responsibility means and about its consequences, as well as their natural reluctance to accept any further constraints on the traditional freedom of the business decision maker.

We have already seen that respondents feel the media have had a powerful impact on business ethics simply by virtue of publicizing unethical conduct. They also feel that "endorsement of 'social responsibility' by the business media" would have the greatest positive influence on corporate social behavior. Altogether, 72% feel that such an endorsement would have a "positive impact," 55% believe that there would be "some positive impact," and 17% believe that the impact

## Exhibit X  Areas of Responsibility

|  | *Degree* |
|---|---|
| Being an efficient user of energy and natural resources | 4.00 |
| Assessing the potential environmental effects flowing from the company's technological advances | 3.96 |
| Maximizing long-run profits | 3.78 |
| Using every means possible to maximize job content and satisfaction for the hourly worker | 3.35 |
| Having your company's subsidiary in another country use the same occupational safety standards as your company does in the United States | 3.05 |
| Acquiescing to State Department requests that the company not establish operations in a certain country | 3.01 |
| Making implementation of corporate Affirmative Action plans a significant determinant of line officer promotion and salary improvement | 2.91 |
| Instituting a program for hiring the hard-core unemployed | 2.28 |
| Contributing to the local United Fund | 2.17 |

*Note:* The ranking is calculated on a scale of 1 (absolutely voluntary) to 5 (absolutely obligatory).

would be "very positive." Only 4% think it would have a "negative impact," while 24% think it would have "zero impact." Clearly executives look to the business media, not only for information and education, but for guidance in areas of uncertainty as well.[8]

About 62% of our respondents also agree that "the equalization of managerial rewards and punishments for social performance with those for financial performance" would have a positive effect in making corporations more socially responsible. This view is corroborated by our earlier observation that most executives support the view that proposals for corporate social action must convincingly show a net economic advantage to the company.

Polling stockholder opinions on sensitive social issues (part of "shareholder democracy"), public interest representation on boards of directors, educating the average citizen to the realities of corporate operations, and corporate social audits have all been advanced, and debated, in business and academic circles. Our respondents' generally positive view toward these measures — no more than a fourth think any of them would have a negative impact — suggests that, if properly conceived and advanced, these measures might also be acceptable to most executives.

This willingness to accept outside inputs does not include input from government, however. Less than one-sixth of our respondents see anything positive in federal chartering of corporations, strongly endorsed by Ralph Nader among others, while 39% feel that such a measure would be deleterious. And our respondents are least sanguine about increased governmental regulation: 64% fear it would have a negative impact and 14% say it would have none, while only 21% feel it might be beneficial.

## Freedom and Criticism

At the outset we posed three basic questions for our study. The generous response of HBR readers has allowed us to answer them in this article. Now a fourth question is in order: "What do the results mean for managers and students of business ethics?"

Our results suggest changes are necessary in two primary areas: managerial outlook and managerial actions.

The four aspects of change in managerial outlook indicated are:

You will face ethical dilemmas, created by value conflicts, for which there may be no totally satisfactory resolution. But don't use this condition to rationalize unethical behavior on your part.

Don't expect ethical codes to help solve all problems. Codes can create a false sense of security and lead to the encouragement of violations.

If you wish to avoid external enforcement of someone else's ethical code, make self-enforcement work.

Don't deceive yourself into thinking you can hide unethical actions.

The five aspects of managerial action suggested are:

Fair dealing with customers and employees is the most direct way to restore confidence in business morality.

Corporate steps taken to improve ethical behavior clearly must come from the top and be part of the reward and punishment system.

If an ethical code is developed and implemented, have an accompanying information system to detect violations. Then treat violators equitably.

Test decisions against what you think is right rather than against what is expedient.

Don't force others into unethical conduct.

It seems to us our respondents are saying that managers facing ethical dilemmas should refer to the familiar maxim, "Would I want my family, friends, and employers to see this decision and its consequences on television?" If the answer is yes, then go ahead. If the answer is no, then additional thought should be given to finding a more satisfactory solution.

Business executives and the companies they serve have a personal and vested interest in the resolution of ethical and social responsibility dilemmas. Our respondents recognize these dilemmas and to some extent appear willing to accept generalized guidance for their resolution in the form of general precept codes and statements from the business media. Although such measures will help in this regard, they are obviously no panacea for the continued strain arising from challenges to business ethics and responsibility. They also are not as action oriented as specific practice codes or government regulation.

The manager appears to prefer uncertainty and tension to the loss of freedom and complications that would accompany these more rigorous measures. In making this choice, he has to realize that he must continue to bear the criticism of the larger society in both the business ethics and corporate social responsibility areas.

## APPENDIX

My interpretation of Professors Brenner's and Molander's data and the signs of the times indicate that business behavior is more ethical than it was 15 years ago, but that the expectations of a better educated and ethically sensitized public have risen more rapidly than the behavior.

This is the sixth, and most creative and extensive, replication of the series of questions I first asked in 1961. Each time the results have been remarkably similar, especially in the respondents' attitude that: I am more ethical than the average manager, and my department and company are more ethical than their counterparts; and a written code of ethics would help to improve business practices in my industry.

It is good to see the evidence that business managers accept the corporation as a social, as well as an economic, entity.

To me the most surprising finding of this study is that the 1,227 respondents rank responsibility to customers ahead of responsibility to stockholders and employees. What has happened to *caveat emptor*? Now it is the government and suppliers who should beware.

Raymond C. Baumhart, S.J.,
President of Loyola University

## NOTES

1. Raymond C. Baumhart, "How Ethical Are Businessmen?" HBR July–August 1961, p. 6.
2. Rabbi Louis Finkelstein, "The Businessman's Moral Failure," *Fortune*, September 1958, p. 116.
3. Milton Friedman, *Capitalism and Freedom* (Chicago: University of Chicago Press, 1962), ch. 8.
4. Henry G. Manne, in Henry G. Manne and Henry C. Wallich, *The Modern Corporation and Social Responsibility* (Washington, D.C.: American Institute for Public Policy Research, 1972), p. 10.
5. George Cabot Lodge, "Top Priority: Renovating Our Ideology," HBR September–October 1970, p. 50.
6. Neil V. Chamberlain, *The Limits of Corporate Responsibility* (New York: Boise Books, 1973), p. 4.
7. Albert Z. Carr, "Can an Executive Afford a Conscience?" HBR July–August 1970, p. 58.
8. The susceptibility of business people to the ideology of the business media has often been noted; see, for example, Norton Long, "The Corporation, Its Satellites, and the Local Community," in *The Corporation in Modern Society*, edited by Edward S. Mason (Cambridge, Massachusetts: Harvard University Press, 1959), p. 210.

# 5

# The Ethical Roots of the Business System

DOUGLAS S. SHERWIN

In George Bernard Shaw's play *Major Barbara*, Undershaft, the old munitions maker, talks with his 24-year-old son about a career. Undershaft asks his son if he is interested in literature, and the young man replies, "No, I have nothing of the artist about me."

"Philosophy then?" his father asks. And the son replies, "Oh, I make no such ridiculous pretension." His father queries him about the army, the church, and the bar. The son disclaims any knowledge of or interest in any of these.

Finally Undershaft asks, "Well come, is there anything you know or care for?" To which the son replies, "I know the difference between right and wrong." "You don't say so!" exclaims Undershaft. "What, no capacity for business, no knowledge of law, no sympathy with art, no pretension to philosophy, only a simple knowledge of the secret that has puzzled all the philosophers, baffled all the lawyers, muddled all the men of business, and ruined most of the artists? The secret of right and wrong—at 24, too."

Probably you have to be 24 to enjoy such certainty. No longer 24, I won't offer any absolute answers, just a point of view.

For many years now, people have argued the question of right and wrong for business. For a long time, they couched the question in terms of social responsibility. More recently, they have asked whether the corporation can or should have a conscience.

Unhappily, the long debate hasn't improved the public's perception of business and business people. Business is criticized for its behavior at almost every interface with the rest of society: for being unresponsive to consumers, employees, its own shareholders, and the public; for enjoying a symbiotic relationship with a government that gives it inordinate power to serve its own interests; for failing to provide employment for all who want to work; for promoting a biased distribution of income; and for plundering the planet with its voracious appetite for resources, which it then dissipates in trivial products.

In these criticisms the implied remedy for such perceived evils is for the corporation to be socially responsible, behave ethically, and have a conscience. If only business people weren't wholly preoccupied with profits, the argument goes, the necessity for these criticisms would disappear.

Unfortunately, what is meant by social responsibility or ethical behavior remains unclear. But if both business and public leaders could come to some accord on what these concepts mean in the context of business, then possibly business performance and the public's expectations for business performance could converge at a higher level of satisfaction for society. So in this article, I will offer a view of what the social responsibility and ethical behavior of business consist of and consider whether the corporation can have a conscience.

## A Concept of Business

Because accepting my view depends on accepting certain premises concerning the purpose of business and the nature of business, I need to describe these ideas first.

### Business as a System

At its core, business is a feedback system.[1] Capital owners, employees, and consumers are the members of the system. They coproduce its output. In the ideal, each member contributes value to the system's processes and requires in return a share of the system's output in proportion to the value of the contribution. Owners risk capital and expect to be paid fair profit. Employees supply energy, knowledge, and imagination in exchange for appropriate monetary and psychological income. Consumers supply the essential revenues out of which come wages and profits. If the system's members don't get what they expect, they reduce the quality or quantity of their contributions.

What is ofttimes not appreciated, even by the members themselves, is that the system's members are *interdependent*. Together, and *only* together, can they produce the output they subsequently share. What each member receives is constrained by what other members require, and no member can in the long run enjoy a disproportionate share.

Besides being interdependent, the members of the system are entirely equal in importance. Business people often claim primacy for capital, perceiving it as the fuel of enterprise, while consumers tend to assume that the whole point of business is to provide them with goods and services. But no member of a system can be primary. Since the contribution of every member is necessary and no contribution is sufficient, the members are equal.

### The Purpose of Business

To the owners of a company, the purpose of business is to yield them profits and appreciation of capital. To employees, its purpose is to afford them a living. Consumers see its purpose as furnishing them goods and services. But like the blind men of Indostan examining the elephant, their points of view do not account for the whole animal.

Public policy circumscribes the activities of the business system. Its rules govern the relationships among the members of the system and between the business system and the rest of society. But society could go further and replace the private, competitive business institution as we know it with a different arrangement altogether—such as socialism, communism, or any centralized and supervised economy. If we aren't convinced of that, we have only to recall Justice Holmes's chilling observation that "it would not be argued today that the power to regulate does not include the power to prohibit."

So business exists at the pleasure of society. But while society has set limits to business's operations, it has also very consciously left a great deal of room among the nation's institutions for these operations to take place. The question is, Why?

The answer tells us what the purpose of business is from society's point of view.

Our society sees potentials in private, competitive business that justify it over alternative methods for producing and distributing goods and services. Society perceives that, because the future is uncertain, the risks to which capital is exposed in production and distribution are unavoidable regardless of the political form. But we believe that the *costs* of risk will be minimized in private, competitive businesses because the persons undertaking the risk, in order to have something left over for profit, will pay more attention to costs than the state would in using someone else's money.

Our society expects that to satisfy customers, competitive enterprise will produce a greater quantity, quality, and variety of goods than a government or another monopoly would. And because profits are what is left after employees, suppliers, creditors, and governments have been paid, we assume that competitive businesses will strive to maximize the productivity of resources and conserve their use. We expect that this conserving of resources and maximizing of productivity will result in lower cost of goods and services for consumers and higher real income for workers than other political production systems would yield.

Society sees these potentials as benefiting the public at large too. Because the risks are borne by volunteers, society is spared the higher costs of collective risk taking and the indiscriminate spread of these costs to the taxpaying public.

The discipline that runs through society's justification for the business system is economy. Lionel Robbins identified the essence of economics in a definition almost all economists now accept. Economic behavior, he wrote, consists of the allocation of scarce means with alternative uses to deserving, competing ends. "The criterion of economy . . . is the securing of given ends with least means."[2]

### The Sphere of Business

Clearly, U.S. public policy did not by mere accident leave a place for private business among the nation's institutions. The decision reflects the pragmatic strategy to define a sphere in which to secure economic efficiency as a social good.

But besides thus implementing society's value that economic efficiency is good, public policy expresses society's sentiment about the value of this social good in relation to that of the many other social goods our society recognizes—equality, justice, health, and quality of life, for example. When society prefers the economic results of business to other social goods, or vice versa, public policy adjusts.

The business institution is society's principal mechanism for producing and distributing economic goods. Since public policy has assigned this realm to business to secure behavior that is uniquely economic, the purpose of business must be to deliver economic performance to society. Economic performance is both the means and the end of the business system: it is the means business uses to conduct its internal affairs, and it is the end society seeks in assigning a sphere to the business system.

Business executives do not usually describe their jobs in economic terms. Fletcher Byrom, retiring CEO of Koppers Company, Inc., does, however. "My function as leader," he said recently in an interview, "is fundamentally to make decisions on the basis of economic criteria."[3]

## Values and Leadership

I have described business as essentially an economic institution. Must it therefore operate without values? It operates according to the values of its leaders.

As citizens we are vitally interested in what the business institution does. What it does is determined by its leaders. And what leaders cause it to do is determined by their values. Deciding what values are "good" is, therefore, the first responsibility of business leadership.

The values that govern the conduct of business must be conditioned by "the why" of the business institution. They must therefore flow from the purpose of business, carry out that purpose, and be constrained by it. If that logic holds, then business leaders have the responsibility of running the businesses in their charge to realize the potential economic performance of each business.

Business leaders' values must rest also on an adequate conception of the nature of the business organism. If, as I have suggested, business can be fairly described as a system of equal, necessary, and interdependent members, then the leaders' values and their management of business operations must faithfully reflect that conception.

They don't always. Understandably, managers identify with the owners of a business and tend to give priority to the owners' profit objectives. But the concept of business as a system of equal, necessary, and interdependent members suggests that this unilateral orientation can be self-defeating. Profit is the purpose the owners have in risking their capital. It is the reward for bearing risk. And the owners' requirement for profit supplies one of the great disciplines that makes business an economic system. But profit is not the purpose of business.

Giving profits priority endangers them, for, ironically, only by giving equal regard to the requirements of all the system's members can a manager in fact maximize profits and the company's market value for the owners. If a manager rewards capital owners at the expense of employees or consumers, those members will reduce the quantity or quality of their contribution and jeopardize future returns to capital.

In a system, managers are driven by the requirements of their task to distribute to the system's members benefits that are commensurate with the members' contributions. And managers must do that even if, say, the owners whose agents they are have no interest in the rewards being distributed to consumers and workers, or if those members care nothing about whether capital owners get adequate returns for risking their capital. On the other hand, if managers do not manage business as a system, some members of the system will reduce the value of their contributions, economic performance will suffer, and society's purpose for the business institution will be compromised.

Management's values govern how the business is run. They must pervade all its operations. It is a key responsibility of business leadership, therefore, to manage these values throughout the organization so that they are effective in every action. This is the hard conclusion that follows: if in any of the business's operations managers do not realize potential economic performance, either the values of the leadership are not congruent with society's value (that economic performance is the good desired from business) or the leadership is failing to extend its own value system throughout the organization.

## The Reach of Ethics

In conversation, when people use the term *ethics*, they mean a set of moral principles or values to guide behavior. Ethical behavior is, then, behavior that conforms to these values.

But *ethics* also has a more fundamental meaning. Ethics is the discipline that considers the justifications people offer for the principles and values they hold.

I am using the term both ways. My main concern in this article is with ethics in the latter sense: to offer a justification for particular values that should govern business behavior. That justification attempts to draw a straight line from the purpose of business and its systemic nature to the values business leaders should adopt. When business behavior violates values that connect with the purpose and nature of business, I call that behavior unethical.

The ethics of a company's leadership (in the first sense) consists of the set of values the leadership holds. But among these many values, business leaders must hold those particular values that are rooted in society's purpose for business. These values are controlling, for they imply a kind of contract between business and society for managers to deliver the benefits for which society justifies the existence of the business system. These values identify economic performance as a good that society desires. And because they do, they impose requirements and set limits on leaders in their conduct of business.

Some people claim that the values of business people are on a par with the general values in American culture—no better and no worse. If that is true, it's too bad. Business leaders, it seems to me, should have more strongly held values than the rest of society because they have a fiduciary responsibility—a position of trust with employees, stockholders, and customers—in short, with society.

Many of the decisions business leaders make under their stewardship reflect a resolution of the different values they hold. Very often, then, this creates a tension between a person's values and the decision taken or contemplated. Sometimes the leader's cultural values and the controlling values society imposes that are rooted in the purpose of business reinforce each other in opposing an action. Other times they may be in opposition—in which case the controlling values have to be those rooted in business's purpose. In either case, though, the greater the pull of values, the more intense will be the leader's search for solutions—and the greater the likelihood of good decisions.

If business leaders hold strong cultural values onto which are superimposed the values rooted in the purpose of business, what guidance do they give to deal with the dilemmas that beset a company? For such leaders, ethical considerations must perforce reach more deeply into a company's internal affairs than perhaps many people realize and will also sometimes require business to do less in its external relationships than its critics ask of it. The following examples illustrate both these situations.

### Within the Company Itself

Setting annual objectives for return on investment and appraising employee performance are of course two common practices in U.S. industry. I have chosen them as examples to discuss in relation to values for three reasons—first, because they are common practices; second, because both examples illustrate the structural, and sometimes obscure, ways in which management can hamper economic performance; and third, because, having faced firsthand some of the problems in these programs, I think they can be made more effective if we take their limitations into account.

**Annual ROI objectives.** Return on investment is usually the primary annual objective for profit center managers. But many activities affecting ROI take time to complete: developing new products, redesigning products, restructuring the organization, broadening sales coverage, expanding capacity, and so forth. In the meantime, such programs penalize current earnings and may increase investment. But profit center managers are often fast-track executives being tested for advancement in short-term assignments. Given this incentive, profit center managers may forgo the very developments on which the sustained economic performance of the business depends.

This tension presents an obvious challenge to the leadership's values. Is it fair to employees to make them choose between the benefits to themselves and to their families, which would follow from a string of short-term successes, and the long-term performance of the company? But even beyond this, is it ethical for the leadership to *institutionalize* an organizational practice that compromises the economic purpose for which society justifies a place for the business system?

Clearly, we need to monitor business performance regularly and to test and measure employee performance. But the conflict of interest inherent in this method threatens long-term economic performance.

In the Phillips Petroleum subsidiary that I headed, the tension between these divergent pulls led us to look for a way to enhance long-term economic performance while still meeting the need for testing managers in short-term assignments. To counter the short-term bias, we adopted an internal audit to assess whether managers of the profit centers had strengthened the fundamentals of the business over the year. Stronger fundamentals, of course, increase the potential for future satisfactory return on investment.

We based the audit on the assumption that the fundamentals of a business unit would be strengthened if certain conditions were met: if the workplace climate improved; if the quality of production machinery approached state-of-the-art; if structure and staffing were strengthened; and so on up to a dozen or so criteria. In this way, we tried to introduce a long-term component into short-term assignments and to convey to profit center managers the necessity for increasing the ability of the business unit to produce future return on investment.

**Performance appraisals and MBO.** An employee contracts with his supervisor to achieve certain objectives; at the end of a period the supervisor compares the results with the objectives and rates and counsels the employee. Performance appraisals and management by objectives are thus inextricably bound together.

When introduced, MBO looked promising. It seemed to meet two clear organizational needs: to move the company toward its business objectives and to evaluate employees' performance fairly and objectively for salary administration. My observations have persuaded me that MBO meets neither need as well as it might. I have struggled to understand why such a simple commonsense notion hasn't fulfilled its great promise and offer these thoughts.[4]

First, as it has evolved, management by objectives has embraced the wrong purpose. When Peter Drucker presented us with this concept 30 years ago, the objectives he referred to were the objectives of the *business*. The objectives in current MBO programs, however, are the objectives managers and employees agree on as the basis for appraising employee performance. Personnel administrators have captured the concept for their own good purposes and made MBO an adjunct to salary administration.

The employee's objectives are either identical with the business's objectives or not. If they are not, an MBO program is not the instrument to move the company toward its objectives and management will have to provide a different instrument for that purpose.

On the other hand, if the objectives assigned to the employee are the business's objectives, MBO programs as currently designed won't accomplish them either. No employee working alone can attain any significant business objective. Reaching a business objective requires the contribution of several cooperating functions. Take a quality control manager. In a typical MBO program, one of his objectives might be to achieve a certain level of rejects or of returns and allowances for the manufacturing unit. He cannot do this by himself. The training and the performance of operators, the design of the product, the condition of the tools and machinery, and factors other functions control come into play.

The false premise that an employee can by himself achieve a company objective has two unsatisfactory consequences. It may result in an employee being rated as having successfully achieved an objective when it would have been impossible without the effective contribution of the other necessary functions. Or the employee may be rated as not meeting the objective when the necessary contributions of others were lacking through no fault of his own. But even more important, the company's objective is not reached and economic performance suffers.

Ethical considerations enter the situation this way. If MBO programs as now practiced cannot properly appraise employee performance, do not advance the company toward its objectives, and thus cause economic performance to suffer, then a business leader's accepting such programs violates both the fairness principle in his set of values and the values rooted in society's purpose for the business institution.

In this case, the leader's cultural values reinforce and are reinforced by the controlling values rooted in business's purpose to create a tension between what is being done and what can possibly be done better. And this tension can motivate managers to seek a way to appraise performance more fairly and at the same time to accomplish the company's objectives.

A way becomes evident as soon as we acknowledge the distinction between the objectives of the business (or business unit) and the contributions employees make toward these objectives. If achieving a business objective requires the functional contributions of several employees, the manager has a fundamental responsibility to identify the functional contributions needed for a given objective and to organize into a team the particular employees who will make those contributions.

That step taken, it becomes possible for managers to appraise what employees are actually doing—and can realistically do. Performance appraisal then becomes a judgment of the employees' effectiveness in making their contributions to the various teams they are members of and, through these teams, of their effectiveness in contributing to the objectives of the business.

Managers face many other seemingly intractable problems. For example, providing for succession to leadership is clearly a condition for the survival of a business, but it is rarely possible without making challenging assignments available to younger executives when older ones are better qualified. Public policy, of course, makes such discrimination unlawful. Managers, trying to make the best of what they regard as impossible situations, may consciously or unconsciously rate the older employees' performance lower and classify them as unpromotable. Discrimination still occurs, but documentation now lets the company do as it needs to without challenge from the EEOC.

Perhaps, though, if the problem is viewed as an ethical issue rather than as a dilemma between a legal solution and an expedient one, a more creative solution might emerge. A leadership determined to hold to its values might even find a way to use the better qualified older employees to help the younger ones.

If viewed from the perspective of values, other problems might yield better solutions: Do we tell the employees of newly acquired companies that there will be no changes? Is there a net justification for "golden parachutes" for top executives when the company is threatened by unfriendly takeovers, or are these executives simply feathering their own nests? When we cut back employment or shut down facilities in a faltering economy, are we just doing what has to be done, or are we correcting mistakes we made earlier? Most business problems seldom have easy answers. What should be sought in such situations is solutions that resist the compromise of leadership values. The resulting tension offers a challenge to creativity and imagination that can produce superior solutions.

### Beyond the Company

Besides having ethical considerations that reach deep into everyday operations, business has critics who require that it take broad social action. Let's see how leadership's values might influence decisions in two cases.

**Conflicting demands on business.** How might management's values prevent the following problem?

"This year's annual stockholders' meeting of Midton [not its real name], one of the largest companies producing baked goods, has just ended with a dramatic confrontation. A group of stockholders, the Whole Life Sisters of Faith, holding 30 of Midton's 66 million shares of common stock, has formally submitted a request to the Midton board that the company establish a corporate policy drastically restricting advertising to children."[5]

Midton's business generated by advertising directly to children has been very profitable. The advertising is not illegal, and the sisters cannot make the company do anything because they cannot possibly get a majority of the stockholders to support their proposal.

Here, rather than considering what Midton's management should do now, let's go back to the strategic planning that resulted in Midton's predicament and ask how, if it had appealed to strongly held values, the leadership might have avoided the dilemma and at the same time added to the economic performance of the business.

Executives in the strategy meeting would probably all have agreed that advertising to children would be effective in increasing sales and profits. They would also undoubtedly have recognized that this strategy would work by making it difficult for parents to deny gratification to their children. Valuing fairness, Midton's leadership might have looked for another course.

But at a more sophisticated level, the strategy they chose rested on an inad-

equate concept of the nature of business. In the business system it isn't possible
to reward one group at the expense of another without diminishing the economic
performance of the whole. In this case, the Whole Life Sisters, acting as surrogates of the company's customers, have caused the company to expend resources to deal with them and then more resources to devise a new strategy to
accommodate the changed situation. Later on, the company might also lose
customers and revenues if parents, sensitized by the sisters to what the company
has done, resolve to patronize other bakers.

Had Midton's leaders felt a tension between its business values and the strategy
it was contemplating, they might have conceived a better strategy. Of course I
am not qualified to say what that strategy might have been. Midton might have
allocated resources to advertising frankly to parents that Midton's products taste
good. Children, after all, do not live by bread alone either. And Midton might
have followed the lead of its successful small competitor, Sunlite Foods, and, by
applying greater resources than Sunlite, catered with new products to the na-
tionwide interest in health and nutrition.

And what of Midton's competitors who advertise directly to children? Would
they gain or lose market share against Midton's different strategy? We cannot
know. But we can be reasonably sure that they would have the Whole Life Sisters
of Faith over there and waste resources dealing with them.

**Business's responsibility to the public.** How should business respond
to some of the concerns and demands of its critics?

Business is asked to cure many of society's ills. Its critics ask it in the cause of
social action, for example, to hire less qualified persons when better qualified
workers are available, to provide workers with psychological income from their
work, to desist from doing business in apartheid South Africa, to internalize the
costs of doing business, and so forth.

When, for example, its critics demand that business internalize the costs of
damaging the environment, their reasoning seems only straightforward and just:
business laid the costs on the public; business ought to pay.

But the issue is not as straightforward as it first seems. Society's purpose for
the business system and its public policy implementing this purpose have to be
taken into account. Public policy determines whether in a given case the environment needs protection beyond the present standards. If it does, public policy
also determines the form the protection will take. Whatever public policy requires
of business, business, of course, must do: reduce pollutants to meet the new
standards, repair the damage afterwards, or pay higher taxes to compensate for
the damage done.

But if business is already conforming to the requirements of public policy,
one can infer that, for that case and for the time being at least, society prefers
the social good of economic performance from business to the social good of
reduced pollution and accepts the existing degree of pollution. If the business
system nevertheless voluntarily internalizes the cost, it is depriving its members
of value and altruistically conferring that value on a public that isn't directly a
part of the system. If society wants economic performance from business in a
sphere it has defined by public policy, such a gift from management thwarts
society's strategy.

One can hardly discuss what managers should and should not do without
thinking of Milton Friedman's arguments. Friedman categorically disqualifies

managers' taking social action on two grounds: first, in complex situations, business managers will probably not know the correct action to take to achieve the "desired" result and, second, by taking social action, managers would be acting as unauthorized civil servants. Because evidence all around us demonstrates that not even the specialists know what actions produce what effects, agreeing with the first reason is easy enough. But because in a sense all citizens are public servants, the second reason is not so easy to accept. It is arguable that, in allowing and even nurturing the business institution, society commissions leaders to achieve its purpose.

Friedman was right to disqualify managers from social action but not, I think, for the right reason. The right reason is simply that social action falls outside the economic sphere that society's public policy has assigned to the business system.

What we managers do, then, when confronted by demands for social action beyond the requirements of public policy is at root an ethical matter for us. If in order to escape visibility managers yield to the pressures of social action interest groups and stray from the system's mission to deliver economic performance, they circumvent society's value that economic performance is good and desired in the given sphere.

There is, nevertheless, a very important counterpoise to these strictures on the behavior of business leaders. Executives must not only lead their businesses; they must accept the responsibility of leading the business institution. The economic results that society seeks from the business system require maximum benefits from minimum consumption of resources. But the operation of the business system unavoidably imposes costs on society that add to the resources consumed and subtract from other social goods. Society, of course, is concerned with the overall good. By adjusting public policy, society continually strives to optimize the balance between the net economic goods the business system delivers and the other social goods it desires.

Business leaders must be concerned about whatever concerns society. And while they should not, in my view, make de facto public policy by unilaterally altering boundaries that public policy has set between economic and other social goods, their responsibility as leaders requires them to join with other social leaders in a dialogue to make public policy affecting business more reflective of the needs and desires of American society.

## Can the Corporation Have a Conscience?

Many students of business have asked whether the corporation can have a conscience and whether it can be made moral, and they usually offer affirmative answers.[6] Society surely has the right to expect moral behavior from business. But the underlying question remains: What is right conduct for the business corporation? We are back to Undershaft's problem. I do not think that the consciences of either business executives or business's critics are dependable guides. The reasoning to support this opinion applies to both parts of the question, since conscience and moral behavior are opposite sides of the same coin.

Moral behavior is behavior conforming to a standard of what is right and good. Conscience is the sense a person has of the moral goodness or blameworthiness of his or her own behavior, together with a feeling of obligation to do right and be good. We want our corporations to do right, but the question whether a corporation can have a conscience seems an empty one to secure that objective for three reasons.

First, a corporation is a construct of the mind and the law; it is a juristic, not a real, person. Society has to look to the corporation's leaders for whatever behavior it wants from the corporation.

Second, asking the wrong question diverts society's attention from its real concern—that is, what business leaders should cause their corporations to do in particular cases and why. Advocates of the idea of corporate conscience generally argue that the responsibilities of real persons and of artificial persons like corporations are not separate; they hold that corporations and real persons should be equally morally responsible, hence that they should do the same right thing. What real persons do depends on their values. But when the real persons are also leaders of a business corporation, the values that must be controlling for them are the values that connect with the purpose for which society justifies a place for private business among its institutions. Private persons do not have this obligation.

And third, conscience, without a justification acceptable to society for the "right conduct" that conscience would enjoin, is too variable, open-ended, and undisciplined for society to depend on. Just as in other people, the conscience of business people can vary from zero to the other extreme where it can also defeat society's aims. So it is the *justification* for right conduct by business leaders that should be the object of scholars' attention rather than conscience, which varies from person to person.

### The Means Are the Ends

What I have attempted to do in this essay is to suggest a justification for a kind of business leadership that is rooted in the purpose of business. American society has purposefully left a place for business among its institutions to secure economic performance in the production and distribution of goods and services. It follows, for me, that business leaders have the responsibility to try to deliver the benefits society seeks through this strategy. The values that govern our leadership must therefore be grounded in this purpose, must implement it, and must be constrained by it.

Society's choice of this strategy expresses the value that in a circumscribed sphere economic efficiency is good. But society always has this strategy on trial; it continually compares it with alternative strategies for securing economic good and monitors it for negative effects that business's economic behavior might have on other social goods it values. The signs are that society is nowhere near satisfied with business performance, governance, leadership, or values. Our society's perception of business seems to parallel Winston Churchill's description of democracy: as "the worst system in the world, excepting all others."

Fortunately, business is not a static institution: it evolves and develops. Public policy governing its operations sometimes fails to translate society's desires and doesn't always reflect the public interest. But, surely, if business leaders and the critics of business behavior agree on the purpose of business and on the values that are rooted in that purpose, by listening to one another, they ought to be able to make business a better instrument for achieving its purpose.

*NOTES*

1. See C. West Churchman, *The Design of Inquiring Systems* (New York: Basic Books, 1971). He identifies nine conditions something has to meet to be considered a system.
2. Lionel Robbins, *An Essay on the Nature and Significance of Economic Science* (London: Macmillan, 1947), p. 145.
3. See "Manager's Journal," *Wall Street Journal*, June 1, 1982.
4. See my article, "Management of Objectives," HBR May–June 1976, p. 149.
5. See Douglas N. Dickson, "Sugar Babies and the Sisterhood — A Business Case Study," *Across the Board*, January 1982, p. 41; and "Sugar Babies Revisited," *Across the Board*, June 1982, p. 36.
6. See Kenneth E. Goodpaster and John B. Matthews, Jr., "Can a Corporation Have a Conscience?" HBR January–February 1982, p. 132.

# 6

# Can a Corporation Have a Conscience?

### KENNETH E. GOODPASTER
### AND JOHN B. MATTHEWS, JR.

During the severe racial tensions of the 1960s, Southern Steel Company (actual case, disguised name) faced considerable pressure from government and the press to explain and modify its policies regarding discrimination both within its plants and in the major city where it was located. SSC was the largest employer in the area (it had nearly 15,000 workers, one-third of whom were black) and had made great strides toward removing barriers to equal job opportunity in its several plants. In addition, its top executives (especially its chief executive officer, James Weston) had distinguished themselves as private citizens for years in community programs for black housing, education, and small business as well as in attempts at desegregating all-white police and local government organizations.

SSC drew the line, however, at using its substantial economic influence in the local area to advance the cause of the civil rights movement by pressuring banks, suppliers, and the local government.

"As individuals we can exercise what influence we may have as citizens," James Weston said, "but for a corporation to attempt to exert any kind of economic compulsion to achieve a particular end in a social area seems to me to be quite beyond what a corporation should do and quite beyond what a corporation can do. I believe that while government may seek to compel social reforms, any attempt by a private organization like SSC to impose its views, its beliefs, and its will upon the community would be repugnant to our American constitutional concepts and that appropriate steps to correct this abuse of corporate power would be universally demanded by public opinion."

Weston could have been speaking in the early 1980s on any issue that corporations around the United States now face. Instead of social justice, his theme might be environmental protection, product safety, marketing practice, or international bribery. His statement for SSC raises the important issue of corporate responsibility. Can a corporation have a conscience?

Weston apparently felt comfortable saying it need not. The responsibilities of ordinary persons and of "artificial persons" like corporations are, in his view, separate. Persons' responsibilities go beyond those of corporations. Persons, he seems to have believed, ought to care not only about themselves but also about the dignity and well-being of those around them—ought not only to care but also to act. Organizations, he evidently thought, are creatures of, and to a degree prisoners of, the systems of economic incentive and political sanction that give them reality and therefore should not be expected to display the same moral attributes that we expect of persons.

Others inside business as well as outside share Weston's perception. One influential philosopher—John Ladd—carries Weston's view a step further:

> It is improper to expect organizational conduct to conform to the ordinary principles of morality. We cannot and must not expect formal organizations, or their representatives acting in their official capacities, to be honest, courageous, considerate, sympathetic, or to have any kind of moral integrity. Such concepts are not in the vocabulary, so to speak, of the organizational language game.[1]

In our opinion, this line of thought represents a tremendous barrier to the development of business ethics both as a field of inquiry and as a practical force in managerial decision making. This is a matter about which executives must be philosophical and philosophers must be practical. A corporation can and should have a conscience. The language of ethics does have a place in the vocabulary of an organization. There need not be and there should not be a disjunction of the sort attributed to SSC's James Weston. Organizational agents such as corporations should be no more and no less morally responsible (rational, self-interested, altruistic) than ordinary persons.

We take this position because we think an analogy holds between the individual and the corporation. If we analyze the concept of moral responsibility as it applies to persons, we find that projecting it to corporations as agents in society is possible.

## Defining the Responsibility of Persons

When we speak of the responsibility of individuals, philosophers say that we mean three things: someone is to blame, something has to be done, or some kind of trustworthiness can be expected. (See the *Exhibit*.)

### Holding Accountable

We apply the first meaning, what we shall call the *causal* sense, primarily to legal and moral contexts where what is at issue is praise or blame for a past action. We say of a person that he or she was responsible for what happened, is to blame for it, should be held accountable. In this sense of the word, *responsibility* has to do with tracing the causes of actions and events, of finding out who is answerable in a given situation. Our aim is to determine someone's intention, free will, degree of participation, and appropriate reward or punishment.

### Rule Following

We apply the second meaning of *responsibility* to rule following, to contexts where individuals are subject to externally imposed norms often associated with some social role that people play. We speak of the responsibilities of parents to children, of doctors to patients, of lawyers to clients, of citizens to the law. What is socially expected and what the party involved is to answer for are at issue here.

### Decision Making

We use the third meaning of *responsibility* for decision making. With this meaning of the term, we say that individuals are responsible if they are trustworthy and reliable, if they allow appropriate factors to affect their judgment; we refer primarily to a person's independent thought processes and decision making, processes that justify an attitude of trust from those who interact with him or her as a responsible individual.

The distinguishing characteristic of moral responsibility, it seems to us, lies in this third sense of the term. Here the focus is on the intellectual and emotional processes in the individual's moral reasoning. Philosophers call this "taking a moral point of view" and contrast it with such other processes as being financially prudent and attending to legal obligations.

To be sure, characterizing a person as "morally responsible" may seem rather vague. But vagueness is a contextual notion. Everything depends on how we fill in the blank in "vague for_____ purposes."

In some contexts the term "six o'clockish" is vague, while in others it is useful and informative. As a response to a space-shuttle pilot who wants to know when to fire the reentry rockets, it will not do, but it might do in response to a spouse who wants to know when one will arrive home at the end of the workday.

We maintain that the processes underlying moral responsibility can be defined and are not themselves vague, even though gaining consensus on specific moral norms and decisions is not always easy.

What, then, characterizes the processes underlying the judgment of a person we call morally responsible? Philosopher William K. Frankena offers the following answer:

A morality is a normative system in which judgments are made, more or less consciously, [out of a] consideration of the effects of actions . . . on the lives of persons . . . including the lives of others besides the person acting. . . . David Hume took a similar position when he argued that what speaks in a moral judgment is a kind of sympathy. . . . A little later, . . . Kant put the matter somewhat better by characterizing morality as the business of respecting persons as ends and not as means or as things. . . .[2]

Frankena is pointing to two traits, both rooted in a long and diverse philosophical tradition:

1. Rationality. Taking a moral point of view includes the features we

usually attribute to rational decision making, that is, lack of impulsiveness, care in mapping out alternatives and consequences, clarity about goals and purposes, attention to details of implementation.

2. Respect. The moral point of view also includes a special awareness of and concern for the effects of one's decisions and policies on others, special in the sense that it goes beyond the kind of awareness and concern that would ordinarily be part of rationality, that is, beyond seeing others merely as instrumental to accomplishing one's own purposes. This is respect for the lives of others and involves taking their needs and interests seriously, not simply as resources in one's own decision making but as limiting conditions which change the very definition of one's habitat from a self-centered to a shared environment. It is what philosopher Immanuel Kant meant by the "categorical imperative" to treat others as valuable in and for themselves.

It is this feature that permits us to trust the morally responsible person. We know that such a person takes our point of view into account not merely as a useful precaution (as in "honesty is the best policy") but as important in its own right.

These components of moral responsibility are not too vague to be useful. Rationality and respect affect the manner in which a person approaches practical decision making: they affect the way in which the individual processes information and makes choices. A rational but not respectful Bill Jones will not lie to his friends *unless* he is reasonably sure he will not be found out. A rational but not respectful Mary Smith will defend an unjustly treated party *unless* she thinks it may be too costly to herself. A rational *and* respectful decision maker, however, notices — and cares — whether the consequences of his or her conduct lead to injuries or indignities to others.

Two individuals who take "the moral point of view" will not of course always agree on ethical matters, but they do at least have a basis for dialogue.

## Projecting Responsibility to Corporations

Now that we have removed some of the vagueness from the notion of moral responsibility as it applies to persons, we can search for a frame of reference in which, by analogy with Bill Jones and Mary Smith, we can meaningfully and appropriately say that corporations are morally responsible. This is the issue reflected in the SSC case.

To deal with it, we must ask two questions: Is it meaningful to apply moral concepts to actors who are not persons but who are instead made up of persons? And even if meaningful, is it advisable to do so?

If a group can act like a person in some ways, then we can expect it to behave like a person in other ways. For one thing, we know that people organized into a group can act as a unit. As business people well know, legally a corporation is considered a unit. To approach unity, a group usually has some sort of internal decision structure, a system of rules that spell out authority relationships and specify the conditions under which certain individuals' actions become official actions of the group.[3]

If we can say that persons act responsibly only if they gather information about the impact of their actions on others and use it in making decisions, we can reasonably do the same for organizations. Our proposed frame of reference for thinking about and implementing corporate responsibility aims at spelling out the processes associated with the moral responsibility of individuals and projecting them to the level of organizations. This is similar to, though an inversion of, Plato's famous method in the *Republic*, in which justice in the community is used as a model for justice in the individual.

Hence, corporations that monitor their employment practices and the effects of their production processes and products on the environment and human health show the same kind of rationality and respect that morally responsible individuals do. Thus, attributing actions, strategies, decisions, and moral responsibilities to corporations as entities distinguishable from those who hold offices in them poses no problem.

And when we look about us, we can readily see differences in moral responsibility among corporations in much the same way that we see differences among persons. Some corporations have built features into their management incentive systems, board structures, internal control systems, and research agendas that in a person we would call self-control, integrity, and conscientiousness. Some have institutionalized awareness and concern for consumers, employees, and the rest of the public in ways that others clearly have not.

As a matter of course, some corporations attend to the human impact of their operations and policies and reject operations and policies that are questionable. Whether the issue be the health effects of sugared cereal or cigarettes, the safety of tires or tampons, civil liberties in the corporation or the community, an organization reveals its character as surely as a person does.

Indeed, the parallel may be even more dramatic. For just as the moral responsibility displayed by an individual develops over time from infancy to adulthood,[4] so too we may expect to find stages of development in organizational character that show significant patterns.

## Evaluating the Idea of Moral Projection

Concepts like moral responsibility not only make sense when applied to organizations but also provide touchstones for designing more effective models than we now have for guiding corporate policy.

Now we can understand what it means to invite SSC as a corporation to be morally responsible both in-house and in its community, but *should* we issue the invitation? Here we turn to the question of advisability. Should we require the organizational agents in our society to have the same moral attributes we require of ourselves?

Our proposal to spell out the processes associated with moral responsibility for individuals and then to project them to their organizational counterparts takes on added meaning when we examine alternative frames of reference for corporate responsibility.

Two frames of reference that compete for the allegiance of people who ponder the question of corporate responsibility are emphatically opposed to this principle of moral projection — what we might refer to as the "invisible hand" view and the "hand of government" view.

### The Invisible Hand

The most eloquent spokesman of the first view is Milton Friedman (echoing many philosophers and economists since Adam Smith). According to this pattern of thought, the true and only social responsibilities of business

organizations are to make profits and obey the laws. The workings of the free
and competitive marketplace will "moralize" corporate behavior quite independently of any attempts to expand or transform decision making via moral projection.

A deliberate amorality in the executive suite is encouraged in the name of
systemic morality: the common good is best served when each of us and our
economic institutions pursue not the common good or moral purpose, advocates
say, but competitive advantage. Morality, responsibility, and conscience reside
in the invisible hand of the free market system, not in the hands of the organizations within the system, much less the managers within the organizations.

To be sure, people of this opinion admit, there is a sense in which social or
ethical issues can and should enter the corporate mind, but the filtering of such
issues is thorough: they go through the screens of custom, public opinion, public
relations, and the law. And, in any case, self-interest maintains primacy as an
objective and a guiding star.

The reaction from this frame of reference to the suggestion that moral judgment be integrated with corporate strategy is clearly negative. Such an integration
is seen as inefficient and arrogant, and in the end both an illegitimate use of
corporate power and an abuse of the manager's fiduciary role. With respect to
our SSC case, advocates of the invisible hand model would vigorously resist
efforts, beyond legal requirements, to make SSC right the wrongs of racial
injustice. SSC's responsibility would be to make steel of high quality at least cost,
to deliver it on time, and to satisfy its customers and stockholders. Justice would
not be part of SSC's corporate mandate.

### The Hand of Government

Advocates of the second dissenting frame of reference abound, but
John Kenneth Galbraith's work has counterpointed Milton Friedman's with insight and style. Under this view of corporate responsibility, corporations are to
pursue objectives that are rational and purely economic. The regulatory hands
of the law and the political process rather than the invisible hand of the marketplace turns these objectives to the common good.

Again, in this view, it is a system that provides the moral direction for corporate
decision making—a system, though, that is guided by political managers, the
custodians of the public purpose. In the case of SSC, proponents of this view
would look to the state for moral direction and responsible management, both
within SSC and in the community. The corporation would have no moral responsibility beyond political and legal obedience.

What is striking is not so much the radical difference between the economic
and social philosophies that underlie these two views of the source of corporate
responsibility but the conceptual similarities. Both views locate morality, ethics,
responsibility, and conscience in the systems of rules and incentives in which the
modern corporation finds itself embedded. Both views reject the exercise of
independent moral judgment by corporations as actors in society.

Neither view trusts corporate leaders with stewardship over what are often
called noneconomic values. Both require corporate responsibility to march to
the beat of drums outside. In the jargon of moral philosophy, both views press
for a rule-centered or a system-centered ethics instead of an agent-centered
ethics. In terms of the *Exhibit*, these frames of reference countenance corporate

rule-following responsibility for corporations but not corporate decision-making responsibility.

### The Hand of Management

To be sure, the two views under discussion differ in that one looks to an invisible moral force in the market while the other looks to a visible moral force in government. But both would advise against a principle of moral projection that permits or encourages corporations to exercise independent, non-economic judgment over matters that face them in their short- and long-term plans and operations.

Accordingly, both would reject a third view of corporate responsibility that seeks to affect the thought processes of the organization itself — a sort of "hand of management" view — since neither seems willing or able to see the engines of profit regulate themselves to the degree that would be implied by taking the principle of moral projection seriously. Cries of inefficiency and moral imperialism from the right would be matched by cries of insensitivity and illegitimacy from the left, all in the name of preserving us from corporations and managers run morally amok.

Better, critics would say, that moral philosophy be left to philosophers, philanthropists, and politicians than to business leaders. Better that corporate morality be kept to glossy annual reports, where it is safely insulated from policy and performance.

The two conventional frames of reference locate moral restraint in forces external to the person and the corporation. They deny moral reasoning and intent to the corporation in the name of either market competition or society's system of explicit legal constraints and presume that these have a better moral effect than that of rationality and respect.

Although the principle of moral projection, which underwrites the idea of a corporate conscience and patterns it on the thought and feeling processes of the person, is in our view compelling, we must acknowledge that it is neither part of the received wisdom, nor is its advisability beyond question or objection. Indeed, attributing the role of conscience to the corporation seems to carry with it new and disturbing implications for our usual ways of thinking about ethics and business.

Perhaps the best way to clarify and defend this frame of reference is to address the objections to the principle found in the ruled insert here. There we see a summary of the criticisms and counterarguments we have heard during hours

---

## Exhibit  Three Uses of the Term *Responsible*

| | |
|---|---|
| *The causal sense* | "He is responsible for this." Emphasis on holding to account for past actions, causality. |
| *The rule-following sense* | "As a lawyer, he is responsible for defending that client." Emphasis on following social and legal norms. |
| *The decision-making sense* | "He is a responsible person." Emphasis on an individual's independent judgment. |

of discussion with business executives and business school students. We believe
that the replies to the objections about a corporation having a conscience are
convincing.

## Leaving the Double Standard Behind

We have come some distance from our opening reflection on Southern
Steel Company and its role in its community. Our proposal—clarified, we hope,
through these objections and replies—suggests that it is not sufficient to draw
a sharp line between individuals' private ideas and efforts and a corporation's
institutional efforts but that the latter can and should be built upon the former.

Does this frame of reference give us an unequivocal prescription for the
behavior of SSC in its circumstances? No, it does not. Persuasive arguments
might be made now and might have been made then that SSC should not have
used its considerable economic clout to threaten the community into desegregation. A careful analysis of the realities of the environment might have disclosed
that such a course would have been counterproductive, leading to more injustice
than it would have alleviated.

The point is that some of the arguments and some of the analyses are or
would have been moral arguments, and thereby the ultimate decision that of an
ethically responsible organization. The significance of this point can hardly be
overstated, for it represents the adoption of a new perspective on corporate
policy and a new way of thinking about business ethics. We agree with one
authority, who writes that "the business firm, as an organic entity intricately
affected by and affecting its environment, is as appropriately adaptive . . . to
demands for responsible behavior as for economic service."[5]

The frame of reference here developed does not offer a decision procedure
for corporate managers. That has not been our purpose. It does, however, shed
light on the conceptual foundations of business ethics by training attention on
the corporation as a moral agent in society. Legal systems of rules and incentives
are insufficient, even though they may be necessary, as frameworks for corporate
responsibility. Taking conceptual cues from the features of moral responsibility
normally expected of the person in our opinion deserves practicing managers'
serious consideration.

The lack of congruence that James Weston saw between individual and corporate moral responsibility can be, and we think should be, overcome. In the
process, what a number of writers have characterized as a double standard—a
discrepancy between our personal lives and our lives in organizational settings
—might be dampened. The principle of moral projection not only helps us to
conceptualize the kinds of demands that we might make of corporations and
other organizations but also offers the prospect of harmonizing those demands
with the demands that we make of ourselves.

---

*Is a Corporation a Morally Responsible "Person"?*
**Objection 1 to the analogy:**

Corporations are not persons. They are artificial legal constructions,
machines for mobilizing economic investments toward the efficient production
of goods and services. We cannot hold a corporation responsible. We can only
hold individuals responsible.

**Reply:**

Our frame of reference does not imply that corporations are persons in a literal sense. It simply means that in certain respects concepts and functions normally attributed to persons can also be attributed to organizations made up of persons. Goals, economic values, strategies, and other such personal attributes are often usefully projected to the corporate level by managers and researchers. Why should we not project the functions of conscience in the same way? As for holding corporations responsible, recent criminal prosecutions such as the case of Ford Motor Company and its Pinto gas tanks suggest that society finds the idea both intelligible and useful.

**Objection 2:**

A corporation cannot be held responsible at the sacrifice of profit. Profitability and financial health have always been and should continue to be the "categorical imperatives" of a business operation.

**Reply:**

We must of course acknowledge the imperatives of survival, stability, and growth when we discuss corporations, as indeed we must acknowledge them when we discuss the life of an individual. Self-sacrifice has been identified with moral responsibility in only the most extreme cases. The pursuit of profit and self-interest need not be pitted against the demands of moral responsibility. Moral demands are best viewed as containments—not replacements—for self-interest.

This is not to say that profit maximization never conflicts with morality. But profit maximization conflicts with other managerial values as well. The point is to coordinate imperatives, not deny their validity.

**Objection 3:**

Corporate executives are not elected representatives of the people, nor are they anointed or appointed as social guardians. They therefore lack the social mandate that a democratic society rightly demands of those who would pursue ethically or socially motivated policies. By keeping corporate policies confined to economic motivations, we keep the power of corporate executives in its proper place.

**Reply:**

The objection betrays an oversimplified view of the relationship between the public and the private sector. Neither private individuals nor private corporations that guide their conduct by ethical or social values beyond the demands of law should be constrained merely because they are not elected to do so. The demands of moral responsibility are independent of the demands of political legitimacy and are in fact presupposed by them.

To be sure, the state and the political process will and must remain the primary mechanisms for protecting the public interest, but one might be forgiven the hope that the political process will not substitute for the moral judgment of the citizenry or other components of society such as corporations.

**Objection 4:**

Our system of law carefully defines the role of agent or fiduciary and makes corporate managers accountable to shareholders and investors for the use of their assets. Management cannot, in the name of corporate moral responsibility, arrogate to itself the right to manage those assets by partially non-economic criteria.

**Reply:**

First, it is not so clear that investors insist on purely economic criteria in the management of their assets, especially if some of the shareholders' resolutions and board reforms of the last decade are any indication. For instance, companies doing business in South Africa have had stockholders question their activities, other companies have instituted audit committees for their boards before such auditing was mandated, and mutual funds for which "socially responsible behavior" is a major investment criterion now exist.

Second, the categories of "shareholder" and "investor" connote wider time spans than do immediate or short-term returns. As a practical matter, considerations of stability and long-term return on investment enlarge the class of principals to which managers bear a fiduciary relationship.

Third, the trust that managers hold does not and never has extended to "any means available" to advance the interests of the principals. Both legal and moral constraints must be understood to qualify that trust—even, perhaps, in the name of a larger trust and a more basic fiduciary relationship to the members of society at large.

**Objection 5:**

The power, size, and scale of the modern corporation—domestic as well as international—are awesome. To unleash, even partially, such power from the discipline of the marketplace and the narrow or possibly nonexistent moral purpose implicit in that discipline would be socially dangerous. Had SSC acted in the community to further racial justice, its purposes might have been admirable, but those purposes could have led to a kind of moral imperialism or worse. Suppose SSC had thrown its power behind the Ku Klux Klan.

**Reply:**

This is a very real and important objection. What seems not to be appreciated is the fact that power affects when it is used as well as when it is not used. A decision by SSC not to exercise its economic influence according to "noneconomic" criteria is inevitably a moral decision and just as inevitably affects the community. The issue in the end is not whether corporations (and other organizations) should be "unleashed" to exert moral force in our society but rather how critically and self-consciously they should choose to do so.

The degree of influence enjoyed by an agent, whether a person or an organization, is not so much a factor recommending moral disengagement as a factor demanding a high level of moral awareness. Imperialism is more to be feared when moral reasoning is absent than when it is present. Nor do we suggest that the "discipline of the marketplace" be diluted; rather, we call for it to be supplemented with the discipline of moral reflection.

**Objection 6:**

The idea of moral projection is a useful device for structuring corporate responsibility only if our understanding of moral responsibility at the level of the person is in some sense richer than our understanding of moral responsibility on the level of the organization as a whole. If we are not clear about individual responsibility, the projection is fruitless.

**Reply:**

The objection is well taken. The challenge offered by the idea of moral projection lies in our capacity to articulate criteria or frameworks of reasoning for the morally responsible person. And though such a challenge is formidable, it is not clear that it cannot be met, at least with sufficient consensus to be useful.

For centuries, the study and criticism of frameworks have gone on, carried forward by many disciplines, including psychology, the social sciences, and philosophy. And though it would be a mistake to suggest that any single framework (much less a decision mechanism) has emerged as the right one, it is true that recurrent patterns are discernible and well enough defined to structure moral discussion.

In the body of the article, we spoke of rationality and respect as components of individual responsibility. Further analysis of these components would translate them into social costs and benefits, justice in the distribution of goods and services, basic rights and duties, and fidelity to contracts. The view that pluralism in our society has undercut all possibility of moral agreement is anything but self-evident. Sincere moral disagreement is, of course, inevitable and not clearly lamentable. But a process and a vocabulary for articulating such values as we share is no small step forward when compared with the alternatives. Perhaps in our exploration of the moral projection we might make some surprising and even reassuring discoveries about ourselves.

**Objection 7:**

Why is it necessary to project moral responsibility to the level of the organization? Isn't the task of defining corporate responsibility and business ethics sufficiently discharged if we clarify the responsibilities of men and women in business as individuals? Doesn't ethics finally rest on the honesty and integrity of the individual in the business world?

**Reply:**

Yes and no. Yes, in the sense that the control of large organizations does finally rest in the hands of managers, of men and women. No, in the sense that what is being controlled is a cooperative system for a cooperative purpose. The projection of responsibility to the organization is simply an acknowledgement of the fact that the whole is more than the sum of its parts. Many intelligent people do not an intelligent organization make. Intelligence needs to be structured, organized, divided, and recombined in complex processes for complex purposes.

Studies of management have long shown that the attributes, successes, and failures of organizations are phenomena that emerge from the coordination of persons' attributes and that explanations of such phenomena require categories of analysis and description beyond the level of the individual. Moral responsibility is an attribute that can manifest itself in organizations as surely as competence or efficiency.

**Objection 8:**

Is the frame of reference here proposed intended to replace or undercut the relevance of the "invisible hand" and the "government hand" views, which depend on external controls?

**Reply:**

No. Just as regulation and economic competition are not substitutes for corporate responsibility, so corporate responsibility is not a substitute for law and the market. The imperatives of ethics cannot be relied on — nor have they ever been relied on — without a context of external sanctions. And this is true as much for individuals as for organizations.

This frame of reference takes us beneath, but not beyond, the realm of external systems of rules and incentives and into the thought processes that interpret and respond to the corporation's environment. Morality is more than merely part of that environment. It aims at the projection of conscience, not the enthronement of it in either the state or the competitive process.

The rise of the modern large corporation and the concomitant rise of the professional manager demand a conceptual framework in which these phenomena can be accommodated to moral thought. The principle of moral projection furthers such accommodation by recognizing a new level of agency in society and thus a new level of responsibility.

**Objection 9:**

Corporations have always taken the interests of those outside the corporation into account in the sense that customer relations and public relations generally are an integral part of rational economic decision making. Market signals and social signals that filter through the market mechanism inevitably represent the interests of parties affected by the behavior of the company. What, then, is the point of adding respect to rationality?

**Reply:**

Representing the affected parties solely as economic variables in the environment of the company is treating them as means or resources and not as ends in themselves. It implies that the only voice which affected parties should have in organizational decision making is that of potential buyers, sellers, regulators, or boycotters. Besides, many affected parties may not occupy such roles, and those who do may not be able to signal the organization with messages that effectively represent their stakes in its actions.

To be sure, classical economic theory would have us believe that perfect competition in free markets (with modest adjustments from the state) will result in all relevant signals being "heard," but the abstractions from reality implicit in such theory make it insufficient as a frame of reference for moral responsibility. In a world in which strict self-interest was congruent with the common good, moral responsibility might be unnecessary. We do not, alas, live in such a world.

The element of respect in our analysis of responsibility plays an essential role in ensuring the recognition of unrepresented or under-represented voices in the decision making of organizations as agents. Showing respect for persons as ends and not mere means to organizational purposes is central to the concept of corporate moral responsibility.

### NOTES

1. See John Ladd, "Morality and the Ideal of Rationality in Formal Organizations," *The Monist*, October 1970, p. 499.
2. See William K. Frankena, *Thinking About Morality* (Ann Arbor: University of Michigan Press, 1980), p. 26.
3. See Peter French, "The Corporation as a Moral Person," *American Philosophical Quarterly*, July 1979, p. 207.
4. A process that psychological researchers from Jean Piaget to Lawrence Kohlberg have examined carefully; see Jean Piaget, *The Moral Judgment of the Child* (New York: Free Press, 1965) and Lawrence Kohlberg, *The Philosophy of Moral Development* (New York: Harper & Row, 1981).
5. See Kenneth R. Andrews, *The Concept of Corporate Strategy*, rev. ed. (Homewood, Ill.: Dow Jones-Irwin, 1980), p. 99.

# 7

# Moral Mazes: Bureaucracy and Managerial Work

## ROBERT JACKALL

Corporate leaders often tell their charges that hard work will lead to success. Indeed, this theory of reward being commensurate with effort has been an enduring belief in our society, one central to our self-image as a people where the "main chance" is available to anyone of ability who has the gumption and the persistence to seize it. Hard work, it is also frequently asserted, builds character. This notion carries less conviction because businessmen, and our society as a whole, have little patience with those who make a habit of finishing out of the money. In the end, it is success that matters, that legitimates striving, and that makes work worthwhile.

What if, however, men and women in the big corporation no longer see success as necessarily connected to hard work? What becomes of the social morality of the corporation—I mean the everyday rules in use that people play by—when there is thought to be no "objective" standard of excellence to explain how and why winners are separated from also-rans, how and why some people succeed and others fail?

This is the puzzle that confronted me while doing a great many extensive interviews with managers and executives in several large corporations, particularly in a large chemical company and a large textile firm. (See the Appendix for more details.) I went into these corporations to study how bureaucracy—

the prevailing organizational form of our society and economy—shapes moral consciousness. I came to see that managers' rules for success are at the heart of what may be called the bureaucratic ethic.

This article suggests no changes and offers no programs for reform. It is, rather, simply an interpretive sociological analysis of the moral dimensions of managers' work. Some readers may find the essay sharp-edged, others familiar. For both groups, it is important to note at the outset that my materials are managers' own descriptions of their experiences.[1] In listening to managers, I have had the decided advantages of being unencumbered with business responsibilities and also of being free from the taken-for-granted views and vocabularies of the business world. As it happens, my own research in a variety of other settings suggests that managers' experiences are by no means unique; indeed they have a deep resonance with those of other occupational groups.

## What Happened to the Protestant Ethic?

To grasp managers' experiences and the more general implications they contain, one must see them against the background of the great historical transformations, both social and cultural, that produced managers as an occupational group. Since the concern here is with the moral significance of work in business, it is important to begin with an understanding of the original Protestant Ethic, the world view of the rising bourgeois class that spearheaded the emergence of capitalism.

The Protestant Ethic was a set of beliefs that counseled "secular asceticism" —the methodical, rational subjection of human impulse and desire to God's will through "restless, continuous, systematic work in a worldly calling."[2] This ethic of ceaseless work and ceaseless renunciation of the fruits of one's toil provided both the economic and the moral foundations for modern capitalism.

On one hand, secular asceticism was a ready-made prescription for building economic capital; on the other, it became for the upward-moving bourgeois class—self-made industrialists, farmers, and enterprising artisans—the ideology that justified their attention to this world, their accumulation of wealth, and indeed the social inequities that inevitably followed such accumulation. This bourgeois ethic, with its imperatives for self-reliance, hard work, frugality, and rational planning, and its clear definition of success and failure, came to dominate a whole historical epoch in the West.

But the ethic came under assault from two directions. First, the very accumulation of wealth that the old Protestant Ethic made possible gradually stripped away the religious basis of the ethic, especially among the rising middle class that benefited from it. There were, of course, periodic reassertions of the religious context of the ethic, as in the case of John D. Rockefeller and his turn toward Baptism. But on the whole, by the late 1800s the religious roots of the ethic survived principally among independent farmers and proprietors of small businesses in rural areas and towns across America.

In the mainstream of an emerging urban America, the ethic had become secularized into the "work ethic," "rugged individualism," and especially the "success ethic." By the beginning of this century, among most of the economically successful, frugality had become an aberration, conspicuous consumption the norm. And with the shaping of the mass consumer society later in this century, the sanctification of consumption became widespread, indeed crucial to the maintenance of the economic order.

Affluence and the emergence of the consumer society were responsible, however, for the demise of only aspects of the old ethic—namely, the imperatives for saving and investment. The core of the ethic, even in its later, secularized form—self-reliance, unremitting devotion to work, and a morality that postulated just rewards for work well done—was undermined by the complete transformation of the organizational form of work itself. The hallmarks of the emerging modern production and distribution systems were administrative hierarchies, standardized work procedures, regularized timetables, uniform policies, and centralized control—in a word, the bureaucratization of the economy.

This bureaucratization was heralded at first by a very small class of salaried managers, who were later joined by legions of clerks and still later by technicians and professionals of every stripe. In this century, the process spilled over from the private to the public sector and government bureaucracies came to rival those of industry. This great transformation produced the decline of the old middle class of entrepreneurs, free professionals, independent farmers, and small independent businessmen—the traditional carriers of the old Protestant Ethic—and the ascendance of a new middle class of salaried employees whose chief common characteristic was and is their dependence on the big organization.

Any understanding of what happened to the original Protestant Ethic and to the old morality and social character it embodied—and therefore any understanding of the moral significance of work today—is inextricably tied to an analysis of bureaucracy. More specifically, it is, in my view, tied to an analysis of the work and occupational cultures of managerial groups within bureaucracies. Managers are the quintessential bureaucratic work group; they not only fashion bureaucratic rules, but they are also bound by them. Typically, they are not just *in* the organization; they are *of* the organization. As such, managers represent the prototype of the white-collar salaried employee. By analyzing the kind of ethic bureaucracy produces in managers, one can begin to understand how bureaucracy shapes morality in our society as a whole.

## Pyramidal Politics

American businesses typically both centralize and decentralize authority. Power is concentrated at the top in the person of the chief executive officer and is simultaneously decentralized; that is, responsibility for decisions and profits is pushed as far down the organizational line as possible. For example, the chemical company that I studied—and its structure is typical of other organizations I examined—is one of several operating companies of a large and growing conglomerate. Like the other operating companies, the chemical concern has its own president, executive vice presidents, vice presidents, other executive officers, business area managers, entire staff divisions, and operating plants. Each company is, in effect, a self-sufficient organization, though they are all coordinated by the corporation, and each president reports directly to the corporate CEO.

Now, the key interlocking mechanism of this structure is its reporting system. Each manager gathers up the profit targets or other objectives of his or her subordinates, and with these formulates his commitments to his boss; this boss takes these commitments, and those of his other subordinates, and in turn makes a commitment to *his* boss. (Note: henceforth only "he" or "his" will be used to allow for easier reading.) At the top of the line, the president of each company makes his commitment to the CEO of the corporation, based on the stated objectives given to him by his vice presidents. There is always pressure from the top to set higher goals.

This management-by-objectives system, as it is usually called, creates a chain of commitments from the CEO down to the lowliest product manager. In practice, it also shapes a patrimonial authority arrangement which is crucial to defining both the immediate experiences and the long-run career chances of individual managers. In this world, a subordinate owes fealty principally to his immediate boss. A subordinate must not overcommit his boss; he must keep the boss from making mistakes, particularly public ones; he must not circumvent the boss. On a social level, even though an easy, breezy informality is the prevalent style of American business, the subordinate must extend to the boss a certain ritual deference: for instance, he must follow the boss's lead in conversation, must not speak out of turn at meetings, and must laugh at the boss's jokes while not making jokes of his own.

In short, the subordinate must not exhibit any behavior which symbolizes parity. In return, he can hope to be elevated when and if the boss is elevated, although other important criteria also intervene here. He can also expect protection for mistakes made up to a point. However, that point is never exactly defined and always depends on the complicated politics of each situation.

### Who Gets Credit?

It is characteristic of this authority system that details are pushed down and credit is pushed up. Superiors do not like to give detailed instructions to subordinates. The official reason for this is to maximize subordinates' autonomy; the underlying reason seems to be to get rid of tedious details and to protect the privilege of authority to declare that a mistake has been made.

It is not at all uncommon for very bald and extremely general edicts to emerge from on high. For example, "Sell the plant in St. Louis. Let me know when you've struck a deal." This pushing down of details has important consequences:

1. Because they are unfamiliar with entangling details, corporate higher echelons tend to expect highly successful results without complications. This is central to top executives' well-known aversion to bad news and to the resulting tendency to "kill the messenger" who bears that news.

2. The pushing down of detail creates great pressure on middle managers not only to transmit good news but to protect their corporations, their bosses, and themselves in the process. They become the "point men" of a given strategy and the potential "fall guys" when things go wrong.

Credit flows up in this structure and usually is appropriated by the highest ranking officer involved in a decision. This person redistributes credit as he chooses, bound essentially by a sensitivity to public perceptions of his fairness. At the middle level, credit for a particular success is always a type of refracted social honor; one cannot claim credit even if it is earned. Credit has to be given, and acceptance of the gift implicitly involves a reaffirmation and strengthening of fealty. A superior may share some credit with subordinates in order to deepen fealty relationships and induce greater future efforts on his behalf. Of course, a different system is involved in the allocation of blame, a point I shall discuss later.

### Fealty to the "King"

Because of the interlocking character of the commitment system, a CEO carries enormous influence in his corporation. If, for a moment, one thinks of the presidents of individual operating companies as barons, then the CEO of the parent company is the king. His word is law; even the CEO's wishes and whims are taken as commands by close subordinates on the corporate staff, who zealously turn them into policies and directives.

A typical example occurred in the textile company last year when the CEO, new at the time, expressed mild concern about the rising operating costs of the company's fleet of rented cars. The following day, a stringent system for monitoring mileage replaced the previous casual practice.

Great efforts are made to please the CEO. For example, when the CEO of the large conglomerate that includes the chemical company visits a plant, the most important order of business for local management is a fresh paint job, even when, as in several cases last year, the cost of paint alone exceeds $100,000. I am told that similar anecdotes from other organizations have been in circulation since 1910; this suggests a certain historical continuity of behavior toward top bosses.

The second order of business for the plant management is to produce a complete book describing the plant and its operations, replete with photographs and illustrations, for presentation to the CEO; such a book costs about $10,000 for the single copy. By any standards of budgetary stringency, such expenditures are irrational. But by the social standards of the corporation, they make perfect sense. It is far more important to please the king today than to worry about the future economic state of one's fief, since if one does not please the king, there may not be a fief to worry about or indeed any vassals to do the worrying.

By the same token, all of this leads to an intense interest in everything the CEO does and says. In both the chemical and the textile companies, the most common topic of conversation among managers up and down the line is speculation about their respective CEOs' plans, intentions, strategies, actions, styles, and public images.

Such speculation is more than idle gossip. Because he stands at the apex of the corporation's bureaucratic and patrimonial structures and locks the intricate system of commitments between bosses and subordinates into place, it is the CEO who ultimately decides whether those commitments have been satisfactorily met. Moreover, the CEO and his trusted associates determine the fate of whole business areas of a corporation.

### Shake-ups and Contingency

One must appreciate the simultaneously monocratic and patrimonial character of business bureaucracies in order to grasp what we might call their contingency. One has only to read the *Wall Street Journal* or the *New York Times* to realize that, despite their carefully constructed "eternal" public image, corporations are quite unstable organizations. Mergers, buy-outs, divestitures, and especially "organizational restructuring" are commonplace aspects of business life. I shall discuss only organizational shake-ups here.

Usually, shake-ups occur because of the appointment of a new CEO and/or division president, or because of some failure that is adjudged to demand retribution; sometimes these occurrences work together. The first action of most new CEOs is some form of organizational change. On the one hand, this prevents the inheritance of blame for past mistakes; on the other, it projects an image of bareknuckled aggressiveness much appreciated on Wall Street. Perhaps most important, a shake-up rearranges the fealty structure of the corporation, placing in power those barons whose style and public image mesh closely with that of the new CEO.

A shake-up has reverberations throughout an organization. Shortly after the new CEO of the conglomerate was named, he reorganized the whole business and selected new presidents to head each of the five newly formed companies of the corporation. He mandated that the presidents carry out a thorough reorganization of their separate companies complete with extensive "census reduction"—that is, firing as many people as possible.

The new president of the chemical company, one of these five, had risen from a small but important specialty chemicals division in the former company. Upon promotion to president, he reached back into his former division, indeed back to his own past work in a particular product line, and systematically elevated many of his former colleagues, friends, and allies. Powerful managers in other divisions, particularly in a rival process chemicals division, were: (1) forced to take big demotions in the new power structure; (2) put on "special assignment"—the corporate euphemism for Siberia (the saying is: "No one ever comes back from special assignment"); (3) fired; or (4) given "early retirement," a graceful way of doing the same thing.

Up and down the chemical company, former associates of the president now hold virtually every important position. Managers in the company view all of this as an inevitable fact of life. In their view, the whole reorganization could easily have gone in a completely different direction had another CEO been named or had the one selected picked a different president for the chemical company, or had the president come from a different work group in the old organization. Similarly, there is the abiding feeling that another significant change in top management could trigger yet another sweeping reorganization.

Fealty is the mortar of the corporate hierarchy, but the removal of one well-placed stone loosens the mortar throughout the pyramid and can cause things to fall apart. And no one is ever quite sure, until after the fact, just how the pyramid will be put back together.

## Success and Failure

It is within this complicated and ambiguous authority structure, always subject to upheaval, that success and failure are meted out to those in the middle and upper middle managerial ranks. Managers rarely spoke to me of objective criteria for achieving success because once certain crucial points in one's career are passed, success and failure seem to have little to do with one's accomplishments. Rather, success is socially defined and distributed. Corporations do demand, of course, a basic competence and sometimes specified training and experience; hiring patterns usually ensure these. A weeding-out process takes place, however, among the lower ranks of managers during the first several years of their experience. By the time a manager reaches a certain numbered grade in the ordered hierarchy—in the chemical company this is Grade 13 out of 25, defining the top 8 ½% of management in the company—managerial competence as such is taken for granted and assumed not to differ greatly from one manager to the next. The focus then switches to social factors, which are determined by authority and political alignments—the fealty structure—and by the ethos and style of the corporation.

### Moving to the Top

In the chemical and textile companies as well as the other concerns I studied, five criteria seem to control a person's ability to rise in middle and upper middle management. In ascending order they are:

1. Appearance and dress. This criterion is so familiar that I shall mention it only briefly. Managers have to look the part, and it is sufficient to say that corporations are filled with attractive, well-groomed, and conventionally well-dressed men and women.

2. Self-control. Managers stress the need to exercise iron self-control and to have the ability to mask all emotion and intention behind bland, smiling, and agreeable public faces. They believe it is a fatal weakness to lose control of oneself, in any way, in a public forum. Similarly, to betray valuable secret knowledge (for instance, a confidential reorganization plan) or intentions through some relaxation of self-control—for example, an indiscreet comment or a lack of adroitness in turning aside a query—can not only jeopardize a manager's immediate position but can undermine others' trust in him.

3. Perception as a team player. While being a team player has many meanings, one of the most important is to appear to be interchangeable with other managers near one's level. Corporations discourage narrow specialization more strongly as one goes higher. They also discourage the expression of moral or political qualms. One might object, for example, to working with chemicals used in nuclear power, and most corporations today would honor that objection. The public statement of such objections, however, would end any realistic aspirations for higher posts because one's usefulness to the organization depends on versatility. As one manager in the chemical company commented: "Well, we'd go along with his request but we'd always wonder about the guy. And in the back of our minds, we'd be thinking that he'll soon object to working in the soda ash division because he doesn't like glass."

Another important meaning of team play is putting in long hours at the office. This requires a certain amount of sheer physical energy, even though a great deal of this time is spent not in actual work but in social rituals—like reading and discussing newspaper articles, taking coffee breaks, or having informal conversations. These rituals, readily observable in every corporation that I studied, forge the social bonds that make real managerial work—that is, group work of various sorts—possible. One must participate in the rituals to be considered effective in the work.

4. Style. Managers emphasize the importance of "being fast on your feet"; always being well organized; giving slick presentations complete with color slides; giving the appearance of knowledge even in its absence; and possessing a subtle, almost indefinable sophistication, marked especially by an urbane, witty, graceful, engaging, and friendly demeanor.

I want to pause for a moment to note that some observers have interpreted such conformity, team playing, affability, and urbanity as evidence of the decline of the individualism of the old Protestant Ethic.[3] To the extent that commentators take the public images that managers project at face value, I think they miss the main point. Managers up and down the corporate ladder adopt the public faces that they wear quite consciously; they are, in fact, the masks behind which the real struggles and moral issues of the corporation can be found.

Karl Mannheim's conception of self-rationalization or self-streamlining is useful in understanding what is one of the central social psychological processes of organizational life.[4] In a world where appearances—in the broadest sense—mean everything, the wise and ambitious person learns to cultivate assiduously the proper, prescribed modes of appearing. He dispassionately takes stock of himself, treating himself as an object. He analyzes his strengths and weaknesses, and decides what he needs to change in order to survive and flourish in his organization. And then he systematically undertakes a program to reconstruct his image. Self-rationalization curiously parallels the methodical subjection of self to God's will that the old Protestant Ethic counseled; the difference, of course, is that one acquires not moral virtues but a masterful ability to manipulate personae.

5. Patron power. To advance, a manager must have a patron, also called a mentor, a sponsor, a rabbi, or a godfather. Without a powerful patron in the higher echelons of management, one's prospects are poor in most corporations. The patron might be the manager's immediate boss or someone several levels higher in the chain of command. In either case the manager is still bound by the immediate, formal authority and fealty patterns of his position; the new—although more ambiguous—fealty relationships with the patron are added.

A patron provides his "client" with opportunities to get visibility, to showcase his abilities, to make connections with those of high status. A patron cues his client to crucial political developments in the corporation, helps arrange lateral moves if the client's upward progress is thwarted by a particular job or a particular boss, applauds his presentations or suggestions at meetings, and promotes the client during an organizational shake-up. One must, of course, be lucky in one's patron. If the patron gets caught in a political crossfire, the arrows are likely to find his clients as well.

### Social Definitions of Performance

Surely, one might argue, there must be more to success in the corporation than style, personality, team play, chameleonic adaptability, and fortunate connections. What about the bottom line—profits, performance?

Unquestionably, "hitting your numbers"—that is, meeting the profit commitments already discussed—is important, but only within the social context I have described. There are several rules here. First, no one in a line position—that is, with responsibility for profit and loss—who regularly "misses his numbers" will survive, let alone rise. Second, a person who always hits his numbers but who lacks some or all of the required social skills will not rise. Third, a person who sometimes misses his numbers but who has all the desirable social traits will rise.

Performance is thus always subject to a myriad of interpretations. Profits matter, but it is much more important in the long run to be perceived as "promotable" by belonging to central political networks. Patrons protect those already selected as rising stars from the negative judgments of others; and only the foolhardy point out even egregious errors of those in power or those destined for it.

Failure is also socially defined. The most damaging failure is, as one middle manager in the chemical company puts it, "when your boss or someone who has the power to determine your fate says: 'You failed.' " Such a godlike pronouncement means, of course, out-and-out personal ruin; one must, at any cost, arrange matters to prevent such an occurrence.

As it happens, things rarely come to such a dramatic point even in the midst of an organizational crisis. The same judgment may be made but it is usually called "nonpromotability." The difference is that those who are publicly labeled as failures normally have no choice but to leave the organization; those adjudged nonpromotable can remain, provided they are willing to accept being shelved or, more colorfully, "mushroomed"—that is, kept in a dark place, fed manure, and left to do nothing but grow fat. Usually, seniors do not tell juniors they are nonpromotable (though the verdict may be common knowledge among senior peer groups). Rather, subordinates are expected to get the message after they have been repeatedly overlooked for promotions. In fact, middle managers interpret staying in the same job for more than two or three years as evidence of a negative judgment. This leads to a mobility panic at the middle levels which, in turn, has crucial consequences for pinpointing responsibility in the organization.

### Capriciousness of Success

Finally, managers think that there is a tremendous amount of plain luck involved in advancement. It is striking how often managers who pride themselves on being hardheaded rationalists explain their own career patterns and those of others in terms of luck. Various uncertainties shape this perception. One is the sense of organizational contingency. One change at the top can create profound upheaval throughout the entire corporate structure, producing startling reversals of fortune, good or bad, depending on one's connections. Another is the uncertainty of the markets that often makes managerial planning simply elaborate guesswork, causing real economic outcome to depend on factors totally beyond organizational and personal control.

It is interesting to note in this context that a line manager's credibility suffers just as much from missing his numbers on the up side (that is, achieving profits higher than predicted) as from missing them on the down side. Both outcomes undercut the ideology of managerial planning and control, perhaps the only bulwark managers have against market irrationality.

Even managers in staff positions, often quite removed from the market, face uncertainty. Occupational safety specialists, for instance, know that the bad publicity from one serious accident in the workplace can jeopardize years of work and scores of safety awards. As one high-ranking executive in the chemical company says, "In the corporate world, 1,000 'Attaboys!' are wiped away by one 'Oh, shit!' "

Because of such uncertainties, managers in all the companies I studied speak continually of the great importance of being in the right place at the right time and of the catastrophe of being in the wrong place at the wrong time. My interview materials are filled with stories of people who were transferred immediately before a big shake-up and, as a result, found themselves riding the crest of a wave to power; of people in a promising business area who were terminated because top management suddenly decided that the area no longer fit the corporate image desired; of others caught in an unpredictable and fatal political battle among their patrons; of a product manager whose plant accidentally produced an odd color batch of chemicals, who sold them as a premium version of the old product, and who is now thought to be a marketing genius.

The point is that managers have a sharply defined sense of the *capriciousness* of organizational life. Luck seems to be as good an explanation as any of why, after a certain point, some people succeed and others fail. The upshot is that many managers decide that they can do little to influence external events in their favor. One can, however, shamelessly streamline oneself, learn to wear all the right masks, and get to know all the right people. And then sit tight and wait for things to happen.

### "Gut Decisions"

Authority and advancement patterns come together in the decision-making process. The core of the managerial mystique is decision-making prowess, and the real test of such prowess is what managers call "gut decisions," that is, important decisions involving big money, public exposure, or significant effects on the organization. At all but the highest levels of the chemical and textile companies, the rules for making gut decisions are, in the words of one upper middle manager: "(1) Avoid making any decisions if at all possible; and (2) if a decision has to be made, involve as many people as you can so that, if things go south, you're able to point in as many directions as possible."

Consider the case of a large coking plant of the chemical company. Coke making requires a gigantic battery to cook the coke slowly and evenly for long periods; the battery is the most important piece of capital equipment in a coking plant. In 1975, the plant's battery showed signs of weakening and certain managers at corporate headquarters had to decide whether to invest $6 million to restore the battery to top form. Clearly, because of the amount of money involved, this was a gut decision.

No decision was made. The CEO had sent the word out to defer all unnecessary capital expenditures to give the corporation cash reserves for other investments. So the managers allocated small amounts of money to patch the battery up until 1979, when it collapsed entirely. This brought the company into a breach of contract with a steel producer and into violation of various Environmental Protection Agency pollution regulations. The total bill, including lawsuits and now federally mandated repairs to the battery, exceeded $100 million. I have heard figures as high as $150 million, but because of "creative accounting," no one is sure of the exact amount.

This simple but very typical example gets to the heart of how decision making is intertwined with a company's authority structure and advancement patterns. As the chemical company managers see it, the decisions facing them in 1975 and 1979 were crucially different. Had they acted decisively in 1975—in hindsight, the only rational course—they would have salvaged the battery and saved their corporation millions of dollars in the long run.

In the short run, however, since even seemingly rational decisions are subject to widely varying interpretations, particularly decisions which run counter to a CEO's stated objectives, they would have been taking a serious risk in restoring the battery. What is more, their political networks might have unraveled, leaving them vulnerable to attack. They chose short-term safety over long-term gain because they felt they were judged, both by higher authority and by their peers, on their short-term performances. Managers feel that if they do not survive the short run, the long run hardly matters. Even correct decisions can shorten promising careers.

By contrast, in 1979 the decision was simple and posed little risk. The corporation had to meet its legal obligations; also it had to either repair the battery the way the EPA demanded or shut down the plant and lose several hundred million dollars. Since there were no real choices, everyone could agree on a course of action because everyone could appeal to inevitability. Diffusion of responsibility, in this case by procrastinating until total crisis, is intrinsic to organizational life because the real issue in most gut decisions is: Who is going to get blamed if things go wrong?

### "Blame Time"

There is no more feared hour in the corporate world than "blame time." Blame is quite different from responsibility. There is a cartoon of Richard Nixon declaring: "I accept all of the responsibility, but none of the blame." To blame someone is to injure him verbally in public; in large organizations, where one's image is crucial, this poses the most serious sort of threat. For managers, blame — like failure — has nothing to do with the merits of a case; it is a matter of social definition. As a general rule, it is those who are or who become politically vulnerable or expendable who get "set up" and become blamable. The most feared situation of all is to end up inadvertently in the wrong place at the wrong time and get blamed.

Yet this is exactly what often happens in a structure that systematically diffuses responsibility. It is because managers fear blame time that they diffuse responsibility; however, such diffusion inevitably means that someone, somewhere is going to become a scapegoat when things go wrong. Big corporations encourage this process by their complete lack of any tracking system. Whoever is currently in charge of an area is responsible — that is, potentially blamable — for whatever goes wrong in the area, even if he has inherited others' mistakes. An example from the chemical company illustrates this process.

When the CEO of the large conglomerate took office, he wanted to rid his capital accounts of all serious financial drags. The corporation had been operating a storage depot for natural gas which it bought, stored, and then resold. Some years before the energy crisis, the company had entered into a long-term contract to supply gas to a buyer — call him Jones. At the time, this was a sound deal because it provided a steady market for a stably priced commodity.

When gas prices soared, the corporation was still bound to deliver gas to Jones at 20¢ per unit instead of the going market price of $2. The CEO ordered one of his subordinates to get rid of this albatross as expeditiously as possible. This was done by selling the operation to another party — call him Brown — with the agreement that Brown would continue to meet the contractual obligations to Jones. In return for Brown's assumption of these costly contracts, the corporation agreed to buy gas from Brown at grossly inflated prices to meet some of its own energy needs.

In effect, the CEO transferred the drag on his capital accounts to the company's operating expenses. This enabled him to project an aggressive, asset-reducing image to Wall Street. Several levels down the ladder, however, a new vice president for a particular business found himself saddled with exorbitant operating costs when, during a reorganization, those plants purchasing gas from Brown at inflated prices came under his purview. The high costs helped to undercut the vice president's division earnings and thus to erode his position in the hierarchy. The origin of the situation did not matter. All that counted was that the vice president's division was steadily losing big money. In the end, he resigned to "pursue new opportunities."

One might ask why top management does not institute codes or systems for tracking responsibility. This example provides the clue. An explicit system of accountability for subordinates would probably have to apply to top executives as well and would restrict their freedom. Bureaucracy expands the freedom of those on top by giving them the power to restrict the freedom of those beneath.

### On the Fast Track

Managers see what happened to the vice president as completely capricious, but completely understandable. They take for granted the absence of any tracking of responsibility. If anything, they blame the vice president for not recognizing soon enough the dangers of the situation into which he was being drawn and for not preparing a defense—even perhaps finding a substitute scapegoat. At the same time, they realize that this sort of thing could easily happen to them. They see few defenses against being caught in the wrong place at the wrong time except constant wariness, the diffusion of responsibility, and perhaps being shrewd enough to declare the ineptitude of one's predecessor on first taking a job.

What about avoiding the consequences of their own errors? Here they enjoy more control. They can "outrun" their mistakes so that when blame time arrives, the burden will fall on someone else. The ideal situation, of course, is to be in a position to fire one's successors for one's own previous mistakes.

Some managers, in fact, argue that outrunning mistakes is the real key to managerial success. One way to do this is by manipulating the numbers. Both the chemical and the textile companies place a great premium on a division's or a subsidiary's return on assets. A good way for business managers to increase their ROA is to reduce their assets while maintaining sales. Usually they will do everything they can to hold down expenditures in order to decrease the asset base, particularly at the end of the fiscal year. The most common way of doing this is by deferring capital expenditures, from maintenance to innovative investments, as long as possible. Done for a short time, this is called "starving" a plant; done over a longer period, it is called "milking" a plant.

Some managers become very adept at milking businesses and showing a consistent record of high returns. They move from one job to another in a company, always upward, rarely staying more than two years in any post. They may leave behind them deteriorating plants and unsafe working conditions, but they know that if they move quickly enough, the blame will fall on others. In this sense, bureaucracies may be thought of as vast systems of organized irresponsibility.

## Flexibility and Dexterity with Symbols

The intense competition among managers takes place not only behind the agreeable public faces I have described but within an extraordinarily indirect and ambiguous linguistic framework. Except at blame time, managers do not publicly criticize or disagree with one another or with company policy. The sanction against such criticism or disagreement is so strong that it constitutes, in managers' view, a suppression of professional debate. The sanction seems to be rooted principally in their acute sense of organizational contingency; the person one criticizes or argues with today could be one's boss tomorrow.

This leads to the use of an elaborate linguistic code marked by emotional neutrality, especially in group settings. The code communicates the meaning one might wish to convey to other managers, but since it is devoid of any significant emotional sentiment, it can be reinterpreted should social relationships or attitudes change. Here, for example, are some typical phrases describing performance appraisals followed by their probable intended meanings:

| Stock Phrase | Probable Intended Meaning |
| --- | --- |
| Exceptionally well qualified | Has committed no major blunders to date |
| Tactful in dealing with superiors | Knows when to keep his mouth shut |
| Quick thinking | Offers plausible excuses for errors |
| Meticulous attention to detail | A nitpicker |
| Slightly below average | Stupid |
| Unusually loyal | Wanted by no one else |

For the most part, such neutered language is not used with the intent to deceive; rather, its purpose is to communicate certain meanings within specific contexts with the implicit understanding that, should the context change, a new, more appropriate meaning can be attached to the language already used. In effect, the corporation is a setting where people are not held to their word because it is generally understood that their word is always provisional.

The higher one goes in the corporate world, the more this seems to be the case; in fact, advancement beyond the upper middle level depends greatly on one's ability to manipulate a variety of symbols without becoming tied to or identified with any of them. For example, an amazing variety of organizational improvement programs marks practically every corporation. I am referring here to the myriad ideas generated by corporate staff, business consultants, academics, and a host of others to improve corporate structure; sharpen decision making; raise morale; create a more humanistic workplace; adopt Theory X, Theory Y, or, more recently, Theory Z of management; and so on. These programs become important when they are pushed from the top.

The watchword in the large conglomerate at the moment is productivity and, since this is a pet project of the CEO himself, it is said that no one goes into his presence without wearing a blue *Productivity!* button and talking about "quality circles" and "feedback sessions." The president of another company pushes a series of managerial seminars that endlessly repeats the basic functions of management: (1) planning, (2) organizing, (3) motivating, and (4) controlling. Aspiring young managers attend these sessions and with a seemingly dutiful eagerness learn to repeat the formulas under the watchful eyes of senior officials.

Privately, managers characterize such programs as the "CEO's incantations over the assembled multitude," as "elaborate rituals with no practical effect," or as "waving a magic wand to make things wonderful again." Publicly, of course, managers on the way up adopt the programs with great enthusiasm, participate in or run them very effectively, and then quietly drop them when the time is right.

### Playing the Game

Such flexibility, as it is called, can be confusing even to those in the inner circles. I was told the following by a highly placed staff member whose work requires him to interact daily with the top figures of his company:

> I get faked out all the time and I'm part of the system. I come from a very different culture. Where I come from, if you give someone your *word*, no one ever questions it. It's the old hard-work-will-lead-to-success ideology. Small community, Protestant, agrarian, small business, merchant-type values. I'm disadvantaged in a system like this.

He goes on to characterize the system more fully and what it takes to succeed within it:

> It's the ability to play this system that determines whether you will rise. . . . And part of the adeptness [required] is determined by how much it bothers people. One thing you have to be able to do is to play the game, but you can't be disturbed by the game. What's the game? It's bringing troops home from Vietnam and declaring peace with honor. It's saying one thing and meaning another.
>
> It's characterizing the reality of a situation with *any* description that is necessary to make that situation more palatable to some group that matters. It means that you have to come up with a culturally accepted verbalization to explain why you are *not* doing what you are doing. . . . [Or] you say that we had to do what we did because it was inevitable; or because the guys at the [regulatory] agencies were dumb; [you] say we won when we really lost; [you] say we saved money when we squandered it; [you] say something's safe when it's potentially or actually dangerous. . . . Everyone knows that it's bullshit, but it's *accepted*. This is the game.

In addition, then, to the other characteristics that I have described, it seems that a prerequisite for big success in the corporation is a certain adeptness at inconsistency. This premium on inconsistency is particularly evident in the many areas of public controversy that face top-ranking managers. Two things come together to produce this situation. The first is managers' sense of beleaguerment from a wide array of adversaries who, it is thought, want to disrupt or impede management's attempts to further the economic interests of their companies. In every company that I studied, managers see themselves and their traditional prerogatives as being under siege, and they respond with a set of caricatures of their perceived principal adversaries.

For example, government regulators are brash, young, unkempt hippies in blue jeans who know nothing about the business for which they make rules; environmental activists—the bird and bunny people—are softheaded idealists who want everybody to live in tents, burn candles, ride horses, and eat berries; workers' compensation lawyers are out-and-out crooks who prey on corporations to appropriate exorbitant fees from unwary clients; labor activists are radical troublemakers who want to disrupt harmonious industrial communities; and the news media consist of rabble-rousers who propagate sensational antibusiness stories to sell papers or advertising time on shows like "60 Minutes."

Second, within this context of perceived harassment, managers must address a multiplicity of audiences, some of whom are considered adversaries. These audiences are the internal corporate hierarchy with its intricate and shifting power and status cliques, key regulators, key local and federal legislators, special publics that vary according to the issues, and the public at large, whose goodwill and favorable opinion are considered essential for a company's free operation.

Managerial adeptness at inconsistency becomes evident in the widely discrepant perspectives, reasons for action, and presentations of fact that explain, excuse, or justify corporate behavior to these diverse audiences.

### Adeptness at Inconsistency

The cotton dust issue in the textile industry provides a fine illustration of what I mean. Prolonged exposure to cotton dust produces in many textile workers a chronic and eventually disabling pulmonary disease called byssinosis or, colloquially, brown lung. In the early 1970s, the Occupational Safety and Health Administration proposed a ruling to cut workers' exposure to cotton dust sharply by requiring textile companies to invest large amounts of money in cleaning up their plants. The industry fought the regulation fiercely but a final OSHA ruling was made in 1978 requiring full compliance by 1984.

The industry took the case to court. Despite an attempt by Reagan appointees in OSHA to have the case removed from judicial consideration and remanded to the agency they controlled for further cost/benefit analysis, the Supreme Court ruled in 1981 that the 1978 OSHA ruling was fully within the agency's mandate, namely, to protect workers' health and safety as the primary benefit exceeding all cost considerations.

During these proceedings, the textile company was engaged on a variety of fronts and was pursuing a number of actions. For instance, it intensively lobbied regulators and legislators and it prepared court materials for the industry's defense, arguing that the proposed standard would crush the industry and that the problem, if it existed, should be met by increasing workers' use of respirators.

The company also aimed a public relations barrage at special-interest groups as well as at the general public. It argued that there is probably no such thing as byssinosis; workers suffering from pulmonary problems are all heavy smokers and the real culprit is the government-subsidized tobacco industry. How can cotton cause brown lung when cotton is white? Further, if there is a problem, only some workers are afflicted, and therefore the solution is more careful screening of the work force to detect susceptible people and prevent them from ever reaching the workplace. Finally, the company claimed that if the regulation were imposed, most of the textile industry would move overseas where regulations are less harsh.[5]

In the meantime, the company was actually addressing the problem but in a characteristically indirect way. It invested $20 million in a few plants where it knew such an investment would make money; this investment automated the early stages of handling cotton, traditionally a very slow procedure, and greatly increased productivity. The investment had the side benefit of reducing cotton dust levels to the new standard in precisely those areas of the work process where the dust problem is greatest. Publicly, of course, the company claims that the money was spent entirely to eliminate dust, evidence of its corporate good citizenship. (Privately, executives admit that, without the productive return, they would not have spent the money and they have not done so in several other plants.)

Indeed, the productive return is the only rationale that carries weight within the corporate hierarchy. Executives also admit, somewhat ruefully and only when their office doors are closed, that OSHA's regulation on cotton dust has been the main factor in forcing technological innovation in a centuries-old and somewhat stagnant industry.

Such adeptness at inconsistency, without moral uneasiness, is essential for executive success. It means being able to say, as a very high-ranking official of the textile company said to me without batting an eye, that the industry has never caused the slightest problem in any worker's breathing capacity. It means, in the chemical company, propagating an elaborate hazard/benefit calculus for appraisal of dangerous chemicals while internally conceptualizing "hazards" as business risks. It means publicly extolling the carefulness of testing procedures on toxic chemicals while privately ridiculing animal tests as inapplicable to humans.

It means lobbying intensively in the present to shape government regulations to one's immediate advantage and, ten years later, in the event of a catastrophe, arguing that the company acted strictly in accordance with the standards of the time. It means claiming that the real problem of our society is its unwillingness to take risks, while in the thickets of one's bureaucracy avoiding risks at every turn; it means as well making every effort to socialize the risks of industrial activity while privatizing the benefits.

## The Bureaucratic Ethic

The bureaucratic ethic contrasts sharply with the original Protestant Ethic. The Protestant Ethic was the ideology of a self-confident and independent propertied social class. It was an ideology that extolled the virtues of accumulating wealth in a society organized around property and that accepted the stewardship responsibilities entailed by property. It was an ideology where a person's word was his bond and where the integrity of the handshake was seen as crucial to the maintenance of good business relationships. Perhaps most important, it was connected to a predictable economy of salvation—that is, hard work will lead to success, which is a sign of one's election by God—a notion also containing its own theodicy to explain the misery of those who do not make it in this world.

Bureaucracy, however, breaks apart substance from appearances, action from responsibility, and language from meaning. Most important, it breaks apart the older connection between the meaning of work and salvation. In the bureaucratic world, one's success, one's sign of election, no longer depends on one's own efforts and on an inscrutable God but on the capriciousness of one's superiors and the market; and one achieves economic salvation to the extent that one pleases and submits to one's employer and meets the exigencies of an impersonal market.

In this way, because moral choices are inextricably tied to personal fates, bureaucracy erodes internal and even external standards of morality, not only in matters of individual success and failure but also in all the issues that managers face in their daily work. Bureaucracy makes its own internal rules and social context the principal moral gauges for action. Men and women in bureaucracies turn to each other for moral cues for behavior and come to fashion specific situational moralities for specific significant people in their worlds.

As it happens, the guidance they receive from each other is profoundly ambiguous because what matters in the bureaucratic world is not what a person is but how closely his many personae mesh with the organizational ideal; not his willingness to stand by his actions but his agility in avoiding blame; not what he believes or says but how well he has mastered the ideologies that serve his corporation; not what he stands for but whom he stands with in the labyrinths of his organization.

In short, bureaucracy structures for managers an intricate series of moral mazes. Even the inviting paths out of the puzzle often turn out to be invitations to jeopardy.

## APPENDIX

### Field Work Details

The field work during 1980 to 1981 encompassed four companies—a large chemical company, one of several operating companies of a diversified conglomerate; a large textile company; a medium-sized chemical company; and a large defense contractor. My access to the latter two businesses was limited to a series of interviews with top executive officers, some observation, and some access to internal company documents. Although many of the themes treated in this article emerged in my work in these two companies, I have for the most part treated these materials as preliminary data.

It is also important to note that I was denied access to 36 companies, an instructive experience in itself. In about half these cases, access was denied after lengthy negotiations involving interviews with various company officials; these materials are also treated as preliminary. In this article, when I claim that something occurs in all the companies that I studied, I mean to include these preliminary materials as well as the more substantive data described here.

I concentrated most of my substantive work in the two companies where my access was broadest—in the large textile company and particularly in the large chemical company. I pursued the research in these companies until mid-1982 and mid-1983, respectively. I draw my analysis principally from these two organizations. My materials from both are rich and detailed; moreover, their size and complexity make them representative of important sectors of American industry. Further, the kinds of problems managers face in these companies—

organizational, regulatory, and personal—are, I think, typical of those confronted more generally.

My methodology in this research was intensive semistructured interviews with managers and executives at every level of management. The interviews usually lasted between two and three hours but, sometimes, especially with reinterviews, went much longer. I interviewed more than 100 people in these two companies alone.

In addition, I gathered material in a number of more informal ways—for example, through nonparticipant observation, over meals, and in attendance at various management seminars. I also had extensive access to internal company documents and publications.

### NOTES

1. There is a long sociological tradition of work on managers and I am, of course, indebted to that literature. I am particularly indebted to the work, both joint and separate, of Joseph Bensman and Arthur J. Vidich, two of the keenest observers of the new middle class. See especially their *The New American Society: The Revolution of the Middle Class* (Chicago: Quadrangle Books, 1971).
2. See Max Weber, *The Protestant Ethic and the Spirit of Capitalism*, translated by Talcott Parsons (New York: Charles Scribner's Sons, 1958), p. 172.
3. See William H. Whyte, *The Organization Man* (New York: Simon & Schuster, 1956), and David Riesman, in collaboration with Reuel Denney and Nathan Glazer, *The Lonely Crowd: A Study of the Changing American Character* (New Haven: Yale University Press, 1950).
4. Karl Mannheim, *Man and Society in an Age of Reconstruction* (London: Paul [Kegan], Trench, Trubner Ltd. 1940), p. 55.
5. On February 9, 1982, the Occupational Safety and Health Administration issued a notice that it was once again reviewing its 1978 standard on cotton dust for "cost-effectiveness." See *Federal Register*, vol. 47, p. 5906. As of this writing (May 1983), this review has still not been officially completed.

# 8

# Why Do Companies Succumb to Price Fixing?

## JEFFREY SONNENFELD AND PAUL R. LAWRENCE

Down the centuries social analysts have frequently charged, "Laws are like spiderwebs, which may catch small flies but let wasps and hornets break through." As more and more corporations have been caught in the web of price-fixing laws, however, this charge has lost its punch. Senior business managers in industries that have never before known these problems, as well as previous offenders, are probably more concerned now about their corporate exposure to being indicted and convicted of price fixing than they were in any other recent period.

The reasons are not hard to find. As federal agencies, the courts, and Congress respond to the heightened post-Watergate expectations of the public, the law enforcement net has been substantially strengthened.[1] Instead of hearing protests over the legal immunity granted to the large and powerful, one now hears the anguish coming from the reverse direction. One can regularly read about prominent individuals and organizations that are overwhelmed by the stiff penalties they have incurred for behavior which may have been customary business practice in the past but which now violates social and legal standards.[2]

The costs of violating price-fixing laws are very high: lawyers' fees, government fines, poor morale, damaged public image, civil suits, and now prison terms. Justice Department statistics indicate that 60% of antitrust felons are sentenced to prison terms.[3] Thus, for very pragmatic reasons as well as for personal convictions, America's top executives are searching for fail-safe ways of meeting legal requirements. While top executives strongly complain about increasing government interference, they also acknowledge, "We operate through a license from society which can be revoked whenever we violate the terms of the license."

Executives in large decentralized organizations, however, find it increasingly difficult to carry through on their intentions. The considerable time and money corporations spend developing positive public images can be wasted by the careless actions of just one or two lower level employees. At the same time that organization size and complexity increase, top executives find that the law imposes on them additional responsibility for the business practices of their subordinates.

Executives tremble over what may be going on in the field despite their internal directives and public declarations. One CEO well expressed the frustration common to executives in convicted companies:

> We've tried hard to stress that collusion is illegal. We point out that anticompetitive practices hurt the company's ethical standards, public image, internal morale, and earnings. Yet we wind up in trouble continually. When we try to find out why employees got involved, they have the gall to say that they "were only looking out for the best interests of the company." They seem to think that the company message is for everyone else but them. You begin to wonder about the intelligence of these people. Either they don't listen or they're just plain stupid.

Some executives we interviewed in researching this article believe with the CEO quoted that their employees who collude in price fixing are just not listening or are plain stupid. In our view it is less likely that the employees are deaf or stupid than that many well-meaning, ethical top managers simply are not getting their message down the line to loyal alert employees.

To better understand this lack of communication as well as other forces contributing to employees committing unlawful acts, we thought that it would be enlightening to look at the unfortunate experience of the forest products and paper industry in the midst of antitrust litigation. Looking just at antitrust cases in 1977, one can see that the paper industry was hit with separate prosecutions for price fixing in consumer paper, fine paper and stationery, multiwall bags, shopping bags, labels, corrugated containers, and folding cartons. In early 1978, over 100 suits have been filed against the industry.

In addition, a U.S. grand jury has been gathering information on competitive practices in the industry at large—which many suspect is part of a probe into industry collusion to restrain supply.[4] In fact, the *Wall Street Journal* recently stated that the paper industry is gaining the reputation as the "nation's biggest price fixer."[5]

The folding-box litigation has, by far, been the most damaging (see Appendix). The Justice Department has described this case as the largest price-fixing one since 1960. It is hard to understand how socially responsible companies could ever have found themselves in such a nightmarish situation. To find out, we discussed the various pressures and conditions in this industry with 40 senior, division, and middle level executives. Our investigation concentrated on the predicament of the large forest products companies that derive about 4% or 5% of their total company sales from folding-carton revenues.

The shock for those companies, with strong, well-publicized ethical positions, is perhaps most severe. In case the reader is skeptical, our interviews with the senior people in these companies left us without a shred of doubt about the sincerity and completeness of their personal commitment to legal compliance. In fact, the top people we spoke to in the major forest products companies desperately want to know how and why they got on the wrong side of the law so that they can be sure it never happens again.

## How It Can Happen

Before we discuss the factors that create a price-fixing prone industry and organization, we would like to point out that the various problematic situations that contributed to this unhappy end are certainly not unique to the paper industry. One can easily draw parallels between the paper industry's difficulties and the situations leading to price fixing in other very different industries. For such a comparison, we will at times glance at the 1960 electrical contractors' conspiracy. We hope too that no one will read this article without reflecting on his or her own company's situation.

### Price-fixing Prone Industry

Many economists would consider the folding-carton industry to be one of the least likely to spawn a price-fixing conspiracy. The industry's very diffuse structure is the complete antithesis of the tight-knit oligopoly, which, economists tell us, breeds collusion. Of the over 450 box-making companies, the larger ones control only from 5% to 7% of the market; only one company controls near 10%.

With this number of companies, one would think that the rivalry among them would be so intense that it would preclude any mutual understandings and tacit agreements. Yet companies representing 70% of the $1.5 billion in annual industry sales were convicted.

In fact, the number of companies in the industry is one of the factors that tempted some businessmen to abandon the rugged competitor role and adopt "a more statesmanlike attitude toward competitors," as one executive euphemistically puts it. The market was, simply, badly crowded. Other pressures toward collusion were the job-order nature of the business and the fact that the products were undifferentiated.

**Crowded and mature market.** In the late 1950s and early 1960s, as the expansion of prepackaged and frozen foods kept the market growing at about 7% a year, the folding-carton business attracted new entrants. With low barriers to entry, competitors of all sizes saw this area as a great opportunity. Traditionally dominated by small family-run box-making shops, the industry became attractive to very large forest products companies, which integrated forward. These large companies first supplied the paperboard for box making, and then began to compete with their customers further down the line in making the actual boxes themselves.

The tendency toward overcapacity in paperboard production tempted these large paper companies to look on folding boxes as a way to unload excesses. Some blamed the softening of the box market on this attitude, claiming that "the big companies did not care about box prices because they were making their profit back at the paperboard mill."

Also harmful to the market in the intervening years was the halt of super-market expansion as well as the growth of the use of substitute containers, such as plastics, which eroded the market share for paper containers. The industry is now very mature and has even suffered revenue as well as profit declines.

These declines place great pressure on middle level managers who are keenly aware that the constant use of existing capital equipment is the way to drive down unit costs. One general manager commented:

> Large volume is important because we didn't make the investment in more efficient equipment we should have years ago. We could have brought on more sophisticated equipment and been more efficient in the use of labor and style of production. However, we can't get the money now. Too much was invested in the paperboard mills and nothing in folding-carton plants. Financial analysts look at these past bad investments and the bad earnings here and refuse to look on this industry with a favorable eye. It's a bad cycle we're caught in.

Some say a shakeout is long overdue; others complain about vicious customers. Some managers in folding-box companies complain of the predatory influence of the large companies they supply. One division manager stated:

> This sector has been ripped off by big customers for a long time. Anything this industry has done has been more in defense than offense. Business is really dwindling, and we are even more dependent on pleasing the big customers we depend on. You really can't do a profitable business with a customer buying $30 million from one carton manufacturer. They will de-stroy you. . . . No one here is making much in this industry anymore. Now the pressures are not to make more money but to keep from going under. Price discussions between competitors are important just to keep from going broke. Our customers should be investigated instead.

When a manager feels his or her division's survival is in question, the cor-poration's standards of business conduct are apt to be sacrificed. In the 1960 electrical contractors case the issue was also survival. A convicted General Electric division vice president explained:

> I think we understood it was against the law. . . . The moral issue didn't seem to be important at that time . . . it was a period of trying to obtain stability, to put an umbrella over the smaller manufacturers . . . I've seen the situation change, primarily due to overcapacity, to almost a situation where people thought it was a survival measure. . . .[6]

**Job-order nature of business.** In the folding-box industry cost-cutting practices are also hampered by the nature of the production process. Boxes are generally manufactured for short job orders. One general manager said: "Those guys up in headquarters think making boxes is like making paper, but paper-making is just following recipes. No two boxes are the same for us. Even with soap boxes, there are diverse product specifications."

Each of these jobs is costed and priced individually. Since each order is custom made, the pricing decisions are made frequently and at low levels of the organization. One salesman illustrated how a job-order business exposes a company to low-level price collusion:

> Every order is a negotiation, even when we've got a contract. Dialogue on prices is always on your mind. Any time I've met with a competitor, whether at a trade association meeting or in a customer's waiting room, one of us will eventually crack a smile and say, "You son of a bitch, you're cutting my prices again. . . ." Sometimes things go on from there and sometimes they don't. I think our company has been stupidly naive. It is impossible not to have talked price at some time.

**Undifferentiated products.** Finally, while job specifications vary greatly between orders, the skills and equipment are fairly undifferentiated between companies. Several executives we interviewed concur with the following state-ment from one vice president:

> Part of the problem is that we're not competing with a unique article here. Our bags and boxes aren't really any better or worse than those of our competitors. You don't really go out and sell the product. Salespeople don't have any special product to sell. The only way to get a buyer is to sell at a lower price. Thus competitors may think that the only way to make it is to get together and fix prices.

With such factors as a crowded and mature market, declining demand, dif-ficulty in cutting costs, and no company product differentiation, it is not sur-prising that profits have been bad. Lately, folding-carton profits, at best, have been running between 3% to 6% of sales. Several companies have folding-carton divisions that have not seen a real profit in years. Just in the period of time in which we conducted this research, three large box makers announced they were either selling out or closing up.

Collusion may then take place despite economists' doubts that it will succeed and despite company statements that legal compliance is mandated.[7] When we try to empathize with someone fighting for the survival of a sick business, we realize that the problem may be greater than employees that don't listen or are just plain stupid. Perhaps these people really believe that they are committed to the company's best interests. We heard one convicted executive explain in a quivering voice:

> The unhealthy state which characterizes this industry has of course afflicted this company as well. We're not vicious enemies in this industry, but rather people in similar binds. I've always thought of myself as an honorable citizen. We didn't do these things for our own behalf. It was presumably done for the betterment of the company.

It seems that the recognition of common goals can be shared within a large group of diverse competitors as well as within a close-knit oligopoly. Certainly not all industries face such adverse conditions. But many other industries face some combination of these circumstances, and management complacency in the face of these conditions could be very costly.

### Price-fixing Prone Organization

Our interviews clearly reveal that not all the factors contributing to price fixing come from the industry, economic, and technical factors we have considered. Some come directly from the companies themselves and the subculture of the industry; some are built into personnel pricing, sales, and legal staff practices.

**Culture of the business.** In the electrical contractors conspiracy, there were strong pressures to enforce the anticompetitive norms. A GE vice president describing the type of coercion placed on an executive who resisted the norms of collusion stated, "We worked him over pretty hard, and I did too; I admit it." One GE executive who was a target of this pressure from his colleagues committed suicide.[8] In one recent folding-box case, some executives threatened others with physical violence if they resisted raising prices.[9]

Executives in the paper industry point out that people in the folding-carton business are not necessarily evil but are just people who have worked in a system with a history of very different ground rules. A convicted executive claimed that price fixing was common practice in his business:

> Price agreements between competitors was a way of life. Our ethics were not out of line with what was being done in this company and, in fact, in this industry for a long time. I've been in this industry for 32 years, and this situation was not just a passing incident. That's just the way I was brought up in the business, right or wrong.

Another factor encouraging price fixing arises when a company with one culture acquires another with a quite different one. In several companies convicted of price fixing, senior executives acknowledge that rapid vertical integration brought their forest products companies into secondary converting businesses, which were little and poorly integrated.[10] One division vice president of a convicted company conceded: "Our folding-carton units were like a bunch of geographic 'left outs.' The geographic separation was fantastic. The 15 individual plants were poorly coordinated and poorly managed. We just came along with our acquisition drive and then sent top management attention elsewhere."

The parent companies often naively assumed that business practice and ethics in the two companies would automatically be congruent even if there were no common heritage. As an illustration of the sort of side practices that may come with a business acquisition, the management of one large forest products company learned to its shock that the box-making company it had just acquired had been running a house of prostitution as a customer service for years. One vice president stated:

> The guys at the core of this conspiracy were acquired people from acquired companies and not part of our culture. That is just not the way we do business. Questions of ethics were never raised. We assumed that people do business ethically at our company. Apparently that was a simple-minded assumption.

**Personnel practices.** On top of any other influences, the personnel practices used in many companies seemed actually to encourage people to engage in price fixing.[11] In a number of the companies convicted, management almost exclusively appraised individual performance on the basis of profits and volume. And not only advancement but also bonuses and commissions, which often exceeded 50% of base salary, were dependent on these measures. A division manager spelled out these practices:

> In the folding-carton division, our local salesmen have all been compensated with a base salary and a commission. Some bonus programs account for 60% of someone's compensation. People have been evaluated on the basis of profit and how forcefully they can execute a price increase. Thus, if he does this by price agreement with competitors, he'll build profit and price credits and get a reward.

So, instead of seeing the top people explicitly and officially acknowledge the difficult industry conditions, many of the lower officials see only strong pressures and inducements to "get the numbers no matter what." As one executive of a convicted company sadly acknowledged, "We've definitely run into some problems from jamming our corporate targets down everyone's throats."

It is not surprising that junior managers perceive such company-induced pressure as conveying top management's intent. One sales manager explained that any other corporate messages that came down from other company executives were only from "staff guys and were not related to my evaluation and advancement. If it is known that the operating chief of your area wants business conducted in a certain way, it seems that is what really counts."

One chief executive officer who spent a lot of time thinking over his company's involvement in the recent conspiracy summed up the effect of these kinds of pressures:

> I think we are particularly vulnerable where we have a salesman with two kids, plenty of financial demands, and a concern over the security of his

job. There is a certain amount of looseness to a new set of rules. He may accept questionable practices feeling that he may just not know the system. There are no specific procedures for him to follow other than what other salesmen tell him.

At the same time, he is in an industry where the acceptance for his product and the level of profitability are clearly dropping. Finally, we add to his pressures by letting him know who will take his job from him if he doesn't get good price and volume levels. I guess this will bring a lot of soul-searching out of an individual.

**Pricing decisions.** Another area that caused vulnerability in companies convicted of price fixing was their decentralized price-setting mechanism. A GE division manager jailed for price fixing made this point before a Senate sub-committee 15 years ago:

> I think decentralization exposed the flanks a great deal more. It made the exposure greater. . . . It has put more pressure on the manager because he has complete responsibility in a smaller organization. Yes, I think de-centralization has certainly contributed to the forces that tend to make [con-spiracies] a reality.[12]

Descriptions of this earlier conspiracy indicate that the job-order nature of this equipment business increased the frequency of these decisions and the degree of competitor contact.

In the paper industry, we found that senior managers assumed pricing was done as it was for commodity products, where any changes were large, rare, and received top management attention. The prices for folding boxes, however, like other job-order business, are heavily influenced by very junior managers and salespeople. This was true even though a general manager was nominally held responsible for pricing. Because managers made pricing decisions frequently, the number of diffuse influences on these decisions are great. As a result, one salesman explained:

> Everyone gets his nose into pricing issues. You're nothing unless you get into the pricing mechanism. There are maybe ten guys that can get involved in every decision, including clerks, plant managers, cost estimators, and salespeople. Yeah, the responsibility rests ultimately with the general man-ager but that's horseshit! Everyone wants a piece of the action and an awful lot of people get their hands into prices unnecessarily.

Thus people can get involved in pricing issues for status reasons alone and can be tempted to use their influence to impress and help friends in other companies. It is also clear that the more decentralized pricing decisions become, the more difficult it will be for top managers to control collusion.

**Trade associations.** Over two centuries ago, Adam Smith, the dean of free market economics, warned: "People of the same trade seldom meet together, even for merriment and diversion, but the conversation ends in a conspiracy against the public, or in some contrivance to raise prices."[13]

In keeping with this prediction, a sales manager of a convicted paper company complained that industry trade association activities can directly contribute to a company's involvement in conspiracy:

> You must limit the occasion of sin. You can't put yourself in a position of contact with competitors. I've dropped contact with personal friends in competing companies since this prosecution started, and I should have dropped such contacts sooner. I don't go to industry meetings at all. Now, finally, this whole company frowns on industry bullshit!

Though many executives will not now talk to old friends in competitive companies, some general managers disagree with these assessments. They feel that there may be truth to the suspicion that these trade meetings give an opportunity for price fixing, but as one manager argued: "Just the same, these associations have a great value, and it's too bad to see them in trouble. A lot of lobbying relevant to the industry happens there. Perhaps participation has been too liberal . . . it's just a big party."

Virtually all the senior managers surveyed agree "that it's hard to talk about the costs of production without discussing prices." An executive at one of the relatively uninvolved companies proudly stated that his company has sharply curtailed the number of company employees participating in trade association meetings:

> I think that trade associations have some value, but the risks are fairly high. We've cut back dramatically and now only one or two people per division attend the meetings. The trade meetings are limited to the top people. Some second echelon employees just loved to go to these meetings and take their wives. They wanted to be entertained. I've always believed that familiarity breeds attempt. For each point on the asset side, trade associations have two points on the liability side.

Similarly, executives in the electrical contractors case condemned the collusionary influence at the trade association meetings. In 1960, a GE vice president stated to a congressional committee: "The way I feel about it now, sir, the way my company . . . has been damaged, the way my associates and their personal careers have been damaged and destroyed, the way my family and myself have been suffering, if I see a competitor on one side of the street, I will walk on the other side, sir."[14]

**Corporate legal staff.** Several corporate lawyers reluctantly acknowledge that their performance was related to their company's convictions. While in many companies antitrust memoranda and periodic legal lectures became more frequent after the landmark 1960 electrical contractors conspiracy, legal departments in the paper companies still tended to react to problems rather than to anticipate them. The corporate counsel at one of the convicted paper companies explained: "In the past, we practiced what we thought was our proper role, and that was to respond to legal questions. We sometimes did big group things like lectures, but we never sat down to talk the subject through with small groups of managers."

Similarly, another vice president of legal affairs conceded that, although his department is quite heavily involved in antitrust education now, "We've only really become anticipatory since the folding-carton case."

Thus the lawyers did not serve as a source for legal advice to avoid problems but allowed people to navigate to the brink of prosecution. A division manager in one of the convicted companies summed this up by giving his impression of the performance of the legal division: "I can tell you that the lawyers here are a damned smart bunch of guys who can get you out of trouble once you've gotten into it. But we sure need more of an active force."

## How to Avoid It

We have examined both the industry and the company factors that contributed to one industry's being so badly caught up in price fixing. It is time to take stock of the implications of our inquiry for managers who are resolved to avoid such traumatic experiences. How should managers respond to this predicament? The lessons are, in fact, fairly easy to perceive but at times very difficult to put into practice.

It is obvious but not trivial to say that managers in competing companies who would be fail-safe should move to the opposite poles from each and every one of the contributing factors we have identified. (The *Exhibit* lists these factors and their opposites.) But, of course, recognizing danger signs provides no more than a start toward solving the problem. Which factors are relatively controllable and which are not? What specific practices have we identified in our study that were helpful? What ideas and concepts can be useful in achieving compliance?

### Managing the Market Conditions

Certainly very little in the market environment is under management's direct control. One may conclude that the conditions of the folding-carton industry are sufficiently hostile that a company would be justified in leaving the business entirely. Since four large companies have left the business over the past year, obviously some involved executives have reached that very conclusion. In our interviews, senior managers at one forest products company expressed sheer relief at being "liberated."

Those who have remained are striving for cost control and product differentiation to allow for longer runs and greater pricing freedom. Only a few have as yet succeeded in this effort. Many executives complain that their company could never remove itself from the brutal paper-carton market unless top management made a really major commitment to a new strategy. Most are unable to free themselves from the tradition of trying to be all things to all people. A vice president of legal affairs in one convicted company pointed to the superficial nature of some attempts to affect the market and shows how they can backfire:

Everyone here is competing for the same sales. We wanted to somehow differentiate ourselves, so through the 1950s and the early 1960s we developed over 300 minor patents. These patents weren't really worth the time, but that was the way we competed then. Customers would insist that at least one other box maker be licensed under the patent so they wouldn't be so dependent on one supplier. That's how we then got involved in pricing discussions. When discussing royalties, prices became important issues.

A sales manager of one of the convicted companies reported that the larger companies did seriously try to segment the market into areas such as frozen food, beverages, cosmetics, and so forth.

But, said this manager, "Some independents would just continue to treat their businesses like general printing shops, and the large companies could never organize the market." Such a market allocation could, of course, still violate antitrust legislation.

Only a handful of companies seems to have succeeded in a product differentiation strategy. But the fact that a few have is not insignificant, and we will return to this point later.

### Managing the Company Culture

As we talked to executives in the forest products industry, we of course asked about their experience with management methods that could help control the price-fixing problem. One of the consistent and early points that came up was the example set for the company by the behavior of top management. We found one of the most frequent approaches senior management uses to encourage legal compliance is to cite its record in regard to social responsibility.

Psychological research on obedience,[15] business research on employee morality, and common sense all indicate that the behavior of those in authority serves as important role models to others.[16] Unless top management projects consistent and sincere company commitment, operating practices will not change.

This commitment, however, is a necessary but not a sufficient factor to ensure compliance. The major forest products companies where we interviewed have a long-standing reputation for the expression of public interest commitment by senior executives. Each company has its own internal maxim for, "We believe that ethics start at the front office." Unfortunately, these statements tend to stop here as well. A vice president of a convicted paper company explained:

> When we were small enough and in a stable environment, people all knew each other by first names. We could communicate informally, and we were successful in molding behavior through modeling. People could resolve gray areas of decision making by reflecting on how their superiors would handle such an issue. But, with our very explosive growth of the last decade and a half, this old approach has become problematic. Can we still communicate corporate standards to a lot of people in the same way we communicated to a few?

A number of companies are actively developing some promising ways to go beyond the example of the front office.

**General management signals.** Some executives talked very explicitly about the problem of changing the culture of a problem division. Having been burned in the past, the financial vice president of a convicted company has adopted a preventive approach. He has communicated new acquisition criteria to his investment brokers. He is now at least as interested in information about a company's ethical practices as in its financial performance. One chief executive officer said that he and his top managers learned the hard way from troubles soon after making an acquisition. He felt that retraining management is helpful:

   Managing these disparate cultures in the face of institutional transition is difficult. You have to change the self-perpetuating norms. Given our hard charging acquisition policy, maintaining our corporate beliefs is hard. We have to move in and go with the old management still in place. Managing newly acquired divisions is like trying to raise adopted kids. An adopted child after age five may still need his new parents to teach him when to go to bed and when to get up.

   Some companies find that just as training acquired personnel is helpful to reorient business practices, training salesmen to sell product features rather than to sell for price alone also helps change practices. If a company manages to develop special mechanical packaging systems, special graphic design abilities, or some other means of differentiation, salesmen must be given the knowledge needed to sell these features. Well-trained salesmen can often find ways to compete in terms of special delivery services, inventory aids, and design suggestions. As one sales manager put it, "Only lazy sales managers rely on commissions to get their salesmen to sell."
   Another tool of general management is the evaluation and rewards system. The companies that were least involved in the price-fixing conspiracy compensate their sales forces on straight salary and evaluate on the basis of volume rather than of price level or profit. Several companies convicted of price fixing have

---

## Exhibit   Danger and Safety Zones of the Factors Contributing to Price Fixing

### Industry characteristics

| Danger zone | Safety zone |
|---|---|
| Overcapacity | Undercapacity |
| Undifferentiated products | Differentiated products |
| Frequent job-order pricing | Infrequent commodity pricing |
| Contact with competitors | No contact with competitors |
| Large, price sensitive customers | Small, price sensitive customers |

### Company characteristics

| Danger zone | Safety zone |
|---|---|
| Collusion culture | Top management modeling and training |
| High rewards for profits | Multidimensional rewards |
| Decentralized pricing decisions | Centralized pricing decisions |
| Widespread trade association participation | Constrained trade association participation |
| Reactive legal staff | Anticipatory legal staff |
| Loose, general ethical rules | Specific ethical codes with auditing |

now adopted this method and are in the process of learning to evaluate people along broader dimensions.

**Price decision procedures.** One of the factors contributing to price fixing we cited previously was the practice in some of the companies studied of allowing specific price decisions to be influenced by salespeople and others below the general management level. In effect, because of bonus and commission arrangements, junior people were acting almost as profit center managers. Since these were the same people who might well see their competitors' sales representatives in the customers' waiting rooms, the scene for illegal action was set.

Some managers in the companies we studied have been reviewing their practices in this regard and making tighter definitions of who can legitimately take part in pricing decisions. It takes careful analysis of the multiple sources of relevant information concerning prices as well as an explicit commitment procedure to make such rules both workable and prudent.

**Code of ethics.** Attempts to move beyond top-level role modeling have led some executives to prepare codes of ethics on company business practices. In some companies this document circulates only at top levels and, again, the word seems to have trouble getting down the line. Even those documents that were sent to all employees seemed to have been broadly written, toothless versions of the golden rule. One company tried to get more commitment by requiring employees to sign and return a pledge. A senior vice president in this company complained that even though a copy of the law is also sent along: "This stuff isn't all that valuable. In the first place you're only sending the employee what the law says and you're not telling him or her anything new. Second, it's not signed in blood! You haven't committed him to any behavior; he just recognizes that he has to sign the card to work."

An employee convicted of price fixing agreed with these comments and questioned the view that price fixers can be helped by ethical statements: "A code of ethics doesn't do anything. I thought I had morals. I still think I do. I didn't understand the laws . . . not morals. What might to me be an ethical practice might have been interpreted differently by a legal scholar. The golden rule might be consistent with both views."

For codes to really work, substantial specificity is important. One executive said his company's method was successful because the code was tied in with an employee's daily routine: "There is a code of business conduct here. To really make it meaningful, you have to get past the stage of endorsing motherhood and deal with the specific problems of policy in the different functional areas. We wrote up 20 pages on just purchasing issues."

**Auditing for compliance.** Once these more specific codes of business conduct are distributed, top managers may want more than a signed statement in return. Individuals can be held responsible if they have been informed on how to act in certain gray areas. The company can show its commitment to the code by checking to see that it is respected and by then disciplining violators.

Several companies are developing ways to implement internal policing. Some executives think that audits could hold people responsible for unusual pricing successes as well as for failures.[17] Market conditions, product specifications, and factory scheduling could be coded, put on tables, and compared to prices. High variations could be investigated. One division vice president also plans to audit expense accounts to see that competitor contact is minimized.

**Legal training.** As we noted earlier, executives in the convicted paper companies acknowledge that the lack of contact between them and company lawyers makes it hard to apply the law. Direct contact between operating managers and members of the legal staff seemed to be less frequent in the companies that were more heavily involved in the conspiracy. There are at least three barriers that the legal division must overcome in order to take this more anticipatory stance.

The first barrier is a negative image. As advisers, lawyers must accept being seen as holier-than-thou naysayers. One general manager complained:

> I'm very critical of legal people in big corporations. Most corporate counsel is negative on any level of risk. They say don't take chances in new areas, when we should. They tell us not to sue, when we should. They don't want us to cause any waves because it's easier for them. If it were up to them, they'd say don't even get out in the market.

This statement indicates how important it is for operating managers to understand the legal constraints on their plans and for the lawyers to be sensitive to the pressures of operating managers. Senior management must take the initiative to legitimize both perspectives.

The second barrier, limited interaction, is a problem for lawyers when they play the detective role, which they must at times. In one convicted company we often heard comments such as: "Lawyers only come around when they're invited. That's only when we're in trouble. We could really use a lot more of a missionary effort from the legal department with more frequent visits." Lawyers also complain that meeting people at infrequent lectures and formal visits rarely gives them the information that they seek.

Part of this problem is owing not only to the frequency of the visit, but also to the level of the people visited. At many companies lawyers often meet with only top level managers who are expected to spread the word through the organization. Unfortunately, the word rarely reaches the people in an organization who are the most vulnerable and who need to hear it most. One convicted sales manager explained:

> If you want to face facts, we never got any indication from above that what we were doing was wrong. I was never asked to attend any of the lectures our legal division gave. I guess only the general managers did. If any applicable information had ever been passed down to me or if there had been any support to ask questions from above, I don't know what I would have done. You can bet that, at the least, I would have begun to ask some questions.

The third barrier, boredom, stems from the educator role that the corporate counsel must assume. One lawyer in one of the convicted companies complained, "We really don't know how to teach this stuff without sending people off to the coffeepot." Another lawyer complained that only now, because the costs of prosecution have been so severe, are people starting to listen.

Some companies have developed successful legal programs by fostering very close contact between the general managers and the legal division. In one such program there are two lawyers who specialize in traveling around and meeting the general managers. The chief legal counsel added:

> Any whistle blowing probably comes through the lawyers. This style of communication is essential in getting the point across. We try to be serious and sincere. Also the approach is important. A lot of smart legal departments used to start off with the first line of vice presidents and work up in their education program. However, these people often think that they're smarter than the lawyer or else they may not have very good communication with their subordinates, so we try to get close to the danger line. If nothing happens in five years, they say we're paranoid, but with top management support we can continue.

Thus even a successful program has problems of its own. If it works, people may not believe it was needed in the first place.[18]

Executives in another company, which was not involved in the conspiracy, agree with the need to tailor a program to the danger line of the organization. Outside counsel is extensively involved on two levels. First, attorneys meet with each salesman on a one-on-one basis. The lawyer digs up expense reports and other files and grills the salesman. This same procedure is then repeated at group and general manager meetings.

At the general manager and vice president levels, the legal staff puts on a simulated grand jury inquiry. In these dramatizations even the president sits on the witness stand to defend himself on the basis of documents prepared by his vice presidents. There is a great deal of tension surrounding these mock trials. The president of this company cited this trial as:

> . . . one of the most important ways we've sought to keep the organization sensitive to legal issues. We identify several hundred people with point-of-sales exposure and talk to a large percentage of that group. We're trying to get the lawyers to prepare a dossier and challenge each of these people. This confessional situation is a very intensive experience.

This procedure helps management spot problems so it can clear up misunderstandings before they become more serious. The possible interpretations of employee words and actions are made very clear. The president said that this sort of investigation on top of the usual lectures is needed to bring the message across: "We've had attorneys giving their fire and brimstone talks to large groups for 10 to 15 years, and we have simply concluded that isn't strong enough medicine for this ailment. Our experiences in other parts of the company convinced us that this thoroughness is vital."

Several members of this same company told us that they feel more comfortable discussing these issues with outside counsel, as this plan provides. They prefer speaking to someone who represents broader legal expertise and who is not immediately tied in with the corporate hierarchy and internal pressure. The interrogation by a fresh outsider seems to bring more reality to the investigation.

Most of the managers in the company believe that communication with counsel is protected by attorney-client privilege, but recent court decisions suggest that should the interests of the corporation differ from those of any executives, it is the corporation, in the name of the shareholders, not management, which really has the right of attorney-client privilege. Unless shareholders abdicate this right, management cannot be categorically protected in such communication.[19] The use of safeguarded channels of communication, however, whether they be lawyers or general ombudsmen, is important for individuals trapped by the questionable practices of superiors.[20]

## Professional Pride

Many industries share the exposures to price fixing we have highlighted. And the problems of ensuring compliance increase in complexity as the list of contributing factors grows. Our review of the specific compliance methods that are being used in the forest products companies with the better records provides a good start toward the development of a fail-safe approach. In our interviews we were also searching for a promising general approach—perhaps a philosophy of management—that could infuse a company and serve as an antibody to thoughts of price collusion.

We believe we did find such a condition in one company. The evidence we saw was largely indirect, but it can probably best be characterized as professional pride. This company is one of the handful that is largely successful in developing a differentiated set of products. It is no accident. Even in the face of all the industry difficulties we have cited there exists a very strong belief that "if we're not smart enough to make reasonable profits without resorting to any form of price fixing, we'll simply get out of the business."

This belief is translated at the individual level into "I'd rather quit than stoop to getting my results that way." In effect, this company's executives are making an old-fashioned distinction between clean, earned profits and rigged, dirty profits. It is literally unthinkable for them to want to make money the latter way. They have too much self-esteem.

Although executives and salespeople in this company widely share the strong code of behavior, it is not clear exactly how it has been disseminated throughout the organization. The best evidence is that when top managers emphasize professional pride and the distinction between clean and dirty profits, the commitment to achieve profits through legal means is clearly driven down the line. Such emphasis cuts out ambiguous signals that lead to junior people second-guessing top management's intentions.

### APPENDIX

#### Costs of Ambiguous Policies

In late 1976, a federal judge imposed fines, probation, or jail terms on 47 of 48 executives in 22 companies charged with and found guilty of price-fixing violations in the folding-carton industry. In terms of the numbers of defendants, this case was the largest price-fixing one since 1964.

Of those convicted, 15, including chief executive officers, were sentenced to brief prison terms, from 5 to 60 days, and were individually fined as much as $35,000. Of the remaining executives, 17 were fined from $500 to $30,000 and placed on probation. The remaining 15 executives were fined between $100 and

$2,500. The 22 companies were initially fined $50,000 each, the maximum fine for a misdemeanor violation. The maximum fine now for a felony violation of antitrust law is $2 million for each violating company.

Following these criminal convictions, the companies faced 45 civil suits filed by customers seeking damages for alleged overcharges. Over the past two years, many of these same companies have been inundated with charges of criminal price fixing involving felony and misdemeanor violations in virtually every one of the converting ends of the business. One chief executive officer reported that his folding-carton division's past five years' earnings had been surpassed by just the legal fees involved in this case. The cost to image and company morale is incalculable.

### NOTES

1. "Carter Trust Busters," *Newsweek*, September 26, 1977.
2. United States v. Park 421 U.S. Court 658 (1975); Tony McAdams and Robert C. Miljus, "Growing Criminal Liability of Executives," HBR March–April 1977, p. 36.
3. Timothy D. Schellhardt, "Price-Fixing Charges Rise in Industry Despite Convictions," *Wall Street Journal*, May 4, 1978, p. 31.
4. "13 Paper Concerns Face Price Fixing Charges," *New York Times*, December 23, 1977, p. D5; "Two Paper Firms are Convicted in Price-Fixing," *Wall Street Journal*, November 27, 1977, p. 3; "Indictment Cites 14 Paper Makers for Price-Fixing," *Wall Street Journal*, January 26, 1978, p. 3; Morris S. Thompson, "Aides of Box-Making Concerns Sentenced to Prison, Fined in Price-Fixing Case," *Wall Street Journal*, December 1, 1976, p. 4.
5. Schellhardt, "Price-Fixing Charges Rise," p. 1.
6. John Herling, *The Great Price Conspiracy* (Washington, D.C.: Luce, 1962), p. 241.
7. W. Bruce Erickson, "Price Fixing Conspiracies, Their Long Term Impact," *Journal of Industrial Economics*, March 1976, p. 200; Almarin Phillips, *Market Structure, Organization and Performance* (Cambridge: Harvard University Press, 1962). The belief is that as the number of companies increases, the probability of mutual understanding and anticompetitive agreement will decrease.
8. Herling, *The Great Price Conspiracy*, p. 249.
9. Schellhardt, "Price-Fixing Charges Rise," p. 1.
10. The recent acquisition spree may exacerbate this problem. See "The Great Takeover Binge," *Business Week*, November 14, 1977, p. 176.
11. Gilbert Geis, "White Collar Crime: The Heavy Electrical Equipment Antitrust Case in 1961," in *Criminal Behavior Systems: A Typology*, eds. Marshall B. Clinard and Richard Quinrey (New York: Holt, Rinehart and Winston, 1967), p. 150. Here it is explained that structural factors are major contributing elements to criminal behavior. Executives who were uncooperative with price-fixing training were transferred by the company. These issues are more fully discussed in: Laura Shill Schrager and James J. Short, Jr., "Toward a Sociology of Organizational Crime," presented at the American Sociological Association meeting, Chicago, August 1977.
12. "Administered Prices," Hearings Before the Subcommittee on Anti-trust and Monopoly of the Committee on the Judiciary, U.S. Senate, April 12 to May 2, 1961, p. 17065.
13. Adam Smith, *The Wealth of Nations*.
14. "Administered Prices," p. 16663.
15. Stanley Milgrim, *Obedience to Authority: An Experimental View* (New York: Harper & Row, 1974).
16. Raymond Baumhart, *An Honest Profit* (New York: Holt, Rinehart and Winston, 1968). This survey, based on 1,710 subscribers responding to an HBR poll, found most subordinates ultimately accept the values of chief executives. See also Archie

B. Carrol, "Managerial Ethics: A Post Watergate View," *Business Horizons*, April 1975, p. 75.

17. William D. Hartley, "More Firms Now Stress In-House Auditing, But It's Old Hat at GE . . . Staff Doesn't Spare Top Brass Keeping Antitrust Vigil," *Wall Street Journal*, August 22, 1977, p. 75.

18. These sorts of frustrations are frequently heard in legal conferences, for example, see Allen D. Choka, "The Role of Corporate Counsel," presentation at the Eighth Annual Corporate Counsel Institute, Northwestern School of Law, October 8 and 9, 1969.

19. Howard E. O'Leary, Jr., "Criminal Antitrust and the Corporate Executive," *American Bar Association Journal*, October 1977, p. 1389; "Attorneys Privilege," *U.S. Law Week*, *Bureau of National Affairs*, February 28, 1978, p. 2435.

20. Helen Dudar, "The Price of Blowing the Whistle," *New York Times Magazine*, October 30, 1977, p. 41.

# 9

# The Parable of the Sadhu

## BOWEN H. McCOY

Last year, as the first participant in the new six-month sabbatical program that Morgan Stanley has adopted, I enjoyed a rare opportunity to collect my thoughts as well as do some traveling. I spent the first three months in Nepal, walking 600 miles through 200 villages in the Himalayas and climbing some 120,000 vertical feet. On the trip my sole Western companion was an anthropologist who shed light on the cultural patterns of the villages we passed through.

During the Nepal hike, something occurred that has had a powerful impact on my thinking about corporate ethics. Although some might argue that the experience has no relevance to business, it was a situation in which a basic ethical dilemma suddenly intruded into the lives of a group of individuals. How the group responded I think holds a lesson for all organizations no matter how defined.

### The Sadhu

The Nepal experience was more rugged and adventuresome than I had anticipated. Most commercial treks last two or three weeks and cover a quarter of the distance we traveled.

My friend Stephen, the anthropologist, and I were halfway through the 60-day Himalayan part of the trip when we reached the high point, an 18,000-foot pass over a crest that we'd have to traverse to reach to the village of Muklinath, an ancient holy place for pilgrims.

Six years earlier I had suffered pulmonary edema, an acute form of altitude sickness, at 16,500 feet in the vicinity of Everest base camp, so we were understandably concerned about what would happen at 18,000 feet. Moreover, the Himalayas were having their wettest spring in 20 years; hip-deep powder and ice had already driven us off one ridge. If we failed to cross the pass, I feared that the last half of our "once in a lifetime" trip would be ruined.

The night before we would try the pass, we camped at a hut at 14,500 feet. In the photos taken at that camp, my face appears wan. The last village we'd passed through was a sturdy two-day walk below us, and I was tired.

During the late afternoon, four backpackers from New Zealand joined us, and we spent most of the night awake, anticipating the climb. Below we could see the fires of two other parties, which turned out to be two Swiss couples and a Japanese hiking club.

To get over the steep part of the climb before the sun melted the steps cut in the ice, we departed at 3:30 A.M. The New Zealanders left first, followed by Stephen and myself, our porters and Sherpas, and then the Swiss. The Japanese lingered in their camp. The sky was clear, and we were confident that no spring storm would erupt that day to close the pass.

At 15,500 feet, it looked to me as if Stephen were shuffling and staggering a bit, which are symptoms of altitude sickness. (The initial stage of altitude sickness brings a headache and nausea. As the condition worsens, a climber may encounter difficult breathing, disorientation, aphasia, and paralysis.) I felt strong, my adrenaline was flowing, but I was very concerned about my ultimate ability to get across. A couple of our porters were also suffering from the height, and Pasang, our Sherpa sirdar (leader), was worried.

Just after daybreak, while we rested at 15,500 feet, one of the New Zealanders, who had gone ahead, came staggering down toward us with a body slung across his shoulders. He dumped the almost naked, barefoot body of an Indian holy man — a sadhu — at my feet. He had found the pilgrim lying on the ice, shivering and suffering from hypothermia. I cradled the sadhu's head and laid him out on the rocks. The New Zealander was angry. He wanted to get across the pass before the bright sun melted the snow. He said, "Look, I've done what I can. You have porters and Sherpa guides. You care for him. We're going on!" He turned and went back up the mountain to join his friends.

I took a carotid pulse and found that the sadhu was still alive. We figured he had probably visited the holy shrines at Muklinath and was on his way home. It was fruitless to question why he had chosen this desperately high route instead of the safe, heavily traveled caravan route through the Kali Gandaki gorge. Or why he was almost naked and with no shoes, or how long he had been lying in the pass. The answers weren't going to solve our problem.

Stephen and the four Swiss began stripping off outer clothing and opening their packs. The sadhu was soon clothed from head to foot. He was not able to walk, but he was very much alive. I looked down the mountain and spotted below the Japanese climbers marching up with a horse.

Without a great deal of thought, I told Stephen and Pasang that I was concerned about withstanding the heights to come and wanted to get over the pass. I took off after several of our porters who had gone ahead.

On the steep part of the ascent where, if the ice steps had given way, I would have slid down about 3,000 feet, I felt vertigo. I stopped for a breather, allowing the Swiss to catch up with me. I inquired about the sadhu and Stephen. They said that the sadhu was fine and that Stephen was just behind. I set off again for the summit.

Stephen arrived at the summit an hour after I did. Still exhilarated by victory, I ran down the snow slope to congratulate him. He was suffering from altitude sickness, walking 15 steps, then stopping, walking 15 steps, then stopping. Pasang accompanied him all the way up. When I reached them, Stephen glared at me and said: "How do you feel about contributing to the death of a fellow man?"

I did not fully comprehend what he meant.

"Is the sadhu dead?" I inquired.

"No," replied Stephen, "but he surely will be!"

After I had gone, and the Swiss had departed not long after, Stephen had remained with the sadhu. When the Japanese had arrived, Stephen had asked to use their horse to transport the sadhu down to the hut. They had refused. He had then asked Pasang to have a group of our porters carry the sadhu. Pasang had resisted the idea, saying that the porters would have to exert all their energy to get themselves over the pass. He had thought they could not carry a man down 1,000 feet to the hut, reclimb the slope, and get across safely before the snow melted. Pasang had pressed Stephen not to delay any longer.

The Sherpas had carried the sadhu down to a rock in the sun at about 15,000 feet and had pointed out the hut another 500 feet below. The Japanese had given him food and drink. When they had last seen him he was listlessly throwing rocks at the Japanese party's dog, which had frightened him.

We do not know if the sadhu lived or died.

For many of the following days and evenings Stephen and I discussed and debated our behavior toward the sadhu. Stephen is a committed Quaker with deep moral vision. He said, "I feel that what happened with the sadhu is a good example of the breakdown between the individual ethic and the corporate ethic. No one person was willing to assume ultimate responsibility for the sadhu. Each was willing to do his bit just so long as it was not too inconvenient. When it got to be a bother, everyone just passed the buck to someone else and took off. Jesus was relevant to a more individualistic stage of society, but how do we interpret his teaching today in a world filled with large, impersonal organizations and groups?"

I defended the larger group, saying, "Look, we all cared. We all stopped and gave aid and comfort. Everyone did his bit. The New Zealander carried him down below the snow line. I took his pulse and suggested we treat him for hypothermia. You and the Swiss gave him clothing and got him warmed up. The Japanese gave him food and water. The Sherpas carried him down to the sun and pointed out the easy trail toward the hut. He was well enough to throw rocks at a dog. What more could we do?"

"You have just described the typical affluent Westerner's response to a problem. Throwing money—in this case food and sweaters—at it, but not solving the fundamentals!" Stephen retorted.

"What would satisfy you?" I said. "Here we are, a group of New Zealanders, Swiss, Americans, and Japanese who have never met before and who are at the apex of one of the most powerful experiences of our lives. Some years the pass is so bad no one gets over it. What right does an almost naked pilgrim who chooses the wrong trail have to disrupt our lives? Even the Sherpas had no interest in risking the trip to help him beyond a certain point."

Stephen calmly rebutted, "I wonder what the Sherpas would have done if the sadhu had been a well-dressed Nepali, or what the Japanese would have done if the sadhu had been a well-dressed Asian, or what you would have done, Buzz, if the sadhu had been a well-dressed Western woman?"

"Where, in your opinion," I asked instead, "is the limit of our responsibility in a situation like this? We had our own well-being to worry about. Our Sherpa guides were unwilling to jeopardize us or the porters for the sadhu. No one else on the mountain was willing to commit himself beyond certain self-imposed limits."

Stephen said, "As individual Christians or people with a Western ethical tradition, we can fulfill our obligations in such a situation only if (1) the sadhu dies in our care, (2) the sadhu demonstrates to us that he could undertake the two-day walk down to the village, or (3) we carry the sadhu for two days down to the village and convince someone there to care for him."

"Leaving the sadhu in the sun with food and clothing, while he demonstrated hand-eye coordination by throwing a rock at a dog, comes close to fulfilling items one and two," I answered. "And it wouldn't have made sense to take him to the village where the people appeared to be far less caring than the Sherpas, so the third condition is impractical. Are you really saying that, no matter what the implications, we should, at the drop of a hat, have changed our entire plan?"

## The Individual versus the Group Ethic

Despite my arguments, I felt and continue to feel guilt about the sadhu. I had literally walked through a classic moral dilemma without fully thinking through the consequences. My excuses for my actions include a high adrenaline flow, a super-ordinate goal, and a once-in-a-lifetime opportunity—factors in the usual corporate situation, especially when one is under stress.

Real moral dilemmas are ambiguous, and many of us hike right through them, unaware that they exist. When, usually after the fact, someone makes an issue of them, we tend to resent his or her bringing it up. Often, when the full import of what we have done (or not done) falls on us, we dig into a defensive position from which it is very difficult to emerge. In rare circumstances we may contemplate what we have done from inside a prison.

Had we mountaineers been free of physical and mental stress caused by the effort and the high altitude, we might have treated the sadhu differently. Yet isn't stress the real test of personal and corporate values? The instant decisions executives make under pressure reveal the most about personal and corporate character.

Among the many questions that occur to me when pondering my experience are: What are the practical limits of moral imagination and vision? Is there a collective or institutional ethic beyond the ethics of the individual? At what level of effort or commitment can one discharge one's ethical responsibilities?

Not every ethical dilemma has a right solution. Reasonable people often disagree; otherwise there would be no dilemma. In a business context, however, it is essential that managers agree on a process for dealing with dilemmas.

The sadhu experience offers an interesting parallel to business situations. An immediate response was mandatory. Failure to act was a decision in itself. Up on the mountain we could not resign and submit our résumés to a headhunter. In contrast to philosophy, business involves action and implementation — getting things done. Managers must come up with answers to problems based on what they see and what they allow to influence their decision-making processes. On the mountain, none of us but Stephen realized the true dimensions of the situation we were facing.

One of our problems was that as a group we had no process for developing a consensus. We had no sense of purpose or plan. The difficulties of dealing with the sadhu were so complex that no one person could handle it. Because it did not have a set of preconditions that could guide its action to an acceptable resolution, the group reacted instinctively as individuals. The cross-cultural nature of the group added a further layer of complexity. We had no leader with whom we could all identify and in whose purpose we believed. Only Stephen was willing to take charge, but he could not gain adequate support to care for the sadhu.

Some organizations do have a value system that transcends the personal values of the managers. Such values, which go beyond profitability, are usually revealed when the organization is under stress. People throughout the organization generally accept its values, which, because they are not presented as a rigid list of commandments, may be somewhat ambiguous. The stories people tell, rather than printed materials, transmit these conceptions of what is proper behavior.

For 20 years I have been exposed at senior levels to a variety of corporations and organizations. It is amazing how quickly an outsider can sense the tone and style of an organization and the degree of tolerated openness and freedom to challenge management.

Organizations that do not have a heritage of mutually accepted, shared values tend to become unhinged during stress, with each individual bailing out for himself. In the great takeover battles we have witnessed during past years, companies that had strong cultures drew the wagons around them and fought it out, while other companies saw executives supported by their golden parachutes, bail out of the struggles.

Because corporations and their members are interdependent, for the corporation to be strong the members need to share a preconceived notion of what is correct behavior, a "business ethic," and think of it as a positive force, not a constraint.

As an investment banker I am continually warned by well-meaning lawyers, clients, and associates to be wary of conflicts of interest. Yet if I were to run away from every difficult situation, I wouldn't be an effective investment banker. I have to feel my way through conflicts. An effective manager can't run from risk either; he or she has to confront and deal with risk. To feel "safe" in doing this, managers need the guidelines of an agreed-on process and set of values within the organization.

After my three months in Nepal, I spent three months as an executive-in-residence at both Stanford Business School and the Center for Ethics and Social Policy at the Graduate Theological Union at Berkeley. These six months away from my job gave me time to assimilate 20 years of business experience. My thoughts turned often to the meaning of the leadership role in any large organization. Students at the seminary thought of themselves as antibusiness. But when I questioned them they agreed that they distrusted all large organizations, including the church. They perceived all large organizations as impersonal and opposed to individual values and needs. Yet we all know of organizations where peoples' values and beliefs are respected and their expressions encouraged. What makes the difference? Can we identify the difference and, as a result, manage more effectively?

The word "ethics" turns off many and confuses more. Yet the notions of shared values and an agreed-on process for dealing with adversity and change —what many people mean when they talk about corporate culture—seem to be at the heart of the ethical issue. People who are in touch with their own core beliefs and the beliefs of others and are sustained by them can be more comfortable living on the cutting edge. At times, taking a tough line or a decisive stand in a muddle of ambiguity is the only ethical thing to do. If a manager is indecisive and spends time trying to figure out the "good" thing to do, the enterprise may be lost.

Business ethics, then, has to do with the authenticity and integrity of the enterprise. To be ethical is to follow the business as well as the cultural goals of the corporation, its owners, its employees, and its customers. Those who cannot serve the corporate vision are not authentic business people and, therefore, are not ethical in the business sense.

At this stage of my own business experience I have a strong interest in organizational behavior. Sociologists are keenly studying what they call corporate stories, legends, and heroes as a way organizations have of transmitting the value system. Corporations such as Arco have even hired consultants to perform an audit of their corporate culture. In a company, the leader is the person who understands, interprets, and manages the corporate value system. Effective managers are then action-oriented people who resolve conflict, are tolerant of ambiguity, stress, and change, and have a strong sense of purpose for themselves and their organizations.

If all this is true, I wonder about the role of the professional manager who moves from company to company. How can he or she quickly absorb the values and culture of different organizations? Or is there, indeed, an art of management that is totally transportable? Assuming such fungible managers do exist, is it proper for them to manipulate the values of others?

What would have happened had Stephen and I carried the sadhu for two days back to the village and become involved with the villagers in his care? In four trips to Nepal my most interesting experiences occurred in 1975 when I lived in a Sherpa home in the Khumbu for five days recovering from altitude sickness. The high point of Stephen's trip was an invitation to participate in a family funeral ceremony in Manang. Neither experience had to do with climbing the high passes of the Himalayas. Why were we so reluctant to try the lower path, the ambiguous trail? Perhaps because we did not have a leader who could reveal the greater purpose of the trip to us.

Why didn't Stephen with his moral vision opt to take the sadhu under his personal care? The answer is because, in part, Stephen was hard-stressed physically himself, and because, in part, without some support system that involved our involuntary and episodic community on the mountain, it was beyond his individual capacity to do so.

I see the current interest in corporate culture and corporate value systems as a positive response to Stephen's pessimism about the decline of the role of the individual in large organizations. Individuals who operate from a thoughtful set of personal values provide the foundation for a corporate culture. A corporate tradition that encourages freedom of inquiry, supports personal values, and reinforces a focused sense of direction can fulfill the need for individuality along with the prosperity and success of the group. Without such corporate support, the individual is lost.

That is the lesson of the sadhu. In a complex corporate situation, the individual requires and deserves the support of the group. If people cannot find such support from their organization, they don't know how to act. If such support is forthcoming, a person has a stake in the success of the group, and can add much to the process of establishing and maintaining a corporate culture. It is management's challenge to be sensitive to individual needs, to shape them, and to direct and focus them for the benefit of the group as a whole.

For each of us the sadhu lives. Should we stop what we are doing and comfort him; or should we keep trudging up toward the high pass? Should I pause to help the derelict I pass on the street each night as I walk by the Yale Club en route to Grand Central Station? Am I his brother? What is the nature of our responsibility if we consider ourselves to be ethical persons? Perhaps it is to change the values of the group so that it can, with all its resources, take the other road.

# PART THREE

# THREE

# Executive Action for Moral Outcomes

The course each person must follow to be a qualified and authoritative analyst and responsible actor in ethically ambiguous situations is at best difficult. In a hostile environment it may become so nearly impossible as to require resignation as an alternative to self-betrayal. The program of action appropriate to a company in which the management has become aware of its problems depends, like most crucial decisions, on the company's industry, history, and character. But though the program cannot be derived from a series of maxims or imitated in detail from other companies, its main outlines will address universal needs and be recognizable, however unique in detail may be the history and tradition of the company and its present ethical condition.

The articles in this part continue to refer to the autonomy and ethical awareness of the individual as the key to the decision to protect the integrity of persons and processes as competitive advantage in the marketplace is pursued. The articles extend the discussion of corporate pressures, intricately disguised by rationalization, to succumb to immorality. But each emphasizes, by implication or direct advice, action that may be taken to resolve ethical conflicts and to carry out policy decisions.

Kenneth Goodpaster's "Ethical Imperatives and Corporate Leadership" comments on the Gellerman and McCoy articles in the course of interpreting the source of shoddy behavior as "teleopathy." This is his word for the imbalance in corporate purposes that makes a narrowly defined purpose (for example, to become number one in market share) the supreme guide for action, to the exclusion of more broadly defined economic goals and of ethical consideration of process and obligations. His typology of different kinds of management thinking sets up a framework within which most of the issues discussed in the articles presented here may be reviewed. The imperatives for corporate leadership are orienting (read *shaping*), institutionalizing, and maintaining consciously understood corporate values.

Thereafter the article is predominantly concerned with action. The allusions to companies may suggest to the readers analogous observations from their own situations. Goodpaster's paper is the product of a long and increasingly successful effort (which I have alluded to before) of a scholarly moral philosopher to bring his discipline to practical application. For those who wish to go more deeply into the moral mazes of philosophy, or even to consider further the ethical irrelevance and missed opportunities for the educational system, his classifications are analytically useful.

David Ewing's "Case of the Rogue Division" is an interesting down-to-earth example of a major scandal in the district office of a large division of a much larger national organization. Readers are asked to put themselves in the shoes of the division president and tell the parent company's vice president what he plans to do. Then, the reader is given the comments of three executives, among them Douglas Sherwin, who later wrote "The Ethical Roots of the Business System" in Part II. Donald N. Scobel's comments bear directly on the level of awareness and searching inquiry required to deal with breaches of trust.

The commentators address the responsibility of top management in the parent company and the division for the illegal behavior taking place in the district. They recommend full disclosure, preparation for taking severe criticism, and a series of steps to prevent a recurrence. The role of obsolete assumptions about employee motivation, the right of management to be investigator, prosecutor, and judge of its own employees without reference to due process, the exemption of high levels of management from accountability for the behavior on lower levels, and the adequacy of routine accounting and control are all challenged. The obsession with profits that either exists or is thought to exist in almost all companies in which public scandal erupts leads Sherwin to rework the threadbare idea that profit maximization for the shareholders is the purpose of business. Employees' objectives have to be met, of course, for profits cannot be sought at the expense of customers or employees without jeopardizing future profits for investors. The instance in the company of what Goodpaster calls teleopathy is striking. It illustrates the stubborn fact that the relation of profit to the means and timing for achieving it poses a permanent riddle to people on the firing line, whose obligation for results may lead to undesired consequences.

I have placed Laura L. Nash's "Ethics without the Sermon," which emphasizes leadership in the war against the hazards of individual vulnerability to organization pressures, in this part for one good reason. Rather than specifying action as such, the essay poses twelve questions with the motive, not of solving complex questions about the general welfare, but of avoiding harm while focusing on limited purposes. The questions are not difficult. They seem to me to initiate at long last the possibility that with the wish and the will, inquiry into the ethical implications in advance of a decision is not so difficult after all. Action becomes much easier if its consequences are contemplated in advance.

The next article, "Can the Best Corporations Be Made Moral?"—more about social responsibility than corporate ethics as such—could well be read as further discussion of the corporation as moral environment. A highly moral and humane chief executive can preside over an amoral organization because the incentive system focuses attention on short-term quantifiable results. This curse is cousin to the obsession for profit at the expense of responsibility. The program of action suggested begins with the incorporation into strategic and operating plans of specific objectives in areas of social concern strategically related to the company's economic activity and community environment. Measurement systems are said to require incorporation of qualitative as well as quantitative measures. When middle managers fall short of their targets, inquiry into the reasons and how to help should precede adverse judgment and penalty. Internal audit should extend its purview beyond financial statements and verification of inventory. The promulgation and enforcement of ethical policy framed in light of the particular vulnerability of industry and company can be a prime subject of internal audit, but bookkeepers cannot then be the audit staff.

The administration of ethical behavior can be as strategic in intention and as concretely supervised, in short, as social responsibility, to which it is related only in the sense that social responsibility, inherently ethical, includes attention to suitable nonfinancial objectives and presumes respect for the needs and rights of others. A study by the Business Roundtable entitled *Corporate Ethics: A Prime Business Asset*, published in 1988, describes the ethical policy and practice in ten companies widely thought of as both economically successful and ethical. The study identifies eight elements influential in sustaining the desired level of ethical performance.

1. Continuity of values in the leadership of successive chief executive officers.

2. Development of a tradition of integrity in the promulgation of standards in all areas where quality is essential.

3. Written statements of belief and policy, perhaps in the form of a credo or code and in crucial cases requiring annual signed statements signifying compliance.

4. Education and training in the meaning of policy and the seriousness of intent.

5. Consideration of ethical performance and interest in community affairs linked to performance evaluation and compensation.

6. Open decision making in which differences of opinion are welcomed and the relevance of ethical standards to proposals is discussed.

7. A control system, fortified by audit, to supplement trust with broad surveillance.

8. Strict and public punishment of identified violations of law or policy.

This agenda does not depart widely from the Sonnenfeld-Lawrence prescription for the folding-carton industry. Product differentiation to avoid price wars and commodity pricing, training to change corporate culture and selling practices, control of pricing by fewer people, development of a code of ethics with recurring audits for compliance, legal training in antitrust issues, and efforts to develop professional pride constitute the program designed to prevent recurrence. Its emphases illustrate how the particular problems of an industry and the vulnerability of a company in it should direct the program of action.

Where there is no tradition to draw on and where (as in the defense industry) a new era must be launched, an ethical turnaround must depend more on explicit training, specific policy, forums for discussion, focused controls, and appropriate rewards and punishment. In this case, announcing decisions taken at the expense of short-term profit to sustain quality or correct mistakes does more than a written policy in maintaining a tradition. The corporation can knowingly exert as much influence in the direction of ethically correct decisions as it sometimes unwittingly does in other direction.

An appropriate coda is Abram T. Collier's "Business Leadership and a Creative Society." So far as I can see, the word *ethics* is hardly mentioned, but the kind of leadership prescribed here is profoundly ethical. Creativity is supported by the goals of happiness, freedom, security, goodness, and truth, but is an even higher value. "The first task of business leaders . . . is to create an environment in which there can flourish not only individual genius but, more important, the collective capacities of other people in the organization."

The concepts on which creativity depends are founded on respect—for differences, between individual and group, for the need for understanding, for the matching of rights to obligations, and for faith in individual growth. This vision of the corporation as a creative society is as far as possible from the narrow view of the corporation as an impersonal profit-maximizing machine with no energy wasted on cultivating other purposes.

The view of leadership presented here cannot possibly make sense to the executive taking counsel on his purpose from the bloodless exponent of the corporation as a profit-maximizing black box. I conclude that as soon as the functions of the corporation are admitted to be carried out by people, whose response to an issue goes beyond their performing routine tasks for market wages, then the cheerless counsel of conventional economic and financial theory becomes mostly inapplicable. The executive who would unleash the collective capacity for achievement of an organization held down by unrecognized bureaucratic constraints and misinterpretation of what is wanted of its members should abandon the amorality of theoretical profit maximization. Stretched too far, the pursuit of self-interest by organizations and the multiple personal concerns by people with no awareness of the means by which self-interest is pursued or of its effect on other contestants rapidly becomes unethical under pressure. As we have seen, this development may be unnoticed because of the capacity to rationalize wrongdoing as justifiable in the light of apparently good results.

The theory of capitalism that self-seeking very lightly supervised by law and by permissive or readily stretched rules of the game will in a free market serve the public interest no longer is credible in an era of bureaucratic corporations and regulated or administered markets. To rely on the theory as on the innate morality thought to be conveyed to the individual by the family, community, and school is evidently foolhardy.

The alternative to a theory left behind by the evolution of the corporation is to accord equal attention to goals for economic performance and goals for developing the means by which the performance is to be achieved and made equal to or better than that of competitors. Developing a strategy that includes what an organization is to become, its aspirations for development of internal capability, and a policy for encouraging and requiring ethical and responsible conduct is as feasible as deciding what products to bring to chosen markets with what profit and growth objectives. If ethics means in part attention to means as well as ends, to fairness, and to respect for individuals, then such a strategy will be ethical, at least in intent.

The influence of the financial community has obscured the vision of leadership that Collier presents. The CEO whose attention is monopolized by the self-styled crusaders for the shareholder in the takeover movement looks to his compensation, to leveraged buy-outs, golden parachutes, and poison pills rather than to creative strategies for better qualified organizations and better performance in the marketplace. His vulnerability to unfriendly takeovers may be the result of unwise growth goals and acquisitions. Not only are the latter usually unsuccessful, but they leave seams in an organization that can lead to its dismemberment and make it attractive to raiders. The financial community, resurrecting financial theory in the name of short-term benefits to the shareholders of companies taken over, has no noticeable interest in the implications of leadership and the development of the capability of the corporation. Such amorality is always on the verge of becoming immoral.

Executives appear, perhaps in the name of survival, to abandon the course they think is right, and indeed their companies, to defensive dismemberment or to takeover. The path to independent judgment comes quickly to an end — either because the strategy in question was ill conceived or poorly implemented or the will was weak. Conventional economic theory, certainly no respecter of persons, remains so powerful as to exact craven behavior from those not really equal to the demands of the economic achievement that ethical aspirations should make possible as that performance keeps raiders from the door.

The prospect for more resolute commitment to the kind of leadership that corporations require as human organizations is at the moment, I fear, not very bright. The opportunity for broader-gauged leadership has been opened by the development of the corporation beyond its role to maximize the shareholders' interests. Whether it is seized will depend upon the caliber of the persons appointed to high office. One of the hallmarks of the successful executive is widely believed to be the capacity to balance the need for continuing present profit with the need for investment in longer term profits. When this tension is not unfairly interfered with, this capacity can be developed in profit centers of appropriate size at an early age. Another hallmark is the ability to reconcile the conflicting demands of economic success and clear-cut ethical standards. This ability can also be observed and encouraged. That equal weight should be given to character and competence is the least that an aspiring executive should expect.

# 1

# Ethical Imperatives and Corporate Leadership

KENNETH E. GOODPASTER

To improve our understanding of the emerging field of business ethics is no small task, given the explosion of interest in the subject during the past decade. Voices are entering the conversation from virtually every quarter of the academy, the business world, and the media.

This new level of attention is a valuable precondition to positive intellectual

*This paper was first presented as the Ruffin Lecture in Business Ethics at the Darden Graduate School of Business Administration, University of Virginia, in April 1988.

and social change and to improved practice. Consider the following developments:

1. Business schools are reaching both outward and inward to address the moral dimensions of their educational mission.

2. Students of business are demonstrating heightened concern about ethical values as they prepare for professional business careers.

3. Corporate leaders and executives are reflecting more than ever before on the ethical aspects of business life.

4. Philosophers and other scholars in the humanities are widening their commitment to constructive social and institutional criticism.

5. The media are expanding the public's understanding of both the conceptual and practical implications of ethical criticism.

This is the good news, as I see it. The not-so-good news is our limited knowledge and our limited focus. With respect to knowledge, we have only begun to appreciate the complexities involved in the application of moral categories to contemporary business life. While the data base has expanded, the knowledge base, in the form of imaginative, coordinated teaching and research programs, has not kept pace. The disciplinary barriers are still strong, making it difficult for academics to communicate with one another, let alone with practitioners.

With respect to focus, there is resistance from those who fear that the new field of business ethics is somehow economically, politically, or educationally subversive. It is variously seen as amateurish, unrealistic, and unteachable. Skeptics damn it when it displays no bottom line, and other critics damn it when it does. This is the state of our art.

In this chapter, I will sketch out some ideas and aspirations about the next act in the unfolding drama. We have developed many of the conceptual tools, and a fair amount of the educational and professional access needed to use them. A period of consolidation is needed, along with cooperative research between disciplines, as business ethics finds its way into professional education and corporate policy. To clarify this suggestion, I offer below some reflections on what I take to be the *normative core* of the emerging field of business ethics. If we can connect our analytical and empirical efforts to a shared perception, we will minimize the risk of a Tower of Babel.

In Part I, the subject is the common ethical challenge faced by both the business professional (as an individual) *and* the business organization. I will argue that meeting this challenge defines the normative core of business ethics. The task of addressing the challenge in theory lies principally with the academy. The task of addressing it in practice lies principally with corporate leadership.

In Part II, I will elicit from the normative core a three-part "moral agenda" for corporate leadership: orienting, institutionalizing, and sustaining shared ethical values. Theoretical and practical reflection on the full implications of this agenda, in my opinion, can provide a touchstone for future teaching and research in business ethics.

## Part I. The Normative Core

The claims of morality, as they operate in human life, present on the face of it a very different appearance from the claims of policy or purpose. They come as a recognized obligation to do or not to do, which is often seen to involve the temporary surrender or restriction of a desire in itself innocent, of a perfectly legitimate purpose. All serious moralists have had to recognize this very obvious and familiar contrast.

J. L. Stocks, 1930

When reflective observers from a striking variety of backgrounds (including psychoanalysis, medicine, law, political and moral philosophy, business administration, and corporate leadership) appear to circle around an idea that has relevance to the field of business ethics, one must take notice and think it through. Let us do just that to introduce and make useful what I am calling the normative core.

### Five Windows on the Core

Twelve years ago, in an insightful but disturbing book entitled *The Gamesman*, psychoanalyst Michael Maccoby described what he called "careerism" as an emotionally self-destructive affliction of many successful executives:

> Obsessed with winning, the gamesman views all of his actions in terms of whether they will help him succeed in his career. The individual's sense of identity, integrity, and self-determination is lost as he treats himself as an object whose worth is determined by its fluctuating market value. Careerism demands [emotional] detachment.[1]

Maccoby's belief was that such emotional detachment corroded integrity — that it led to disintegration of character because it did not allow for a proper balance between what he referred to as traits of the "head" (e.g., initiative, cooperativeness, flexibility, coolness under stress) in contrast to traits of the "heart" (e.g., honesty, friendliness, compassion, generosity, idealism).

The problem, in his view, was that management needed qualities of the heart fully as much as qualities of the head — but modern corporations tended to reinforce careerism instead. Companies (and other institutions) often systematically select against the wholeness needed for managers and leaders, Maccoby argued. Most executives writing to *Fortune* magazine in 1977, after the initial publication of these ideas, confirmed Maccoby's diagnosis. Recent events do not suggest that the problem has disappeared.

Maccoby, drawing on the work of Eric Fromm, identified a central psychological risk of business life. But when we look closely at the traits or virtues to which he paid attention in his study (traits of "head" and "heart"), I think we can see that this psychological view harbors at its core an *ethical* view. For it is the moral integrity as well as the mental health of business professionals that is behind the scenes in Maccoby's study. The question his work posed was whether the moral point of view was systematically "selected against" in the context of modern business life in large organizations.

In a series of *New Yorker* articles that appeared about the same time as Maccoby's work, political theorist and philosopher Hannah Arendt wrote about the "banality of evil," the utter thoughtlessness of wrongdoing, in contrast to our often dramatic preconceptions. The context of Arendt's remarks was her observation of the mindset of Adolf Eichmann during his trial in Jerusalem in the early 1960s:

> The question that imposed itself was, could the activity of thinking as such, the habit of examining whatever happens to come to pass or to attract

attention, regardless of the results and the specific content of the activity—could this activity be among the conditions that make men abstain from evildoing, or even actually "condition" them against it? The very word "conscience," at any rate, points in that direction, insofar as it means "to know with and by myself," a kind of knowledge that is actualized in every thinking process.[2]

Arendt's idea—that evil resides in a kind of thoughtlessness—is not only compatible with, but reinforces, Maccoby's reflections on head and heart. Both see integrity as demanding balance and participation by the whole person in decisions and actions.

Arendt and Maccoby each help us to understand the meaning of psychological and moral integrity. It is a kind of wholeness or balance that refuses to truncate or close off both thoughtfulness and the qualities of the heart—that refuses to anesthetize our humanity in the face of what can sometimes be strong temptations to do so, as when people's lives are affected by business decisions in adverse ways. To quote Arendt again:

Clichés, stock phrases, adherence to conventional, standardized codes of expression and conduct have the socially recognized function of protecting us against reality; that is, against the claim on our thinking attention which all events and facts make by virtue of their existence.[3]

Also in the late 1970s, an essay written several years earlier by philosopher John Ladd began to attract the attention of scholars in business ethics. Ladd described corporations (and formal organizations generally) as rationality-driven machines in which:

the interests and needs of the individuals concerned, as individuals, must be considered only insofar as they establish limiting operating conditions. Organizational rationality dictates that these interests and needs must not be considered in their own right or on their own merits. If we think of an organization as a machine, it is easy to see why we cannot reasonably expect it to have any moral obligations to people or for them to have any to it.[4]

Later in the same essay, Ladd described the consequence for the decision maker as "moral schizophrenia." His argument, in my opinion, went too far by grounding substantive moral criticism on logic alone, implying that amorality in business settings was *a matter of necessity* rather than a matter of observation. But the value of Ladd's insight should not be minimized. He was identifying a malaise that had deep linkages to the perspectives of Maccoby and Arendt. He too provided a window on the normative core.

More recently, against the backdrop of these thoughts of the 1970s, Saul Gellerman, dean of the University of Dallas Graduate School of Management, wrote a perceptive article in the *Harvard Business Review* entitled "How 'Good' Managers Make Bad Ethical Choices." Gellerman suggested the phenomenon of "rationalization" as a key to understanding the principal source of unethical conduct in business. Focusing on a number of well-publicized cases (Manville, Continental Illinois Bank, and E.F. Hutton), Gellerman wrote:

In my view, the explanations go back to four rationalizations that people have relied on through the ages to justify questionable conduct: believing that the activity is not "really" illegal or immoral; that it is in the individual's or the corporation's best interest; that it will never be found out; or that because it helps the company the company will condone it.[5]

Granting that executives have "a right to expect loyalty from employees against competitors and detractors," Gellerman immediately added "but not loyalty against the law, or against common morality, or against society itself."

In 1982, the *Harvard Business Review* established an award "for the best original article written by a corporate manager" that would "inform and expand executives' consideration of ethical problems in business." Our fifth and final window on the normative core comes from the first winner of this award, an essay entitled "The Parable of the Sadhu."

The article was an autobiographical reflection by Bowen H. McCoy, managing director of Morgan Stanley & Co. It described a mountain-climbing experience in which a group of climbers, intent on reaching the summit, faced a painful decision. At 15,500 feet in the Himalayas, they came upon an Indian holy man, a sadhu, who had somehow gotten lost and was in danger of dying from exposure. The group had to decide whether to take the sadhu to safety or to continue toward the summit. Time and circumstances did not permit both. McCoy described the rationalization and eventual continuation toward the summit and then added:

I felt and continue to feel guilt about the sadhu. I had literally walked through a classic moral dilemma without fully thinking through the consequences. My excuses for my actions include a high adrenaline flow, a superordinate goal, and a once-in-a-lifetime opportunity — factors in the usual corporate situation, especially when one is under stress.[6]

McCoy applied the parable to individual managers as well as to corporations. He saw in his mountain-climbing experience a symptom and a symbol of an ethical problem in contemporary business life:

Organizations that do not have a heritage of mutually accepted, shared values tend to become unhinged during stress, with each individual bailing out for himself. In the great takeover battles we have witnessed during past years, companies that had strong cultures drew the wagons around them and fought it out, while other companies saw executives supported by their golden parachutes, bail out of the struggles. . . . Because corporations and their members are interdependent, for the corporation to be strong the members need to share a preconceived notion of what is correct behavior, a "business ethic," and think of it as a positive force, not a constraint.

The phenomena that Maccoby, Arendt, Ladd, Gellerman, and McCoy are attending to (detachment, thoughtlessness, moral schizophrenia, rationalization, singleness of group purpose) display a recurrent pattern. It is striking enough to be given a label and to serve as a paradigm, not only in our thinking about individuals in a *corporate* environment but also about corporations in *their* environment.

## Teleopathy

We can see through these five "windows" an all-too-frequent modern malaise. It is not a sickness that appears in medical or psychiatric manuals. Nor does it appear in the manuals of twentieth-century moral philosophy, preoccupied as these have been with conceptual analysis in contrast to normative ethics. Nor again is it part of most discussions in the literature of management studies or business administration.

I shall refer to the malaise or problem at the normative core as *teleopathy*, combining Greek roots for "goal or purpose" and "disease or sickness." If there were manuals for character disorders in ethics as there are for physical and emotional disorders in medicine, I submit that teleopathy would be a candidate as central in its manual as heart disease and depression are, respectively, in theirs.

For philosophers, teleopathy can be understood as a habit of character that values limited purposes as supremely action-guiding, to the relative exclusion not only of larger ends, but also moral considerations about means, obligations, and duties. It is the unbalanced pursuit of goals or purposes by an individual or group.

Teleopathy in its most abstract form is a suspension of "on-line" moral judgment as a practical force in the life of an individual or group. It substitutes for the call of conscience the call of decision criteria from other sources: winning the game, achieving the goal, following the rules laid down by a framework external to ethical reflection. These other sources generally involve self-interest, peer acceptance, group loyalty, and institutional objectives that themselves may have broad social justification.

Teleopathy is not so much a theory as it is a *condition*. And while we might be inclined to assume that it is a rare condition, I suggest that it is not only common, but even encouraged by the professional climate and culture of modern life. In the business environment, it is evidently widespread. Indeed, it is hard to look at the record of the past decade, including as it does insider trading, industrial espionage, falsifying labor figures on government contracts, ignoring plant safety, deceptive marketing, and insensitivity to employee rights, without a growing recognition that the "bracketing" of moral reflection, both at the level of the individual and at the level of the organized group, is a key part of the explanation.

This is not to say that teleopathy always takes the form of unethical business behavior. But in the vicinity of most unethical business behavior (individual or corporate), we are likely to find teleopathy in one or another of its forms.

Whatever may be the philosophical outcome of the debate over "the moral status of corporations," if we can agree that the normative core of business ethics is similar whether the unit of analysis be the individual in the corporate context or the corporation in the wider social context, we are taking a step forward. I am suggesting that an appreciation of the phenomenon of teleopathy — over-emphasis on limited purposes by individuals and corporations — illuminates a fundamental unity in the multilevel and complex field of business ethics.

Moreover, if I am right, this account of the normative core helps explain why the problems of business ethics *in practice* are so persistent. For, as with their virtues, the pathologies of individuals are both transmitted *to* organizations and reinforced *by* them through the self-perpetuating dynamics of career progression, leadership, management discipline, and corporate culture.

If we add to this organizational dynamic the competitive pressures on the integrity of firms, it is not hard to see how the prospect of reducing teleopathy in the business system can seem overwhelming.

### In Search of Type 3 Management

To clarify further the meaning of teleopathy, let me briefly describe four ways of thinking about ethics in business that may prove useful.

**Type 1 thinking: ethics as a guide to self-interest.** We can imagine an individual holding that his basic value is to look out for himself in a rational way, and that one way of doing so is to be respectful of other persons most of the time. I will refer to this as Type 1 thinking. Organizations might exhibit a similar mindset. The belief would be that respecting others, like honesty, is usually "the best policy."

Type 1 thinking is present wherever ethical values are managed solely with an eye to rational self-interest as the overarching value. It is important to emphasize, however, that this need not mean *ignoring* others in the ordinary sense of that phrase. Some interpretations of "issues management" and "public relations," for example, seem to fit the Type 1 pattern because of the purely self-interested principles behind them, even though they appear on the surface to involve independent concern for others.

**Type 2 thinking: ethics as a systemic constraint.** This type of thinking incorporates ethical norms not through the logic of self-interest but through systemic constraints on the choice of business goals. There are two distinct subtypes. The first looks primarily to market forces as surrogates for morality; the second, to political and legal forces.

**The invisible hand pattern (type 2a).** Some accord importance to ethical norms in business decision making, but quickly add that they are already built into the competitive system. This makes special management attention to ethics redundant. It is what we shall call, remembering Adam Smith, the invisible hand pattern. Nobel laureate Milton Friedman often seems to endorse this way of thinking. The suggestion is that whatever ethical values the business system needs are already programmed in, making supplementary efforts foolish, even morally suspect.

**The hand-of-the-law pattern (type 2b).** This type of thinking relies on noneconomic forces outside the organization to secure the value of, say, environmental protection without direct managerial involvement (a more "visible" than "invisible" hand). Externalizing moral judgment in this way does not mean simply subordinating ethics (as a means) to self-interest. But it does mean placing responsibility for moral judgment outside the manager's principal (economic) concerns. We might say that Type 2b leaders acknowledge authority, but not accountability, when it comes to ethical values.

**Type 3 thinking: ethics as an authoritative guide.** According to this type of thinking, securing respect for others by the invisible hand — and even by more visible hands external to the marketplace, such as government, labor, and the media — is insufficient. Corporate self-interest is not ignored, and neither are competition and the law, but respect for the rights and concerns of affected parties is given independent force in the leader's operating consciousness. Type 3 thinking not only refuses to see ethics as merely a means, it also rejects surrogates for conscience in the form of systemic constraints. Managerial accountability for ethics goes hand in hand with a recognition of its authority.

If we reflect upon the typology just presented, we can see that only Type 3 thinking captures the full meaning of both individual and corporate conscience. For while it is true that the other types espouse ethical values in one way or another, only Type 3 embraces moral obligations *directly*. The others do so *conditionally*: in the case of Type 1, subject to self-interest; and in the case of Types 2a and 2b, subject to institutional structures or systems (the market and the law), which themselves require ethical vigilance both in principle and in operation.

It is with Type 3 thinking that the *balanced* pursuit of purpose gets a normative foothold through what scholars in ethics have called the moral point of view. The full discipline implied by the moral point of view is not part of the definition of Type 3 thinking, but a basic principle of respect for the freedom and welfare of human beings is certainly at the center.

Worries about ethical relativism in connection with Type 3 thinking are natural, of course, and deserve patient attention from both philosophers and managers, especially in the context of multinational business operations. In this chapter, however, I will simply state baldly that these concerns are not insuperable. The moral point of view is not a monolith, but it is a practical perspective that takes all human beings seriously. It seems reasonable to expect that the balance implicit in avoiding teleopathy is also a balance that can tell good judgment from intolerance and dogmatism. In the words of philosopher Mary Midgley: Moral judgment is not a luxury, not a perverse indulgence of the self-righteous. It is a necessity. . . . Morally as well as physically, there is only one world, and we all have to live in it.[7]

In summary, there are four principal ways in which ethical values are acknowledged in the business mindset. Each can *espouse* values like honesty, concern for others, fidelity to contracts, and so forth. But each connects these values to business decision making using a different logic. The diagram below shows the typology in the form of a matrix. Type 1, like Type 3, is an internal or actor-centered action guide, while Types 2a and 2b are external or system-centered action guides.

To embrace, consciously or not, either Type 1 or Type 2 thinking as against Type 3, I believe, sets the stage for either individual or corporate teleopathy. For it suspends the balancing role of direct moral reflection in management in favor of constrained or unconstrained purposes.

In each of Gellerman's explanations of recent corporate scandals, we can see either Type 1 or Type 2 thinking. Teleopathy is at the core of each rationalization, along with echoes of Maccoby's notion of careerism, Arendt's talk about thoughtlessness, Ladd's remarks about organizational rationality, and McCoy's concern about the sadhu left behind on the mountain.

It is also important to observe that *all four* of the patterns in the typology can recognize the conventional notion of stakeholders or "constituencies" in the business environment: government, consumers, suppliers, shareholders, and employees. The difference lies in the *kind* of attention that each gives to them. Type 1 thinking can see attention to stakeholders as attention to factors that might affect self-interest. Type 2a thinking can regard stakeholders as so many markets

## Depiction of the Typology in a 2×2 Matrix

|  | EXTERNAL |  |
|---|---|---|
| Type 2a: | | Type 2b: |
| Market Ethic | | Law Ethic |
| **COMPETITIVE** | | **COOPERATIVE** |
| | INTERNAL | |
| Type 1: | | Type 3: |
| Self-Interested | | Ethic of |
| Rationality | | Respect |

within which companies must operate for profit. Concern for each is seen as built into the market system. Type 2b thinking can regard stakeholders as non-market checks on market reasoning: socio-political limits on the exercise of economic rationality. Only Type 3 thinking views stakeholders apart from their instrumental, economic, or political clout. It refuses to see them merely as what Ladd called "limiting operating conditions" on management attention.

One must conclude, I think, that the notion of a "stakeholder" (originally a play on the word "stockholder") is not, by itself, at the normative core of business ethics — at least not if we accept an interpretation of that core in terms of personal and organizational teleopathy. An examination of the four types of thinking above suggests that, while all four can accommodate the stakeholder idea, only one type (Type 3) embraces the moral point of view as an authoritative guide.

If the perspective outlined above (Part I) is on track, then what are some of the challenges it presents to the field of business ethics? I believe we can discern several, under two broad headings:

(A) Gaining a philosophical understanding of Type 3 leadership

Can we reach a reasonable consensus on a set of moral virtues and *prima facie* obligations that represent the minimal output of Type 3 thinking?

Can we interpret the fiduciary and other role-related obligations of corporate leadership (e.g., to employees and consumers) in terms of the balance of purpose required by Type 3 thinking?

(B) Gaining an administrative understanding of Type 3 leadership

Can we offer practical suggestions and techniques for making this vision part of the corporate leadership agenda?

Can we relate Type 3 virtues and obligations to the conventional functional areas of business administration (marketing, finance, accounting, production, human resource management, strategic planning, and so forth)?

Part II will focus on the second pair of questions, out of a conviction that unless our philosophical conception of a "normative ethic" is tied to the administrative point of view, it is profoundly incomplete. But I will touch on the first pair of questions before concluding Part II, as some paradoxes emerge. It is through the dynamics of leadership that persons influence organizations and organizations affect society. In the heart and mind of the corporate leader, principle touches practice.

If there is a new openness among both business leaders and the general public to the idea of independent moral judgment guiding business conduct (and there is evidence for this in courts, boardrooms, academic studies, and public opinion research), then we need to improve our understanding of the full implications of making Type 3 thinking part of the very definition of leadership.

## Part II. Three Imperatives for Corporate Leadership

Why were we so reluctant to try the lower path, the ambiguous trail? Perhaps because we did not have a leader who could reveal the greater purpose of the trip to us. For each of us the sadhu lives. What is the nature of our responsibility if we consider ourselves to be ethical persons? Perhaps it is to change the values of the group so that it can, with all its resources, take the other road.

— Bowen H. McCoy

A fundamental goal of the study of business ethics is to interpret the leadership implications of balancing the pursuit of purpose — what we have called Type 3 thinking. The more conventional value of organizational rationality often profoundly narrows the vision of corporate leaders. Adding respect to rationality can be seen from the leader's point of view as introducing *conscience* into the corporate mindset, inasmuch as conscience balances a person's pursuit of purpose with a recognition of moral obligations to those who are affected.

We can organize the leader's moral agenda under three broad imperatives—

orienting, institutionalizing, and sustaining corporate values. The first two deal with placing moral considerations in a position of authority alongside considerations of profitability and competitive strategy in the corporate mindset. The third imperative (sustenance) has to do with passing on the spirit of this effort in two directions: to future leaders of the organization and to the wider network of organizations and institutions that make up the social system as a whole. In the sections that follow, I will try to clarify each of the imperatives and then identify some of the ways in which they invite deeper reflection and research from students and practitioners of business ethics.

### Orienting

Leaders must first identify and then, where needed, attempt to modify their organization's shared values. Such a prescription cannot be followed without first performing a kind of moral inventory. What is needed is a sounding process sophisticated enough to get behind the natural cautions, defenses, and espoused values of subordinates. The leader must listen to and understand his or her organization in ways that reach its character strengths and defects. Such a process is relatively easy in a small organization because behavior is observable daily and communication is direct. But in a large divisionalized and diversified corporation, the task is much more complex, almost different in kind.

The objective is to discern the dominant ethical values of the company. Survey and questionnaire instruments may provide an initial scan. Such scans are only a first pass, however. More qualitative, clinical methods are needed to identify moral victories, defeats, and dilemmas that operating managers experience as they do their work and pursue their careers in the organization. In what circumstances are they willing to follow conscience, even when it might be economically costly? In what circumstances is there a tendency toward teleopathy, toward putting results ahead of ethical concerns when conflicts occur? Are there company policies or practices that have unintended negative ethical implications?

In a divisionalized or diversified firm, are there some business units that tend to have more problems than others? Can we tell why—and whether shared experiences and processes might help? Are there problems relating to international business operations that are more (or less) difficult than in domestic operations? Selective sounding out of outside parties is also important: suppliers, customers, regulators, neighbors, creditors, shareholders. Exit interviews with departing employees can also provide helpful insight into company values.

The result of such sounding efforts will be an inventory of attributions, issues, responses, and concerns that can serve as a preliminary map for leadership initiatives. Is this a Type 3 organization? If not, how and where could policies and practices be changed to improve ethical awareness? What can and should be done (and where) in terms of management development? Can the company create its own set of case studies for management education that emerges from the ethical sounding? If a corporate code or credo would be helpful, what should it contain in order to make contact with the strengths and weaknesses that the sounding has uncovered?

In one large manufacturing company that I studied, the sounding was minimal and the resulting ethical communications to employees from senior management were regarded as Sunday school sermons. Little contact was made with the organizational mindset in its operational reality. The leader wanted to orient corporate conscience, but never really located it to begin with. "Getting there from here" is wishful thinking when "here" is a mystery.

In another company, a multinational service firm, the commitment to a sounding was much more in evidence. In an initial workshop session with office managers from around the world, strengths were identified in certain client relationships; policies were identified that enabled managers to avoid conflicts of interest; practices were highlighted that ensured great attention to the accuracy of company reports. Weaknesses were acknowledged in specific personnel practices that seemed unfair and discriminatory.

The CEO did not stop there, however. Plans have been laid to focus the sounding at lower levels and horizontally by type of service rather than just geographical location. The board of directors then intends to articulate a statement of values and to take steps — as yet undetermined — toward institutionalizing and sustaining the strengths and eliminating or reducing the weaknesses that are meaningful to managers and staff throughout the company.

When orienting values is approached in this way, the sounding can be a device not only for gathering information, but for raising awareness and tracking future ethical problems and issues. It can actually become part of the institutionalization process.

### Institutionalizing

Once corporate leadership has identified characteristic values and value conflicts — and has clarified the direction it wants to take in whole or in part — the process of institutionalization becomes paramount. How can these values be made part of the operating consciousness of the company? How can they gain the attention and the allegiance of middle management and other employees? The answers lie in three areas: decisive *actions*, a statement of *standards* with regular *audits*, and appropriate *incentives*.

**Actions.** Since "actions speak louder than words," a major factor in the process of institutionalizing corporate values is leadership activity that has both wide visibility and clear ethical content. Such actions serve as large-scale demonstrations to the rank and file of the seriousness and importance that senior management attaches to ethical values.

It is hard to overstate, for example, the significance of James Burke's decisiveness in his handling of the Tylenol poisonings. It sent a powerful message to employees and customers alike regarding the operating values of Johnson & Johnson.

Another example comes from a case study of the Duke Power Company. In 1974, when Bill Lee was faced with a layoff involving 1,500 construction workers, he had to decide between inverse seniority as a criterion and a mechanism that would permit the retention of many recently employed minorities. The company's affirmative action gains were at stake at a point in its history when past injustices could not be ignored. Lee's conviction led him to protect minorities with less seniority and to face criticisms of reverse discrimination.

In 1980, there was another contraction of the company's work force. Because of Lee's courage in 1974, affirmative action gains were not at stake. Lee shared the following reflections on the importance of his original decision for institutionalizing the core value of racial justice:

> Having bit the bullet in 1974, and being careful in subsequent restaffing, in 1980 we were able to lay off in inverse seniority without affecting minority percentage employment. The 1974 experience gave a positive signal throughout all departments of the company that we really care about affirmative action. I believe this helped set the stage of acceptance of upward mobility for minorities and females as one of our published corporate performance goals. Achievement of these goals would result in some financial reward to all employees at every level. It receives wide publicity and monthly progress reports to all employees.[8]

The institutionalization of ethical values depends first and foremost on leadership conviction expressed in action. But there is more to the story than this. For while highly visible examples of values in action give energy to the process, employees need to learn how less visible, but equally important, ethical decisions fall within their own spans of control.

**Standards and audits.** Every company will, because of its special history, industry, and culture, address ethical values somewhat differently. Nevertheless, certain elements will be common to the process of institutionalization in any firm. A statement of standards along with a monitoring process is one of these common elements.

In 1976, Jack Ludington, CEO of Dow Corning Corporation, asked four senior corporate managers to serve as a Business Conduct Committee (BCC), reporting to the Audit and Social Responsibility Committee of the board of directors. The BCC was charged with developing guidelines that would help communicate ethical standards to company sites around the world and a workable process for monitoring, reporting, and improving the business practices. Once a corporate code was drafted, "it was sent to area managers with instructions that they develop their own codes, paying particular attention to their unique concerns. The only constraint was that area codes not conflict with the corporate code."

Ludington thus did an informal scan or "sounding" of top managers and key outside sources as he identified corporate values. He even involved line management further by asking for area-specific codes consistent with the (more general) corporate code. But he did not stop there.

The code of business conduct was reviewed every two or three years, with an eye to improving its coverage of issues that either corporate or area management thought important. The principal vehicle for this process was a series of regular "Business Conduct Audits" that senior corporate managers undertook on a rotating basis at company offices worldwide.

Area managers were asked to prepare for the audits by using "worksheets" that encouraged concreteness and detail regarding each of the topics raised by the code of conduct. In effect, "cases" were being reported in real time for review by the BCC. Particularly serious issues that emerged from these sessions — issues like questionable payments and abuse of proprietary information — were presented for discussion by the BCC annually to the Audit and Social Responsibility Committee of the board.

In this way, corporate leadership informed both itself and the relevant employees of the specific nature and extent of the company's ethical concerns. Regularly those concerns involved what I have called teleopathy: How will we let competitive pressure lead us in this kind of situation? What about our "technically legal" practices in that situation? Two-way communication made the implications of the code of business conduct quite concrete. There was, in other words, an attempt at a thoughtful balancing of purpose.[9]

**Incentives.** Are actions at the top and audits throughout the organization enough? No, they are not. Kenneth Andrews emphasizes the impotence of even the strongest convictions when they are not tied to structural and cultural incentives:

> It is quite possible . . . and indeed quite usual, for a highly moral and humane chief executive to preside over an "amoral organization"—one made so by processes developed before the liberalization of traditional corporate economic objectives. The internal force which stubbornly resists efforts to make the corporation compassionate (and exacting) toward its own people and responsible (as well as economically efficient) in its external relationships is the incentive system forcing attention to short-term quantifiable results.[10]

Without a willingness to reward performance based on contributions to the "quality" as much as the quantity of profits, the audit process will accomplish very little. It will not do to encourage ethical behavior simply by denying promotions or bonuses to those who cut moral corners. Removing disincentives to ethical behavior may be as important as, if not more important than instituting positive rewards and punishments.

I have characterized the ethical challenge to corporate leadership as involving three imperatives—orienting, institutionalizing, and sustaining shared ethical values. Since the efforts of even the best leaders to act on the first two of these imperatives are subject to a kind of winding down, we must say a word about sustaining corporate values over time.

### Sustaining

To sustain Type 3 values is to communicate them to the next generation of managers as well as to the wider social system. The objective is what Chester Barnard referred to as "fit"—between the mindset of the organization and the mindsets of both its future leaders ("microfits") and its various communities ("macrofits"). Without some degree of ethical fit or congruence, the corporate mindset simply cannot survive or replicate itself.

Microfits involve such issues as management selection and development, executive succession, and even (in the case of large corporations) acquisition and divestiture of business units. Macrofits involve public communication, government relations, and international business activities.

**Microfits.** I am aware of one chief executive of a *Fortune* 100 company who approaches the challenge of sustaining corporate values with great care and self-awareness. Not only does he monitor personally and regularly the progress of seventy-five key managers in his corporation, he does so with explicit attention to the congruence between their beliefs and attitudes and the overall corporate value system. In one case, an otherwise very strong executive who was considered in line to be CEO was asked to resign for reasons related directly to his cynicism about the company's stated philosophy of human values. It should be added that the decision was made with the full understanding, counsel, and support of the board of directors.

Another chief executive officer has worked with his board of directors in developing a set of criteria for appraising the character traits and qualifications of candidates for leadership roles in the corporation. The criteria include not only experience, intelligence, and economic performance, but also integrity, maturity, balance, and community service.

**Macrofits.** Stabilizing a corporate mindset pattern also requires a reasonable fit in the direction of the larger network of organizations and institutions that we refer to collectively as "society." Corporate values within the social system, like individual values within the organization, can have influence. But when they don't, and the company becomes part of the problem rather than the solution, there may be no alternative to withdrawal.

Corporate signatories to the Sullivan Principles in South Africa sought to resolve the dilemma of disinvesting entirely or contributing to social injustice. Some companies decided that they could not or would not seek such influence. IBM, however, refused for many years to close down its operations in South Africa, reaffirming a policy of working for social change from within, both independently and through its commitment to the Sullivan Principles. In 1986, IBM sold its subsidiary, but continued to sell products through the newly independent South African company. Other companies have pulled out entirely, believing that their continued business activity there only served to reinforce the status quo. In any case, a considered decision is necessary.

### Three Paradoxes: Research Needed

In the moral domain the leader guides the decision-making patterns of the corporation as a whole in the direction of Type 3 thinking. Beyond this, the leader must influence persons within the organization as well as the social system outside it toward accommodation or fit with that mindset. In Chester Barnard's words, "the distinguishing mark of executive responsibility" is "not merely conformance to a complex code of morals but also the creation of moral codes for others."[11]

This agenda, however, carries with it a number of serious challenges. Business ethics research is needed, both philosophical and empirical, on each front. For each of the three imperatives (orienting, institutionalizing, and sustaining ethical values) harbors a kind of paradox. And coming to terms with these paradoxes is what gives substance to the moral agenda of corporate leadership. They can be formulated as follows:

1. *The Paradox of Legitimacy.* It seems essential, yet somehow illegitimate, to *orient* corporate strategy by values that go beyond not only pure self-interest, but also conventional economic and legal frameworks.

Leaders must face the fact that the market and the law seem paradoxically definitive and insufficient for corporate responsibility. How far can the responsible leader go beyond the norms defining legitimacy? Can a solid baseline of reasonable ethical principles be identified for public use, even in our pluralistic society? Can a clear understanding of fiduciary obligations to shareholders be given that relates to them?

2. *The Paradox of Motivation.* It seems essential, yet curiously inappropriate, to seek to *institutionalize* ethical motivation in a company by the use of appeals to simple self-interest.

Commonly used management techniques for strategy implementation— various incentives, rewards, and punishments—may appear somewhat incongruous when ethics is the goal. Most of us wonder about, if we do not recoil from, the idea of a bonus for being good. The leader who is mindful of this will want to approach the task of policy implementation in ethics with a special kind of circumspection. Incentives will be important, but just as important will be example, role modeling, open dialogue, and appeals to deeper motives. Like the first paradox, this challenges our conventional understanding of the role of management.

3. *The Paradox of Paternalism.* It seems essential for *sustaining* a group conscience, yet coercive, to seek to influence the value orientation of others, whether inside the corporation or outside.

Ethical values must be communicated in a way that secures maximum adherence among both management (internally) and society (externally). Yet such a demand may seem dogmatic, contrary to the very spirit of the values it seeks to sustain. Imposing morality on employees and society appears to be both intolerant and inescapable. Resolving this paradox in practice may be one of the chief tests of responsible leadership.

If we reflect on these paradoxes, we can begin to appreciate that the three leadership imperatives will be addressed differently if the shared values of an organization involve Type 3 thinking, rather than Type 1 or Type 2. The process by which leadership orients, institutionalizes, and sustains ethical values must be consistent with the content of those values. The moral point of view must play as central a role in the leadership actions that aim to make ethics a reality, as in the clarification of the reality to be aimed at. The implications of this demand for consistency between moral content and moral process are very important and deserve patient study.

These challenges are real. They account for much of the reluctance of top executives to pursue business ethics beyond rhetoric and rule books. They call into question deeply entrenched beliefs about corporate governance, human resource management, and the appropriate use of economic power. But unless leaders can learn to manage them, our business institutions will become increasingly mired in a reactive, externally driven approach to ethical responsibility, or worse.

What is striking about these challenges, in my opinion, is that they call for a variety of skills in their resolution. Clearly each paradox has philosophical dimensions. But just as clearly, there are dimensions that call for the methods of psychology, sociology, corporate law, and management studies. They provide a formidable agenda not only to corporate leaders, but also to those of us who would seek to advance the emerging field of business ethics.

### Summary and Conclusion

In Part I of this paper, I described and defended what I take to be the normative core of business ethics: the avoidance of teleopathy at both the level of the individual and the level of the organization as a whole. More positively, this was interpreted as encouraging Type 3 thinking in business settings, emphasizing the difference between this and popular versions of the stakeholder idea.

Then, since the leader was seen to be the key to aligning the values of the individual and the organization, in Part II I suggested three broad imperatives as the moral agenda of corporate leadership. Reflecting on the implications of these imperatives, three corresponding paradoxes were revealed, paradoxes that call for the philosophical and empirical attention of the academy as well as the managerial attention of corporate leaders.

I have not tried to relate either the normative core or the leadership agenda to the subject of professional education. To do so would require more than a few paragraphs. Suffice it to say here by way of conclusion that the implications are profound. Value-neutral education is a myth and always has been, despite its twentieth-century dominance as an espoused theory. Education-in-action inevitably conveys ethical content, by omission or commission. Emory University president James T. Laney put it nicely:

> In many academic disciplines there has been a retreat from the attempt to relate values and wisdom to what is being taught. Not long ago, Bernard Williams, the noted British philosopher, observed that philosophers have been trying all this century to get rid of the dreadful idea that philosophy ought to be edifying. Philosophers are not the only ones to appreciate the force of that statement. . . . How can society survive if education does not attend to those qualities which it requires for its very perpetuation?[12]

As the field of business ethics develops, it is my hope not only that philosophical and empirical research will be aimed more toward the leadership agenda, but that the business school agenda will serve as a bridge. For if ethics is not integrated into business education (and I am talking about more than simply the addition of a *course*), the academy runs the risk of encouraging (rather than discouraging) teleopathy in its hidden curriculum. The next generation of leadership, after all, is always in school at any given moment.

### NOTES

1. Michael Maccoby, "The Corporate Climber Has to Find His Heart," *Fortune*, December 1976, p. 101.
2. Hannah Arendt, "Thinking," *New Yorker*, November 21, 1977, pp. 65–140; November 28, 1977, pp. 135–216; December 5, 1977, pp. 135–216.
3. Ibid.
4. John Ladd, "Morality and the Ideal of Rationality in Formal Organizations," *The Monist*, October 1970, p. 507.
5. See pp. 18–26 for the full text of Gellerman's article.
6. See pp. 201–207 for the full text of McCoy's article.
7. Mary Midgley, *Heart and Mind* (New York: St. Martin's Press, 1981), pp. 72, 75.
8. Source: Letter to author from Bill Lee, September 7, 1983.
9. See "Dow Corning Corporation: Business Conduct and Global Values" (HBS Case Services, 9-385-018 and 019).
10. See pp. 257–266 for the full text of Andrews's article.
11. Chester Barnard, *The Functions of the Executive* (Cambridge: Harvard University Press, 1938), p. 279.
12. James T. Laney, "The Education of the Heart," *Harvard Magazine*, September–October 1985, pp. 23–24.

## 2

# Case of the Rogue Division

### DAVID W. EWING

*Rumors of improper business conduct move through the grapevine like fire through August wheat, yet company executives are often slow in responding to them. The media, of course, are quick to bite at news of payoffs, kickbacks, and suicides. If caught off guard, companies can feel pressed to defend themselves before they have even established whether the allegations are true.*

*The top managers of one U.S. corporation found themselves struggling to save face for the organization, which was at the center of a scandal involving legislators and rate-making officials. Disguised in the case presented here, the company's situation tests the thinking and judgment of even the most experienced business leaders. HBR asked three executives—Joseph T. Nolan, Donald N. Scobel, and Douglas S. Sherwin—to discuss their reactions to the company's predicament. Read the case and compare your diagnosis and prescription with those of the three commentators.*

*Mr. Nolan is Monsanto's vice president for public affairs. Mr. Scobel is director and founder of the Creative Worklife Center in Mentor, Ohio and was formerly manager of employee relations development for the Eaton Corporation. Mr. Sherwin is board chairman of Duraco Products, Inc. in Streamwood, Illinois and until recently was president of Phillips Products Company, Inc., a subsidiary of Phillips Petroleum (Duraco was organized to acquire Phillips Products from Phillips).*

*The scene is the office of E.J. ("Brad") Bradenhoff, president of North Central Power Company, a division of Trans-National Power Corporation. With Bradenhoff are Alvin H. Tillman, director of public relations; Beverly Walensa, director of personnel; Richard Rinehart, chief legal counsel; and Louis Hyde, vice president of Trans-National. Hyde has just arrived from corporate headquarters in Pittsburgh.*

**Hyde:** Brad, why don't you bring me up to date on the bidding. I've only heard bits and pieces about this thing, and being in Europe most of the past month doesn't help.

**Bradenhoff:** About eight months ago, Lou, I heard about improprieties in some of the district offices. I can't say it was the first time I had heard the rumors, because it wasn't. But in my year here I've had a lot to learn, and I had other problems to work out first. So I asked Rich to investigate. His people went about it as discreetly as they could, but the upshot was they found a mess in one district. It happens to be the Reardon-St. Thomas district up to the north, Lou. Well, there were payoffs to city and town officials, contracts with relatives, some pretty extravagant entertainment going on—you name it, they found it. So I suspended Martin Adams and Gordon Gilby, the two managers who were most involved. After further investigation, I terminated Adams, and then he brought suit against us.

**Hyde:** This was after Gilby—

**Bradenhoff:** After Gilby committed suicide, yes.

**Hyde:** That was when the media got excited.

**Bradenhoff:** And then Adams, you see, began talking to reporters, claiming he was being made the scapegoat. That fueled the fire.

**Hyde:** This story from the *Herald*, now. Is this the kind of thing the papers are saying?

---

### Adams Says North Central Ordered Payoffs, Favors

**Midwest City**—A former employee of North Central Power Co. charged today that he had been ordered to make payments to designated political candidates and do favors for members of the state legislature.

"I dared to resist corporate rapacities," stated Martin Adams, who was fired from his job as Midwest district manager in June. "I didn't like what they were doing, and they decided the best way to shut me up was to get rid of me."

Adams claimed that he and other executives at the department head and division levels were given pay raises that included $1,500 a year to cover political contributions. Also, he said that the company routinely asked managers to make out false expense vouchers so that illegal payments could be made to legislators and municipal officials.

One city mayor, he said, sold more than $80,000 of supplies to the company after presiding over power rate hearings and voting for an increase. A city councilman, said Adams, did more than $165,000 of business with an affiliate of North Central.

Gordon Gilby, Adams's boss and a vice president of the company, also was a victim of the company's retaliation, Adams claimed. Gilby committed suicide last May 19. His estate is joining suit with Adams in charging the company with slander.

The legislature has appointed a subcommittee to look into charges that the company influenced legislators and rate-making officials. The subcommittee will begin hearings Wednesday.

When contacted, officers of Trans-National Power, the parent organization in Pittsburgh, offered no comment.

---

**Bradenhoff:** That's typical, yes. I don't believe Adams has told them much that they haven't reported.

**Hyde:** Pretty one-sided, isn't it? I would've expected better than this from the press out here, but maybe I'm naive. Everybody's so antibusiness these days.

**Walensa:** Actually, the press has treated us OK. In general, anyway.

**Bradenhoff:** It's just that you've got that combination of suicide, which was front-page news because of who Gilby was—his family and everything— and Adams taking potshots at us at every chance—

**Tillman:** And with rates going up all the time, who likes a power company?

**Hyde:** So when the trial starts, I suppose that'll light a fire under it all over again.

**Bradenhoff:** We're in a very awkward position, you know. In order to defend ourselves, we've got to demonstrate what Rich found in his investigation of Adams and Gilby. All of which of course plays right into the hands of the reporters.

**Hyde:** What's the worst that can happen? Just so there won't be any surprises.

**Bradenhoff:** What do you think, Rich? What's the worst that can happen?

**Rinehart:** The Adams-Gilby suit is for slander, and $6.5 million is being asked in damages. It will be alleged by plaintiff Adams that his termination was a retaliatory act because of his knowing too much, with the further motive of discreditation. It will be asserted by Adams that the investigation of his and Gilby's activities was initiated upon our being apprised of their critical stance, a kind of de facto whistleblowing, if you will, and that Gilby *in extremis*—

**Hyde:** Holy cow, what language is this? I'm a country boy from Radcliff, Kentucky and all this day facto and streemus business—

**Walensa:** Rich is our scholar. How many years of Latin did you have at Princeton, Rich?

**Rinehart:** Please, Pennsylvania.

**Hyde:** Anyway, you were saying about Gilby?

**Rinehart:** The suicide was committed in acute anguish.

**Tillman:** Brought on by Gilby's fears that the company was out to get him, Rich means.

**Hyde:** Thank you. So Gilby—or rather, Gilby's widow—and Adams, they're going to be telling us we sat on them to make them swallow the whistle?

**Bradenhoff:** Right. I mean wrong, because of course it isn't true; we didn't do that. The fact is we didn't start the probe until rumors came to us about their improprieties. And at the time we had no knowledge that Adams was critical of the company.

**Hyde:** Can that timing be established?

**Rinehart:** I believe it can be documented, yes. No word of criticism was heard from Gilby, so far as we know, until the writing of his suicide note. As for the plaintiff, Adams, to the best of our knowledge, no allegations against the company were made until after his termination by Brad, which was later still.

**Hyde:** And Mrs. Gilby, the widow, is suing for the same thing as Adams?

**Rinehart:** In essence, yes, although more damages are claimed by her. In addition, the same or similar witnesses will be offered by both plaintiffs. It is anticipated that testimony will be concerned largely with the attempted influence by management in respect to rate-making officials and legislators. This, it is alleged, Adams and Gilby were threatening to disclose and were therefore penalized.

**Hyde:** Former employees testifying against us? I don't like the sound of that.

**Rinehart:** The irony is that comparable testimony will be proffered by our own witnesses, only with regard to the plaintiffs' malfeasance, not management at large.

**Hyde:** Slander is it? Why not just damages for the suspension?

**Bradenhoff:** It's a kind of Catch-22, Lou. To investigate the rumors about Adams and Gilby's conduct, we had to ask many employees about their activities. So the grapevine got to work, you know. There was no way to keep it from buzzing. Most everyone learned early on that Adams and Gilby were under suspicion. So the whole investigation was loaded like a pistol.

**Rinehart:** When Adams was terminated, after the Gilby suicide, the implication clearly was "guilty as charged." Adams is an ambitious man. As he sees it, his career is ruined.

**Hyde:** So you'll be parading witnesses at the trial, Rich, who will lay this out? And what's the bottom line? I mean, what side of the law are we trying to land on?

**Rinehart:** Essentially, what is said by the law is that if North Central did what would have been done by any reasonable employer in similar circumstances, it is on solid ground.

**Hyde:** And you're not worried about proving that?

**Rinehart:** I believe it can be documented that our inquiries were discreet, appropriate, timely, and when the evidence was in, our actions could only be called judicious. Not to have acted would have been a breach of responsibility.

**Hyde:** Will it be a long trial?

**Rinehart:** According to our best estimate, on the order of two to four weeks.

**Hyde:** Two to four weeks! Two to four weeks of parading witnesses in and out to testify about kickbacks, payoffs, sex —

**Tillman:** Why didn't we try to settle?

**Rinehart:** As you know, I took a strong position against that. A settlement would have been tantamount to a tacit admission of guilt, in the public mind if not legally, and *a fortiori* a generous settlement, as demanded by the plaintiffs.

**Hyde:** Does this man ever speak in ordinary words?

**Bradenhoff:** Only when he scuffs a golf shot.

**Walensa:** Anyway, settling out of court tends to leave people in the dark about what really happened.

**Tillman:** Pittsburgh doesn't want a settlement either? I mean, would a settlement be in the realm of possibility there?

**Hyde:** As I understand it, Rich convinced Pittsburgh not to go that route. But of course it's never too late; we could change our minds. You *could* still ask for a postponement and dicker for a settlement, right, Rich?

**Rinehart:** But why let such a dangerous precedent be set? And as I have already said, we will not be let off cheap by these plaintiffs. At the least, a demand of two million will be made.

**Hyde:** I'm not recommending a settlement. I'm just saying that theoretically it's a possibility.

**Tillman:** Two million, that's not so bad. I mean, two million might be cheap compared to what we lose in rate increases. Can you imagine the effect on the legislature and rate commission of two to four weeks of dragging out the dirty linen in court? Officials wined and dined, weekends at hunting lodges at company expense, women, business contracts — why, we'll be lucky to get a tenth of the increase we ask for! The repercussions will last for years!

**Bradenhoff:** Just off the cuff, every percentage in rate increase is worth three-quarters of a million dollars to us every month. Now, we're asking for 11% more in April and hoping to get at least half of it. So that settlement cost could be paid for quickly.

**Hyde:** That's one of the interesting things, you know. You've put your finger on something that fascinates me, Al. Here we've got this rogue division, this renegade company. Over at headquarters, hell, they've worried about it for ages. But the earnings! Damn, if only the other divisions could earn like this one has.

**Rinehart:** Thanks to the state.

**Hyde:** What do you mean, "Thanks to the state"?

**Rinehart:** A decentralized state agency, conflicting jurisdictions between state and municipal, gaps in control, regulation *de minimis* —

**Hyde:** Regulation what?

**Rinehart:** Minimal regulation.

**Tillman:** It may not be so loose after the trial. I've got a feeling there's going to be a lot of tightening up by the legislature after this imbroglio.

**Hyde:** If we've got such a strong case, Rich, why can't we knock it out in a week, get it over with?

**Rinehart:** Because at least a week will be consumed by the plaintiffs in setting forth their side, and about a week will be required by us in defense presentation. It's a case of double whistleblowing, you might say, and in addition to establishing that the requirements of just cause were met by the company, the equitableness of our procedure must be proved. Also, there are some complexities. When a quarter of a million was spent by Gilby to remodel his offices — that was accomplished, by the way, by dividing the contract into small jobs that did not have to be reviewed by the controller — several thousand dollars' worth of improvements were included by Gilby for his home in Maplewood. Actual payment for the home improvements was performed by the architect; then Gilby had an equivalent sum added to the architect's fee. Our case is documented, but the details must be set forth one by one, and more time will be consumed in cross-examination.

**Tillman:** We spend years building up good relations with the legislature, then a shoot-out like this happens. Pow! Everything gone. Any time the rate commission goes along with us after this, they'll be suspect. Did we buy them out again? What favors did we give them? There goes all that hard-earned trust!

**Bradenhoff:** I don't think it's as bad as all that, Al. Don't forget that we've got an asset of 37,000 employees living in cities and towns around the state. They're voters, they're buyers, and what's more, they can be spokespeople. Now, I've seen it happen, because we did it back when I was in Des Moines, you know. We educated the employees and told them what our problem was, and they went out like battalions. They rang doorbells, they took speaking engagements, they went to hearings. We can do that here. We have people who can go to Rotary clubs and speak. We have people who can write for their local newspapers. Some of them would appear on talk shows. We're not helpless, that's what I'm saying. We can fight.

**Walensa:** Sounds terrific. But how do you start the ball rolling?

**Bradenhoff:** With information. You always start with information.

**Tillman:** Like, every day we could summarize the previous day's proceedings in court. One page of facts, a copy on every desk. Every day we could set the record straight, put what Adams says in one column and refute it with the truth in the next column. Salvo! We could send our fact sheets to the legislators, to the media. Every employee would go out armed with a good summary, and whoever they talk to, they would have the answer at their fingertips.

**Bradenhoff:** Bev, show Lou that employee summary you made up. Lou, that shows part of my problem—how do you get a little discipline when the troops are spread out in 63 different places? But there's a plus side, too. See, we've got people in most every club and association and bowling league you ever heard of. Call it people power or whatever you want, there's a lot of weight there.

**Rinehart:** It's not all that transparent to me. Can we be assured that all of those 37,000 are waiting for marching orders, ready to go out and spread the word? If you want the truth, a lot of them regard anything from management with great skepticism. Why not let our talking be done for us by the verdict? Let our day in court be had and many doubts will be put to rest. What is more, a large proportion of employees are in distant and outlying cities and towns, with their own problems to worry about.

**Tillman:** That's fine if you can get people to withhold judgment, but they won't. Every day this goes on, more bombardment from the media—parties, payoffs, hanky-panky. Why, already Channel Three's putting together a show on suicide, and you know what they'll focus on? The Gilby case. They'll intimate that he killed himself in despair when he learned the company would discredit him in order to shut him up. And somebody from *Time* called me about it this morning. I'm telling you, it's very hairy!

**Bradenhoff:** Al's our excitable one.

**Hyde:** It's no wonder. We're sitting on a volcano.

**Bradenhoff:** Still, we've got options, influence, and don't forget those employees, Lou.

**Hyde:** But how can you get them to think with us? Being a country boy myself, I know what it's like to be remote. "Man," you say to yourself, "I'm way out here, and there's nobody going to tell *me* what to do."

**Bradenhoff:** Well, we're going to work on it. One of the things I came here for is to put more coherence in this outfit, knit it closer together.

**Hyde:** Bev, you've been quiet.

**Walensa:** I was just wondering. I worry about trying to manage the news. I kind of agree with Rich that what we say is suspect. But I also agree with Al that we don't want to leave a vacuum for the media to fill. It'll be all sensationalism coming from them.

**Hyde:** So?

**Walensa:** Why not put the complete record of the previous day's trial on every person's desk in the morning? No editing, no commentary, nothing. Just give it to them, lock, stock, and barrel.

**Tillman:** Are you joking?

**Walensa:** I didn't mean to be.

**Tillman:** What about all the testimony that's not true? And what about the embarrassments—people who got promoted by Adams and Gilby for sexual favors, people who saw what was going on and looked the other way? They'll all be named in the proceedings, weird accusations and all. Let all that hang out?

**Hyde:** We've got to be careful of morale. Let's not hurt too many feelings.

**Bradenhoff:** If we're the subject of such hot news, maybe we could get Channel Three to put one of our people on every few days and give our side of the story.

**Hyde:** That sounds kind of defensive. I wonder if it'd be convincing.

**Tillman:** Whatever we do, we seem to lose. Adams and Mrs. Gilby clobber us when they open the case, our own witnesses clobber us when we give our side. Coming and going, we get it.

**Walensa:** I still think that if we could inform every employee completely and be credible, it could be a learning experience.

**Hyde:** We'll learn how to eat crow.

**Bradenhoff:** Intellectually I agree with Rich, you know, but emotionally I can't. I can't resign myself to sitting here watching it happen. And I get a feeling the public will respect us more if we fight.

**Walensa:** Yes, but there really isn't any way to win it, is there? Except legally, maybe. So all we can do is work ahead for the next round.

**Tillman:** The trouble is it's good managers who were the wrongdoers. Hell's bells, Gilby was a fair-haired boy. They said he could go to the top, if he wanted to. And Adams worked his way up from scratch. He started as a cost analyst and ended up running the whole northern area. It's not a case of those guys always wearing the black hats.

**Hyde:** Well, there's a bunch of alternatives for you, Brad, but they all seem to lead downhill, as they are. Do you want to keep your head below the grass or get out and fight? Well, each way there are implications. I don't have to go back till tonight, so you don't have to decide anything right now, but I've got to have something to tell Pittsburgh. I don't say they're going to argue with you, just that they're breathing a little hard out there wondering what's going to happen. So that's what I've got to know. What do you say we meet here again this afternoon at, oh, about 4 o'clock?

Query to readers: *Putting yourself in the shoes of E.J. Bradenhoff, what would you tell Lou Hyde you plan to do? After you have decided, compare your opinions with those that follow.*

In general, the three executives invited by HBR to comment on the case agree that:

Top management has failed to do its job well.

The heads of North Central Power should investigate their own possible contribution to the imbroglio before trying to make corrections in policy and structure.

Management should level immediately with the public about what has happened and why.

However it acts with regard to the current situation, the company will take a beating. Yet management can take many steps to prevent a recurrence of such a crisis. These steps range from enacting codes of conduct for employees to setting up better accounting systems.

Because our three commentators are lucid and articulate, I shall let them do most of the "talking" from here on. They take strong stands on this case, and HBR readers should find their comments rewarding.

### Taking the Blows

The ebullient Joseph T. Nolan makes a forceful case for management's leveling right away with the public:

"New York retailer Nathan Ohrbach said it best. 'I've got a terrific gimmick,' he confided to his advertising colleagues. 'Let's just tell the truth.' That's not only the best course for North Central Power Company but very likely the only one left.

"An out-of-court settlement of the lawsuits would not put off the day of reckoning since a state legislative subcommittee is planning to open public hearings momentarily. Besides, Martin Adams has already gone public with his version of events and can be expected to say even more.

"As Watergate demonstrated so clearly, the best way to prolong an unpleasant situation like this is to follow the 'limited hangout' strategy—to tell only part of the story. North Central should come clean and offer its wholehearted cooperation to authorities to track down any wrongdoing.

"Telling the truth should come easy for Brad Bradenhoff. After all, he has been president of North Central for barely one year. When he heard rumors of improprieties in the district offices, he launched an investigation. As soon as he had the facts, he took the initiative in suspending those managers who were implicated.

"What he should do now is make a forthright statement to the effect that as a matter of policy North Central does not condone payoffs or special deals with public officials and that it has established strict internal controls to prevent a recurrence of such practices.

"Bradenhoff should acknowledge right up front that the company made some mistakes in the past. He should take the blame for not communicating his policy as effectively as he could have. And he should start immediately to make sure all managers understand that the company is committed to achieving its commercial objectives in a manner fully consistent with the applicable laws and regulations of the state and communities in which it does business.

"This ought to be done *not* through a shower of memoranda but through personal visits to all company locations. What better opportunity to enlist the support of North Central's 37,000 employees around the state?"

Nolan harbors no illusions that such a full-disclosure stance will be painless. He continues:

"Will the company come up for criticism as a result of the public hearing and court trial? Certainly. Given the facts of the case, there is no way to avoid such criticism. All Bradenhoff can hope to do is limit the damage.

"If the damage control techniques are handled well, the harm to North Central's reputation should be both moderate and short-lived. A few years ago, when scores of U.S. companies were accused of making improper payments abroad, the ones that fared best were those that readily admitted their guilt, promised to make amends, and followed through on those promises. That's what North Central should do now."

Donald N. Scobel takes a dim view of Brad Bradenhoff's role to date. Putting himself in Bradenhoff's position, Scobel says he would resign:

"I would not be able to live with my ineptness in this case. When I first heard the rumors about the Reardon-St. Thomas district, I perceived it mostly as a legal problem. I failed to involve my human resource management experts. Then when the evidence came in, I blindly accepted it without asking questions or sensing the broader implications. Still I did not seek other perspectives. I suspended a vice president and one of his employees without giving them the chance to explain things—no chance for a hearing, no chance to refute the evidence. But my greatest sin was when Gilby took his life; I let Rinehart convince me this was de facto proof of guilt and crassly terminated Adams. That is when I laid the company open for public scrutiny.

"I paid no attention to Gilby's complaints about North Central in his suicide note. I still didn't foresee the broader implications. Not even a man taking his life shook me into giving Adams a chance to defend himself. I went ahead and fired him knowing full well that he could bring suit against the company and make this a public issue.

"Adams worked for Gilby. His easiest defense would be that he did nothing that wasn't approved or even ordered by his now deceased boss. Yet even in today's discussion, I'm not asking why Adams isn't taking this simple defense.

"Adams has joined Gilby's widow in the suit to say that both of them were scapegoats for a general company malignancy. Would Adams take this far harder tack if he had no evidence at all? As Bradenhoff I would say, 'I am sorry, Mr. Hyde, but my mismanagement and insensitivity to human resource affairs has already caused this company far more damage than the alleged acts of Gilby and Adams. I urge that we try to settle this out of court in order to give the company time to get its house in order under a little less public limelight. As a first step in that building process, I urge you to accept my resignation. I cannot stay on. I feel I even have a death on my hands.' "

It's unlikely, however, that the real Bradenhoff will take this suggestion, says Scobel. A division president in a no-win situation who opines that "the public will respect us more if we fight" isn't about to say farewell. Accordingly, Scobel puts it up to Louis Hyde, the corporate vice president:

"So that leaves it up to Mr. Hyde. Now if I were he, I wouldn't be feeling so hot either, but accountability in this case does rest more squarely on the president of North Central Power. Assuming I have the authority, and in keeping with my country-boy vernacular, my first inclination would be to 'fire Bradenhoff's ass.'

"But that would be denying Bradenhoff what he wrongly denied others—due process. I would ask him to take a week off and think about his future with the company. If he still wanted to stay, I would try to work out an arrangement whereby both perspectives could be presented to an impartial outsider with the assurance that the company would give substantial weight to his or her recommendation."

Although, as Nolan points out, the possibility of a settlement seems to have been ruled out, Douglas S. Sherwin agrees with Scobel that a strong effort should be made to reopen this route. Sherwin argues:

"Litigation will be painful, embarrassing, and very expensive for all parties. Whenever I am angry about something and think of suing, I am rescued by remembering Judge Learned Hand's caution about lawsuits, 'As a litigant, I should dread a lawsuit beyond almost anything else short of sickness and death.'

"No one can emerge a winner from this suit. That fact offers hope that the parties can find a way to meet their objectives without exposing themselves to the drawbacks of a court trial.

"The company should try to settle the case out of court not to cover up any questionable practices that the trial might disclose but to minimize further impairment of the company's ability to serve its customers, employees, and investors.

"A straight financial settlement is one option the company could consider. But if it can understand the needs that led Adams and Mrs. Gilby to sue, North Central may be able to combine certain other benefits with financial concessions as an alternative to a purely financial settlement.

"Mrs. Gilby, for example, probably wants to divert blame from her husband so as to preserve his (and her) name, to replace lost family income, and to salve her anger over the loss of her husband. Her chances of winning the suit, however, appear minimal, and if she loses, her legal expenses will be high. In any event, all the illegal and unethical actions her husband committed will be dragged through the court and his reputation will be permanently soiled. His estate might even be subject to a stockholders' suit to recover the company funds he diverted to the Gilby residence.

"Adams's interests are probably to restore his income, resume his rising career, and salvage as much of his reputation as possible. His suit has only moderate probability of success and, if lost, would be very costly. In addition, the trial would make his unethical actions a matter of public record—damaging his reputation. If testimony reveals illegal acts, he might subsequently be indicted on civil or criminal charges.

"The company could offer to say whatever positive things it could about Mr. Gilby, underwrite his spouse's legal costs to date, and out of appreciation for his service to the company, set up an annuity for Mrs. Gilby. It could offer several conciliatory benefits to Adams, such as extending his salary and providing him with an office and a secretary for a year or more while he seeks new employment, underwriting career counseling services and professional resumé preparation, paying his attorney's fees to date, and agreeing to emphasize to prospective employers the talents that enabled him to work his way up to executive status."

### Getting the House in Order

Turning now to actions that would help in the longer run, our commentators strongly urge North Central Power's management to begin with a hard look at its role in the scandal. Sherwin has this to say:

"The company must first get the facts about its own involvement and activities. For instance, is it unequivocally and incontrovertibly true that the company began the probe only when it heard the rumors of improprieties? Were the improprieties limited to the Reardon-St. Thomas district? What basis in fact did the criticisms contained in Gilby's suicide note have? Is there any evidence or potential testimony that Adams resisted corporate rapacities? Did the company in fact give pay raises that included amounts to cover political contributions? Did it ask managers to make out false expense vouchers to cover illegal payments to legislators and municipal officials? Did the company in fact get unjustifiably large increases from the regulatory bodies?

"The answers to these and other questions will determine the company's posture. For example, demonstrating that the probe came after the rumors would undercut Adams's claim that the dismissal was retaliatory. And if the improprieties were found to be limited to the Reardon-St. Thomas district, the activities in that district could be portrayed as an aberration.

"On the other hand, proof that the company gave pay raises to cover political contributions and asked managers to fill out false vouchers for that purpose would be taken as prima facie evidence that the leadership would support other attempts by its executives to influence rate making. The company needs to establish the absolute truth of these matters; it cannot stand any surprises."

Sherwin also thinks that North Central is guilty of several significant leadership failures. To set its own house in order, management needs to know why it made so many mistakes:

"By declining to offer comment when given the opportunity by the newspaper, the company betrayed its lack of foresight and preparation.

"When Bradenhoff took over the division's presidency, he should have received or written a statement of the goals of the division and the business areas in which high performance was necessary to meet these goals. It would have enabled him to get on top of his job faster.

"The company allowed the investigation of improprieties to drag on for eight months before dealing with the matter.

"The fact that Bradenhoff suspended two employees and fired Adams after Gilby had committed suicide without beforehand assessing the probable consequences of these acts suggests that the company's leadership appointed a man who was not yet ready for the assignment or that it failed to alert him to the most sensitive aspects of the new assignment. It should have been understood that the subordinate manager was to seek higher management's counsel when unusual situations arose.

"Management must discipline employees who have committed improper acts. But first it must articulate what constitutes improper behavior. That was Gilby's responsibility to Adams, Bradenhoff's to Gilby, Hyde's to Bradenhoff—and this duty extends right up to the directors of the company. This is especially important in regulated industries because of the sensitive and temptation-laden relationships with government officials.

"Where were the auditors? Were they inept or were their reports quashed?

"One has to question what it is about the climate that could induce a manager with Gilby's prospects to resort to such measures. Perhaps there was a precedent for Gilby's behavior."

On a broader scale, Sherwin takes corporate management to task for its apparent obsession with profits:

"Trans-National Power simply loves the profits that were coming out of the division and, if it didn't know, didn't *want* to know how they were being generated. The pursuit of profit is an indispensable internal discipline in giving private business its unique capability for economic performance. Profit is the objective investors have in risking their capital; profit commensurate with the risk undertaken is their just reward.

"But the objectives employees have in giving the company their energies and ideas and the objectives customers have in providing revenues out of which come wages and profits have to be met as well. It is only by giving equal regard to all these objectives that a manager can in fact maximize profit for the investors. For if profits are sought at the expense of employees or customers, they will in the long run, just as they have in this case, jeopardize justifiable profits for investors in the future."

Scobel believes that management must change some of its assumptions about employees. The dialogue shows him that the executives are embracing such questionable ideas as that:

1. "Employees have a pawn-like company loyalty that can be executively marshaled.

2. "Management can be prosecutor, investigator, and judge of its own employees without internal checks, balances, or due process.

3. "In the handling of human resource problems there is no real need to drive hard for truth.

4. "High levels in the organization are hardly at all accountable for the behavior of lower levels."

This executive group has some major self-corrections to make, Scobel argues. As he points out:

"Almost a third of the dialogue in this case is on the subject of manipulating employee thoughts and actions. Though some participants resist the notion, the president and PR director feel that they can move the masses with a flick. They perceive themselves as living in the Orwellian 1984. This notion of mass control is actually a vestige of serfdom.

"Another problem: most of the executives feel that decision responsibility rests at high levels yet that accountability for misjudgment or misconduct belongs down there someplace (or even out there someplace with an overzealous government, biased media, or an uninformed public). Misconduct is acknowledged, but how does it arise? What is the perceived policy or expectation? In what milieu does it flourish? The executives in this case can't face the question, Does some of the responsibility for this dilemma rest with the seats of organizational direction?

"A most perplexing part of this dialogue for me is how uninterested these executives seem to be in searching out truth in the broader sense. There is nothing very probing in vice president Hyde's inquiries. The dialogue invites an almost endless list of questions.

"Did anyone investigate the complaints against the company expressed in Gilby's suicide note? What is the validity of Adam's accusations quoted in the newspaper?

"What is the status of the legislative subcommittee investigation? Is it likely to press forward?

"Rinehart says Adams will focus on broad management efforts to influence rate-making officials. How broad? What evidence might he have?

"Why has headquarters worried about this 'rogue' and 'renegade' division for years?

"Has anyone tried to find out if similar problems exist in other districts?

"The list could go on and on, but it is clear that the participants are not curious. They blithely accept the premise that truth is precisely what lawyer Rinehart and his investigators say it to be. They have locked themselves into their own parochial version of truth, which they must now defend unswervingly."

### Preventing a Recurrence

What steps and changes in policy and organization would help North Central Power avoid getting caught in no-win situations like this one?

Nolan thinks management should issue a code of conduct for employees. He looks to Bradenhoff to do this by supplementing his personal visits to company offices with a written statement:

"Bradenhoff should promulgate a new policy statement on business conduct that prohibits the use of company funds for any unlawful purpose and requires every key employee to annually sign a certificate of compliance with this policy."

Scobel urges the company to establish mechanisms allowing employees to speak up and defend themselves when attacked. He decries the lack of any procedure for clearing the air and resolving suspicions:

"The 'discreet' inquiry into rumored improprieties was cursory at best. There is no evidence that any employee, including Gilby and Adams, had any chance to respond to the contentions of fellow employees. There was no hearing, no protection against partiality, very little evidence of factual corroboration, no opportunity for cross-questioning, and no seeking of an impartial opinion. Even the contention that a quarter of a million dollars was sneaked through in small contracts begs more questions than the investigation answers.

"In today's world, organizations need internal mechanisms for due process. If companies are not motivated by the fairness of due process, they should at least realize that employees have many avenues for disputing employer acts and that the old system for unilateral investigations and judgments is no longer viable. This case makes that clear."

Sherwin calls for revisions in accounting control and the board of directors:

"The company should review and provide for the adequacy of its system of internal accounting and management controls. It should immediately develop and issue a 'code of ethical behavior' to its managers. The company should undertake a careful review of the composition, size, and structure of its board of directors to determine whether it needs, among other things, additional out-side directors and an audit committee of board members. There is a lot being written these days about the governance of corporations, and the company should incorporate the best of it into its bylaws and policies."

Sherwin believes further that management should work with state officials in scrutinizing the rate-making process and considering possible reforms:

"The case testimony suggests that profits and prices *are* higher than normal. The crucial question is why. It is conceivable that the employees' improprieties were an insignificant factor compared with the effects of the decentralized state agency, the conflicting jurisdictions between state and municipal responsibilities, loopholes in control, and so forth. If that is the case, the legislative subcommittee members should focus their attention and recommendations on correcting these structural problems.

"The company should make conciliatory moves toward citizen and consumer groups. In addition to detailing for them the steps it is taking to prevent a recurrence of improper acts by its employees, the company can legitimately point out that to a large extent its employees were in effect lured by the uneven administration of the rate-making process and the islands of arbitrary power they had to deal with. Since consumer groups are mainly interested in the service they get for their money, they are likely to prefer a general solution of the problem to ad hoc punishment of the company.

"By instigating a program to repair structural defects in the regulatory process, the company may be paving the way for a reduction in rates for itself. But the company should take a stand on the right side. To avoid punitive prices, it must be willing to settle for fair prices. When the company can no longer reap profits not warranted by the risks to which the investors' capital is exposed, as it had been doing by taking advantage of structural defects in the rate-making process and the cupidity of public servants, it will redirect its efforts to more responsible avenues for increasing its economic performance."

Finally, perhaps the executives in our case could turn the traumatic trial proceedings to the company's long-term advantage. The testimony—even the most compromising sections of it—might be converted to a forceful educational tool. Scobel says:

"I only hope Hyde and Bradenhoff have the good grace to follow Beverly Walensa's advice and keep employees fully and truthfully informed and at least start to build a credibility base for tomorrow. She is right when she says there isn't any way to win except legally, maybe. She speaks with integrity but doesn't seem to have Bradenhoff's ear. Obviously, she was not asked to play much of a role in this important human resource problem. The investigation, the discussion with headquarters, and probably the decision making were handled mostly by the chief counsel."

I would go further. I wonder if Walensa wasn't working on a potent idea when Tillman discouraged her. She was suggesting it might be useful to let every employee have the whole record every day of the previous day's proceedings in court, dirt and all. If, as Bradenhoff and Hyde maintain, management wants to develop higher standards for employees in this rogue division, that trial record could have a chastening effect. Reading the daily transcripts, employees could see for themselves the embarrassment, humiliation, compromises, and other costs that accumulate in an overly "permissive" environment.

"I don't want to end up in a transcript like this" would be a normal reaction. Management ought then to get plenty of cooperation in attempts to institute codes of conduct, as Nolan suggests, sharper accounting systems, as Sherwin suggests, and corporate due process, as Scobel suggests.

Further, daily distribution of the trial record would arm employees with all the information pro and con so that they would never be at a disadvantage in discussing the event with outsiders. I wonder if there is anything quite so denigrating to employees as to have to learn from the media what is going on in their own organization. The message from top management seems to be all too clear: "You only work here."

# 3

# Ethics without the Sermon

### LAURA L. NASH

As if via a network TV program on the telecommunications satellite, declarations such as these are being broadcast throughout the land:

*Scene 1.* Annual meeting, Anyproducts Inc.; John Q. Moneypockets, chairman and CEO, speaking: "Our responsibility to the public has always come first at our company, and we continue to strive toward serving our public in the best way possible in the belief that good ethics is good business. . . . Despite our forecast of a continued recession in the industry through 1982, we are pleased to announce that 1981's earnings per share were up for the twenty-sixth year in a row."

*Scene 2.* Corporate headquarters, Anyproducts Inc.; Linda Diesinker, group vice president, speaking: "Of course we're concerned about minority development and the plight of the inner cities. But the best place for our new plant would be Horsepasture, Minnesota. We need a lot of space for our operations and a skilled labor force, and the demographics and tax incentives in Horse-pasture are perfect."

*Scene 3.* Interview with a financial writer; Rafe Shortstop, president, Any-products Inc., speaking: "We're very concerned about the state 'of American business and our ability to compete with foreign companies. . . . No, I don't think we have any real ethical problems. We don't bribe people or anything like that."

*Scene 4.* Jud McFisticuff, taxi driver, speaking: "Anyproducts? You've got to be kidding! I wouldn't buy their stuff for anything. The last thing of theirs I bought fell apart in six months. And did you see how they were dumping wastes in the Roxburg water system?"

*Scene 5.* Leslie Matriculant, MBA '82, speaking: "Join Anyproducts? I don't want to risk my reputation working for a company like that. They recently acquired a business that turned out to have ten class-action discrimination suits against it. And when Anyproducts tried to settle the whole thing out of court, the president had his picture in *Business Week* with the caption, 'His secretary still serves him coffee'."

Whether you regard it as an unchecked epidemic or as the first blast of Gabriel's horn, the trend toward focusing on the social impact of the corporation is an inescapable reality that must be factored into today's managerial decision making. But for the executive who asks, "How do we as a corporation examine our ethical concerns?" the theoretical insights currently available may be more frustrating than helpful.

As the first scene in this article implies, many executives firmly believe that corporate operations and corporate values are dynamically intertwined. For the purposes of analysis, however, the executive needs to uncoil the business-ethics helix and examine both strands closely.

Unfortunately, the ethics strand has remained largely inaccessible, for business has not yet developed a workable process by which corporate values can be articulated. If ethics and business are part of the same double helix, perhaps we can develop a microscope capable of enlarging our perception of both aspects of business administration — what we do and who we are.

## Sidestepping Triassic Reptiles

Philosophy has been sorting out issues of fairness, injury, empathy, self-sacrifice, and so on for more than 2,000 years. In seeking to examine the ethics of business, therefore, business logically assumes it will be best served by a "consultant" in philosophy who is already familiar with the formal discipline of ethics.

As the philosopher begins to speak, however, a difficulty immediately arises; corporate executives and philosophers approach problems in radically different ways. The academician ponders the intangible, savors the paradoxical, and embraces the peculiar; he or she speaks in a special language of categorical imperatives and deontological viewpoints that must be taken into consideration before a statement about honesty is agreed to have any meaning.

Like some Triassic reptile, the theoretical view of ethics lumbers along in the far past of Sunday School and Philosophy 1, while the reality of practical business concerns is constantly measuring a wide range of competing claims on time and resources against the unrelenting and objective marketplace.

Not surprisingly, the two groups are somewhat hostile. The jokes of the liberal intelligentsia are rampant and weary: "*Ethics and Business* — the shortest book in the world." "Business and ethics — a subject confined to the preface of business books." Accusations from the corporate cadre are delivered with an assurance that rests more on an intuition of social climate than on a certainty of fact: "You do-gooders are ruining America's ability to compete in the world." "Of course, the cancer reports on ———— [choose from a long list] were terribly exaggerated."

What is needed is a process of ethical inquiry that is immediately comprehensible to a group of executives and not predisposed to the utopian, and sometimes anticapitalistic, bias marking much of the work in applied business philosophy today. So I suggest, as a preliminary solution, a set of 12 questions that draw on traditional philosophical frameworks but that avoid the level of abstraction normally associated with formal moral reasoning.

I offer the questions as a first step in a very new discipline. As such, they form a tentative model that will certainly undergo modifications after its parts are given some exercise. The *Exhibit* poses the 12 questions.

To illustrate the application of the questions, I will draw especially on a program at Lex Service Group, Ltd., whose top management prepared a statement of financial objectives and moral values as a part of its strategic planning process.[1] Lex is a British company with operations in the United Kingdom and the United States. Its sales total about $1.2 billion. In 1978 its structure was partially decentralized, and in 1979 the chairman's policy group began a strategic planning process. The intent, according to its statement of values and objectives, was "to make explicit the sort of company Lex was, or wished to be."

Neither a paralegal code nor a generalized philosophy, the statement consisted of a series of general policies regarding financial strategy as well as such aspects of the company's character as customer service, employee-shareholder responsibility, and quality of management. Its content largely reflected the personal values of Lex's chairman and CEO, Trevor Chinn, whose private philanthropy is well known and whose concern for social welfare has long been echoed in the company's personnel policies.

In the past, pressure on senior managers for high-profit performance had obscured some of these ideals in practice, and the statement of strategy was a way of radically realigning various competing moral claims with the financial objectives of the company. As one senior manager remarked to me, "The values seem obvious, and if we hadn't been so gross in the past we wouldn't have needed the statement." Despite a predictable variance among Lex's top executives as to the desirability of the values outlined in the statement, it was adopted with general agreement to comply and was scheduled for reassessment at a senior managers' meeting one year after implementation.

## The 12 Questions

### 1. Have you defined the problem accurately?

How one assembles the facts weights an issue before the moral examination ever begins, and a definition is rarely accurate if it articulates one's loyalties rather than the facts. The importance of factual neutrality is readily seen, for example, in assessing the moral implications of producing a chemical agent for use in warfare. Depending on one's loyalties, the decision to make the substance can be described as serving one's country, developing products, or killing babies. All of the above may be factual statements, but none is neutral or accurate if viewed in isolation.

Similarly, the recent controversy over marketing U.S.-made cigarettes in Third World countries rarely noted that the incidence of lung cancer in underdeveloped nations is quite low (from one-tenth to one-twentieth the rate for U.S. males) due primarily to the lower life expectancies and earlier predominance of other diseases in these nations. Such a fact does not decide the ethical complexities of this marketing problem, but it does add a crucial perspective in the assignment of moral priorities by defining precisely the injury that tobacco exports may cause.

Extensive fact gathering may also help defuse the emotionalism of an issue. For instance, local statistics on lung cancer incidence reveal that the U.S. tobacco industry is not now "exporting death," as has been charged. Moreover, the substantial and immediate economic benefits attached to tobacco may be providing food and health care in these countries. Nevertheless, as life expectancy and the standards of living rise, a higher incidence of cigarette-related diseases appears likely to develop in these nations. Therefore, cultivation of the nicotine habit may be deemed detrimental to the long-term welfare of these nations.

According to one supposedly infallible truth of modernism, technology is so complex that its results will never be fully comprehensible or predictable. Part

## Exhibit  Twelve Questions for Examining the Ethics of a Business Decision

1   Have you defined the problem accurately?

2   How would you define the problem if you stood on the other side of the fence?

3   How did this situation occur in the first place?

4   To whom and to what do you give your loyalty as a person and as a member of the corporation?

5   What is your intention in making this decision?

6   How does this intention compare with the probable results?

7   Whom could your decision or action injure?

8   Can you discuss the problem with the affected parties before you make your decision?

9   Are you confident that your position will be as valid over a long period of time as it seems now?

10  Could you disclose without qualm your decision or action to your boss, your CEO, the board of directors, your family, society as a whole?

11  What is the symbolic potential of your action if understood? If misunderstood?

12  Under what conditions would your allow exceptions to your stand?

---

of the executive's frustration in responding to question 1 is the real possibility that the "experts" will find no grounds for agreement about the facts.

As a first step, however, defining fully the factual implications of a decision determines to a large degree the quality of one's subsequent moral position. Pericles' definition of true courage rejected the Spartans' blind obedience in war in preference to the courage of the Athenian citizen who, he said, was able to make a decision to proceed in full knowledge of the probable danger. A truly moral decision is an informed decision. A decision that is based on blind or convenient ignorance is hardly defensible.

One simple test of the initial definition is the question:

*2. How would you define the problem if you stood on the other side of the fence?*

The contemplated construction of a plant for Division X is touted at the finance committee meeting as an absolute necessity for expansion at a cost saving of at least 25%. With plans drawn up for an energy-efficient building and an option already secured on a 99-year lease in a new industrial park in Chippewa County, the committee is likely to feel comfortable in approving the request for funds in a matter of minutes.

The facts of the matter are that the company will expand in an appropriate market, allocate its resources sensibly, create new jobs, increase Chippewa County's tax base, and most likely increase its returns to the shareholders. To the residents of Chippewa County, however, the plant may mean the destruction of a customary recreation spot, the onset of severe traffic jams, and the erection of an architectural eyesore. These are also facts of the situation, and certainly more immediate to the county than utilitarian justifications of profit performance and rights of ownership from an impersonal corporation whose headquarters are 1,000 miles from Chippewa County and whose executives have plenty of acreage for their own recreation.

The purpose of articulating the other side, whose needs are understandably less proximate than operational considerations, is to allow some mechanism whereby calculations of self-interest (or even of a project's ultimate general beneficence) can be interrupted by a compelling empathy for those who might suffer immediate injury or mere annoyance as a result of a corporation's decisions. Such empathy is a necessary prerequisite for shouldering voluntarily some responsibility for the social consequences of corporate operations, and it may be the only solution to today's overly litigious and anarchic world.

There is a power in self-examination: with an exploration of the likely consequences of a proposal, taken from the viewpoint of those who do not immediately benefit, comes a discomfort or an embarrassment that rises in proportion to the degree of the likely injury and its articulation. Like Socrates as gadfly, who stung his fellow citizens into a critical examination of their conduct when they became complacent, the discomfort of the alternative definition is meant to prompt a disinclination to choose the expedient over the most responsible course of action.

Abstract generalities about the benefits of the profit motive and the free market system are, for some, legitimate and ultimate justifications, but when unadorned with alternative viewpoints, such arguments also tend to promote the complacency, carelessness, and impersonality that have characterized some of the more injurious actions of corporations. The advocates of these arguments are like the reformers in Nathaniel Hawthorne's short story "Hall of Fantasy" who "had got possession of some crystal fragment of truth, the brightness of which so dazzled them that they could see nothing else in the whole universe."

In the example of Division X's new plant, it was a simple matter to define the alternate facts; the process rested largely on an assumption that certain values were commonly shared (no one likes a traffic jam, landscaping pleases more than an unadorned building, and so forth). But the alternative definition often underscores an inherent disparity in values or language. To some, the employment of illegal aliens is a criminal act (fact #1); to others, it is a solution to the 60% unemployment rate of a neighboring country (fact #2). One country's bribe is another country's redistribution of sales commissions.

When there are cultural or linguistic disparities, it is easy to get the facts wrong or to invoke a pluralistic tolerance as an excuse to act in one's own self-interest: "That's the way they do things over there. Who are we to question their beliefs?" This kind of reasoning can be both factually inaccurate (many generalizations about bribery rest on hearsay and do not represent the complexities of a culture) and philosophically inconsistent (there are plenty of beliefs, such as those of the environmentalist, which the same generalizers do not hesitate to question).

### 3. How did this situation occur in the first place?

Lex Motor Company, a subsidiary of Lex Service Group, Ltd., had been losing share at a 20% rate in a declining market; and Depot B's performance was the worst of all. Two nearby Lex depots could easily absorb B's business, and closing it down seemed the only sound financial decision. Lex's chairman, Trevor Chinn, hesitated to approve the closure, however, on the grounds that putting 100 people out of work was not right when the corporation itself was not really jeopardized by B's existence. Moreover, seven department managers, who were all within five years of retirement and had had 25 or more years of service at Lex, were scheduled to be made redundant.

The values statement provided no automatic solution, for it placed value on both employees' security and shareholders' interest. Should they close Depot B? At first Chinn thought not: Why should the little guys suffer disproportionately when the company was not performing well? Why not close a more recently acquired business where employee service was not so large a factor? Or why not wait out the short term and reduce head count through natural attrition?

As important as deciding the ethics of the situation was the inquiry into its history. Indeed, the history gave a clue to solving the dilemma: Lex's traditional emphasis on employee security *and* high financial performance had led to a precipitate series of acquisitions and subsequent divestitures when the company had failed to meet its overall objectives. After each rationalization, the people serving the longest had been retained and placed at Depot B, so that by 1980 the facility had more managers than it needed and a very high proportion of long-service employees.

So the very factors that had created the performance problems were making the closure decision difficult, and the very solution that Lex was inclined to favor again would exacerbate the situation further!

In deciding the ethics of a situation it is important to distinguish the symptoms from the disease. Great profit pressures with no sensitivity to the cycles in a particular industry, for example, may force division managers to be ruthless with employees, to short-weight customers, or even to fiddle with cash flow reports in order to meet headquarters' performance criteria.

Dealing with the immediate case of lying, quality discrepancy, or strained labor relations — when the problem is finally discovered — is only a temporary solution. A full examination of how the situation occurred and what the traditional solutions have been may reveal a more serious discrepancy of values and pressures, and this will illuminate the real significance and ethics of the problem. It will also reveal recurring patterns of events that in isolation appear trivial but that as a whole point up a serious situation.

Such a mechanism is particularly important because very few executives are outright scoundrels. Rather, violations of corporate and social values usually occur inadvertently because no one recognizes that a problem exists until it becomes a crisis. This tendency toward initial trivialization seems to be the biggest ethical problem in business today. Articulating answers to my first three questions is a way of reversing that process.

### 4. To whom and what do you give your loyalties as a person and as a member of the corporation?

Every executive faces conflicts of loyalty. The most familiar occasions pit private conscience and sense of duty against corporate policy, but equally frequent are the situations in which one's close colleagues demand participation (tacit or explicit) in an operation or a decision that runs counter to company policy. To whom or what is the greater loyalty — to one's corporation? superior? family? society? self? race? sex?

The good news about conflicts of loyalty is that their identification is a workable way of smoking out the ethics of a situation and of discovering the absolute values inherent in it. As one executive in a discussion of a Harvard case study put it, "My corporate brain says this action is O.K., but my noncorporate brain keeps flashing these warning lights."

The bad news about conflicts of loyalty is that there are few automatic answers for placing priorities on them. "To thine own self be true" is a murky quagmire when the self takes on a variety of roles, as it does so often in this complex modern world.

Supposedly, today's young managers are giving more weight to individual than to corporate identity, and some older executives see this tendency as being ultimately subversive. At the same time, most of them believe individual integrity is essential to a company's reputation.

The U.S. securities industry, for example, is one of the most rigorous industries in America in its requirements of honesty and disclosure. Yet in the end, all its systematic precautions prove inadequate unless the people involved also have a strong sense of integrity that puts loyalty to these principles above personal gain.

A system, however, must permit the time and foster the motivation to allow personal integrity to surface in a particular situation. An examination of loyalties is one way to bring this about. Such an examination may strengthen reputations but also may result in blowing the whistle (freedom of thought carries with it the risk of revolution). But a sorting out of loyalties can also bridge the gulf between policy and implementation or among various interest groups whose affiliations may mask a common devotion to an aspect of a problem — a devotion on which consensus can be built.

How does one probe into one's own loyalties and their implications? A useful method is simply to play various roles out loud, to call on one's loyalty to family and community (for example) by asking, "What will I say when my child asks me why I did that?" If the answer is "That's the way the world works," then your loyalties are clear and moral passivity inevitable. But if the question presents real problems, you have begun a demodulation of signals from your conscience that can only enhance corporate responsibility.

### 5. What is your intention in making this decision?

### 6. How does this intention compare with the likely results?

These two questions are asked together because their content often bears close resemblance and, by most calculations, both color the ethics of a situation.

Corporation Buglebloom decides to build a new plant in an underdeveloped minority-populated district where the city has been trying with little success to encourage industrial development. The media approve and Buglebloom adds another star to its good reputation. Is Buglebloom a civic leader and a supporter of minorities or a canny investor about to take advantage of the disadvantaged? The possibilities of Buglebloom's intentions are endless and probably unfathomable to the public; Buglebloom may be both canny investor and friend of minority groups.

I argue that despite their complexity and elusiveness, a company's intentions *do* matter. The "purity" of Buglebloom's motives (purely profit-seeking or purely altruistic) will have wide-reaching effects inside and outside the corporation — on attitudes toward minority employees in other parts of the company, on the wages paid at the new plant, and on the number of other investors in the same area — that will legitimize a certain ethos in the corporation and the community.

Sociologist Max Weber called this an "ethics of attitude" and contrasted it with an "ethics of absolute ends." An ethics of attitude sets a standard to ensure a certain action. A firm policy at headquarters of not cheating customers, for example, may also deter salespeople from succumbing to a tendency to lie by omission or purchasers from continuing to patronize a high-priced supplier when the costs are automatically passed on in the selling price.

What about the ethics of result? Two years later, Buglebloom wishes it had never begun Project Minority Plant. Every good intention has been lost in the realities of doing business in an unfamiliar area, and Buglebloom now has dirty hands: some of those payoffs were absolutely unavoidable if the plant was to open, operations have been plagued with vandalism and language problems, and local resentment at the industrialization of the neighborhood has risen as charges of discrimination have surfaced. No one seems to be benefiting from the project.

The goodness of intent pales somewhat before results that perpetrate great injury or simply do little good. Common sense demands that the "responsible" corporation try to align the two more closely, to identify the probable consequences and also the limitations of knowledge that might lead to more harm than good. Two things to remember in comparing intention and results are that knowledge of the future is always inadequate and that overconfidence often precedes a disastrous mistake.

These two precepts, cribbed from ancient Greece, may help the corporation keep the disparities between intent and result a fearsome reality to consider continuously. The next two questions explore two ways of reducing the moral risks of being wrong.

### 7. Whom could your decision or action injure?

The question presses whether injury is intentional or not. Given the limits of knowledge about a new product or policy, who and how many will come into contact with it? Could its inadequate disposal affect an entire community? two employees? yourself? How might your product be used if it happened to be acquired by a terrorist radical group or a terrorist military police force? Has your distribution system or disposal plan ensured against such injury? Could it ever?

If not, there may be a compelling moral justification for stopping production. In an integrated society where business and government share certain values, possible injury is an even more important consideration than potential benefit. In policymaking, a much likelier ground for agreement than benefit is avoidance of injury through those "universal nos"—such as no mass death, no totalitarianism, no hunger or malnutrition, no harm to children.

To exclude *at the outset* any policy or decision that might have such results is to reshape the way modern business examines its own morality. So often business formulates questions of injury only after the fact in the form of liability suits.

### 8. Can you engage the affected parties in a discussion of the problem before you make your decision?

If the calculus of injury is one way of responding to limitations of knowledge about the probable results of a particular business decision, the participation of affected parties is one of the best ways of informing that consideration. Civil rights groups often complain that corporations fail to invite participation from local leaders during the planning stages of community development projects and charitable programs. The corporate foundation that builds a tennis complex for disadvantaged youth is throwing away precious resources if most children in the neighborhood suffer from chronic malnutrition.

In the Lex depot closure case I have mentioned, senior executives agonized over whether the employees would choose redundancy over job transfer and which course would ultimately be more beneficial to them. The managers, however, did not consult the employees. There were more than 200 projected job transfers to another town. But all the affected employees, held by local ties and uneasy about possibly lower housing subsidies, refused relocation offers. Had the employees been allowed to participate in the redundancy discussions, the company might have wasted less time on relocation plans or might have uncovered and resolved the fears about relocating.

The issue of participation affects everyone. (How many executives feel that someone else should decide what is in *their* best interest?) And yet it is a principle often forgotten because of the pressure of time or the inconvenience of calling people together and facing predictably hostile questions.

### 9. Are you confident that your position will be as valid over a long period of time as it seems now?

As anyone knows who has had to consider long-range plans and short-term budgets simultaneously, a difference in time frame can change the meaning of a problem as much as spring and autumn change the colors of a tree. The ethical coloring of a business decision is no exception to this generational aspect of decision making. Time alters circumstances, and few corporate value systems are immune to shifts in financial status, external political pressure, and personnel. (One survey now places the average U.S. CEO's tenure in office at five years.)

At Lex, for example, the humanitarianism of the statement of objectives and values depended on financial prosperity. The values did not fully anticipate the extent to which the U.K. economy would undergo a recession, and the resulting changes had to be examined, reconciled, and fought if the company's values were to have any meaning. At the Lex annual review, the managers asked themselves repeatedly whether hard times were the ultimate test of the statement or a clear indication that a corporation had to be able to "afford" ethical positions.

Ideally, a company's articulation of its values should anticipate changes of fortune. As the hearings for the passage of the Foreign Corrupt Practices Act of 1977 demonstrated, doing what you can get away with today may not be a secure moral standard, but short-term discomfort for long-term sainthood may require irrational courage or a rational reasoning system or, more likely, both. These 12 questions attempt to elicit a rational system. Courage, of course, depends on personal integrity.

Another aspect of the ethical time frame stretches beyond the boundaries of question 9 but deserves special attention, and that is the timing of the ethical inquiry. When and where will it be made?

We do not normally invoke moral principles in our everyday conduct. Some time ago the participants in a national business ethics conference had worked late into the night preparing the final case for the meeting, and they were very anxious the next morning to get the class under way. Just before the session began, however, someone suggested that they all donate a dollar apiece as a gratuity for the dining hall help at the institute.

Then just as everyone automatically reached into his or her pocket, another person questioned the direction of the gift. Why tip the person behind the counter but not the cook in the kitchen? Should the money be given to each person in proportion to salary or divided equally among all? The participants laughed uneasily—or groaned—as they thought of the diversion of precious time from the case. A decision had to be made.

With the sure instincts of efficient managers, the group chose to forgo further discussion of distributive justice and, yes, appoint a committee. The committee doled out the money without further group consideration, and no formal feedback on the donation was asked for or given.

The questions offered here do not solve the problem of making time for the inquiry. For suggestions about creating favorable conditions for examining corporate values, drawn from my field research, see *Appendix*.

### 10. Could you disclose without qualm your decision or action to your boss, your CEO, the board of directors, your family, or society as a whole?

The old question, "Would you want your decision to appear on the front page of the *New York Times*?" still holds. A corporation may maintain that there's really no problem, but a survey of how many "trivial" actions it is reluctant to disclose might be interesting. Disclosure is a way of sounding those submarine depths of conscience and of searching out loyalties.

It is also a way of keeping a corporate character cohesive. The Lex group, for example, was once faced with a very sticky problem concerning a small but profitable site with unpleasant (though in no way illegal) working conditions, where two men with 30 years' service worked. I wrote up the case for a Lex senior managers' meeting on the promise to disguise it heavily because the executive who supervised the plant was convinced that, if the chairman and the personnel director knew the plant's true location, they would close it down immediately.

At the meeting, however, as everyone became involved in the discussion and the chairman himself showed sensitivity to the dilemma, the executive disclosed the location and spoke of his own feelings about the situation. The level of mutual confidence was apparent to all, and by other reports it was the most open discussion the group had ever had.

The meeting also fostered understanding of the company's values and their implementation. When the discussion finally flagged, the chairman spoke up. Basing his views on a full knowledge of the group's understanding of the problem, he set the company's priorities. "Jobs over fancy conditions, health over jobs," Chinn said, "but we always *must disclose*." The group decided to keep the plant open, at least for the time being.

Disclosure does not, however, automatically bring universal sympathy. In the early 1970s, a large food store chain that repeatedly found itself embroiled in the United Farm Workers (UFW) disputes with the Teamsters over California grape and lettuce contracts took very seriously the moral implications of a decision whether to stop selling these products. The company endlessly researched the issues, talked to all sides, and made itself available to public representatives of various interest groups to explain its position and to hear out everyone else.

When the controversy started, the company decided to support the UFW boycott, but three years later top management reversed its position. Most of the people who wrote to the company or asked it to send representatives to their local UFW support meetings, however, continued to condemn the chain even after hearing its views, and the general public apparently never became aware of the company's side of the story.

### 11. What is the symbolic potential of your action if understood? if misunderstood?

Jones Inc., a diversified multinational corporation with assets of $5 billion, has a paper manufacturing operation that happens to be the only major industry in Stirville, and the factory has been polluting the river on which it is located. Local and national conservation groups have filed suit against Jones Inc. for past damages, and the company is defending itself. Meanwhile, the corporation has adopted plans for a new waste-efficient plant. The legal battle is extended and local resentment against Jones Inc. gets bitter.

As a settlement is being reached, Jones Inc. announces that, as a civic-minded gesture, it will make 400 acres of Stirville woodland it owns available to the residents for conservation and recreation purposes. Jones's intention is to offer a peace pipe to the people of Stirville, and the company sees the gift as a symbol of its own belief in conservation and a way of signaling that value to Stirville residents and national conservation groups. Should Jones Inc. give the land away? Is the symbolism significant?

If the symbolic value of the land is understood as Jones Inc. intends, the gift may patch up the company's relations with Stirville and stave off further disaffection with potential employees as the new plant is being built. It may also signal to employees throughout the corporation that Jones Inc. places a premium on conservation efforts and community relations.

If the symbolic value is misunderstood, however, or if completion of the plant is delayed and the old one has to be put back in use—or if another Jones operation is discovered to be polluting another community and becomes a target of the press—the gift could be interpreted as nothing more than a cheap effort to pay off the people of Stirville and hasten settlement of the lawsuit.

The Greek root of our word *symbol* means both signal and contract. A business decision—whether it is the use of an expense account or a corporate donation—has a symbolic value in signaling what is acceptable behavior within the corporate culture and in making a tacit contract with employees and the community about the rules of the game. How the symbol is actually perceived (or misperceived) is as important as how you intend it to be perceived.

### 12. Under what conditions would you allow exceptions to your stand?

If we accept the idea that every business decision has an important symbolic value and a contractual nature, then the need for consistency is obvious. At the same time, it is also important to ask under what conditions the rules of the game may be changed. What conflicting principles, circumstances, or time constraints would provide a morally acceptable basis for making an exception to one's normal institutional ethos? For instance, how does the cost of the strategy to develop managers from minority groups over the long term fit in with short-term hurdle rates? Also to be considered is what would mitigate a clear case of employee dishonesty.

Questions of consistency—if you would do X, would you also do Y?—are yet another way of eliciting the ethics of the company and of oneself, and can be a final test of the strength, idealism, or practicality of those values. A last example from the experience of Lex illustrates this point and gives temporary credence to the platitude that good ethics is good business. An article in the Sunday paper about a company that had run a series of racy ads, with pictures of half-dressed women and promises of free merchandise to promote the sale of a very mundane product, sparked an extended examination at Lex of its policies on corporate inducements.

One area of concern was holiday giving. What was the acceptable limit for a gift—a bottle of whiskey? a case? Did it matter only that the company did not *intend* the gift to be an inducement, or did the mere possibility of inducement taint the gift? Was the cut-off point absolute? The group could agree on no halfway point for allowing some gifts and not others, so a new value was added to the formal statement that prohibited the offering or receiving of inducements.

The next holiday season Chinn sent a letter to friends and colleagues who had received gifts of appreciation in the past. In it he explained that, as a result of Lex's concern with "the very complex area of business ethics," management had decided that the company would no longer send any gifts, nor would it be appropriate for its employees to receive any. Although the letter did not explain Lex's reasoning behind the decision, apparently there was a large untapped consensus about such gift giving: by return mail Chinn received at least 20 letters from directors, general managers, and chairmen of companies with which Lex had done business congratulating him for his decision, agreeing with the new policy, and thanking him for his holiday wishes.

## The "Good Puppy" Theory

The 12 questions are a way to articulate an idea of the responsibilities involved and to lay them open for examination. Whether a decisive policy is also generated or not, there are compelling reasons for holding such discussions:

The process facilitates talk as a group about a subject that has traditionally been reserved for the privacy of one's conscience. Moreover, for those whose consciences twitch but don't speak in full sentences, the questions help sort out their own perceptions of the problem and various ways of thinking about it.

The process builds a cohesiveness of managerial character as points of consensus emerge and people from vastly different operations discover that they share common problems. It is one way of determining the values and goals of the company, and that is a key element in determining corporate strategy.

It acts as an information resource. Senior managers learn about other parts of the company with which they may have little contact.

It helps uncover ethical inconsistencies in the articulated values of the corporation or between these values and the financial strategy.

It helps uncover sometimes dramatic differences between the values and the practicality of their implementation.

It helps the CEO understand how the senior managers think, how they handle a problem, and how willing and able they are to deal with complexity. It reveals how they may be drawing on the private self to the enhancement of corporate activity.

In drawing out the private self in connection with business and in exploring the significance of the corporation's activities, the process derives meaning from an environment that is often characterized as meaningless.

It helps improve the nature and range of alternatives.

It is cathartic.

The process is also reductive in that it limits the level of inquiry. For example, the 12 questions ask what injury might result from a decision and what good is intended, but they do not ask the meaning of *good* or whether the result is "just."

Socrates asked how a person could talk of pursuing the good before knowing what the good is; and the analysis he visualized entailed a lifelong process of learning and examination. Do the 12 short questions, with their explicit goal of simplifying the ethical examination, bastardize the Socratic ideal? To answer this, we must distinguish between personal philosophy and participation as a corporate member in the examination of a *corporate* ethos, for the 12 questions assume some difference between private and corporate "goodness."

This distinction is crucial to any evaluation of my suggested process for conducting an ethical inquiry and needs to be explained. What exactly do we expect of the "ethical," or "good," corporation? Three examples of goodness represent prevailing social opinions, from that of the moral philosopher to the strict Friedmaniac.

     1. The most rigorous moral analogy to the good corporation would be the "good man." An abstract, philosophical ideal having highly moral connotations, the good man encompasses an intricate relation of abstractions such as Plato's four virtues (courage, godliness or philosophical wisdom, righteousness, and prudence). The activities of this kind of good corporation imply a heavy responsibility to collectively know the good and to resolve to achieve it.

     2. Next, there is the purely amoral definition of good, as in a "good martini"—an amoral fulfillment of a largely inanimate and functional purpose. Under this definition, corporate goodness would be best achieved by the unadorned accrual of profits with no regard for the social implications of the means whereby profits are made.

     3. Halfway between these two views lies the good as in "good puppy"—here goodness consists primarily of the fulfillment of a social contract that centers on avoiding social injury. Moral capacity is perceived as present, but its potential is limited. A moral evaluation of the good puppy is possible but exists largely in concrete terms; we do not need to identify the puppy's intentions as utilitarian to understand and agree that its "ethical" fulfillment of the social contract consists of not soiling the carpet or biting the baby.

It seems to me that business ethics operates most appropriately for corporate man when it seeks to define and explore corporate morality at the level of the good puppy. The good corporation is expected to avoid perpetrating irretrievable social injury (and to assume the costs when it unintentionally does injury) while focusing on its purpose as a profit-making organization. Its moral capacity does not extend, however, to determining by itself what will improve the general social welfare.

The good puppy inquiry operates largely in concrete experience; just as the 12 questions impose a limit on our moral expectations, so too they impose a limit (welcome, to some) on our use of abstraction to get at the problem.

The situations for testing business morality remain complex. But by avoiding theoretical inquiry and limiting the expectations of corporate goodness to a few rules for social behavior that are based on common sense, we can develop an ethic that is appropriate to the language, ideology, and institutional dynamics of business decision making and consensus. This ethic can also offer managers a practical way of exploring those occasions when their corporate brains are getting warning flashes from their noncorporate brains.

*APPENDIX*

Shared Conditions of Some Successful Ethical Inquiries

| | |
|---|---|
| **Fixed time frame** | Understanding and identifying moral issues takes time and causes ferment, and the executive needs an uninterrupted block of time to ponder the problems. |
| **Unconventional location** | Religious groups, boards of directors, and professional associations have long recognized the value of the retreat as a way of stimulating fresh approaches to regular activities. If the group is going to transcend normal corporate hierarchies, it should hold the discussion on neutral territory so that all may participate with the same degree of freedom. |
| **Resource person** | The advantage of bringing in an outsider is not that he or she will impose some preconceived notion of right and wrong on management but that he will serve as a midwife for bringing the values already present in the institution out into the open. He can generate closer examination of the discrepancies between values and practice and draw on a wider knowledge of instances and intellectual frameworks than the group can. The resource person may also take the important role of arbitrator—to ensure that one person does not dominate the session with his or her own values and that the dialogue does not become impossibly emotional. |
| **Participation of CEO** | In most corporations the chief executive still commands an extra degree of authority for the intangible we call corporate culture, and the discussion needs the perspective of and legitimization by that authority if it is to have any seriousness of purpose and consequence. One of the most interesting experiments in examining corporate policy I have observed lacked the CEO's support, and within a year it died on the vine. |
| **Credo** | Articulating the corporation's values and objectives provides a reference point for group inquiry and implementation. Ethical codes, however, when drawn up by the legal department, do not always offer a realistic and full representation of management's beliefs. The most important ethical inquiry for management may be the very formulation of such a statement, for the *process* of articulation is as useful as the values agreed on. |
| **Homegrown topics** | In isolating an ethical issue, drawing on your own experience is important. Philosophical business ethics has tended to reflect national social controversies, which though relevant to the corporation may not always be as relevant—not to mention as easily resolved—as some internal issues that are shaping the character of the company to a much |

greater degree. Executives are also more likely to be informed on these issues.

| | |
|---|---|
| **Resolution** | In all the programs I observed except one, there was a point at which the inquiry was slated to have some resolution: either a vote on the issue, the adoption of a new policy, a timetable for implementation, or the formulation of a specific statement of values. The one program observed that had no such decision-making structure was organized simply to gather information about the company's activities through extrahierarchical channels. Because the program had no tangible goals or clearly articulated results, its benefits were impossible to measure. |

### NOTE

1. The process is modeled after ideas in Kenneth R. Andrews's book *The Concept of Corporate Strategy* (Homewood, Ill.: Richard D. Irwin, 1980, revised edition) and in Richard F. Vancil's article "Strategy Formulation in Complex Organizations," *Sloan Management Review*, Winter 1976, p. 4.

## 4

# Can the Best Corporations Be Made Moral?

## KENNETH R. ANDREWS

The concept of corporate social responsibility has made steady progress during the past 40 years. The words mean in part voluntary restraint of profit maximization. More positively, they mean sensitivity to the social costs of economic activity and to the opportunity to focus corporate power on objectives that are possible but sometimes less economically attractive than socially desirable. The term includes:

The determination of a corporation to reduce its profit by voluntary contributions to education and other charities.

The election of an ethical level of operations higher than the minimum required by law and custom.

The choice between businesses of varying economic opportunity on grounds of their imputed social worth.

The investment for reasons other than (but obviously still related to) economic return in the quality of life within the corporation itself.

This doctrine of corporate social responsibility is vigorously opposed honestly and openly by conservative lawyers and economists and covertly by the adherents of business as usual. Milton Friedman, the conservative economist of the University of Chicago, denounces the concern for responsibility as "fundamentally subversive" to a free society. He argues that "there is one and only one social responsibility of business—to use its resources and engage in activities designed to increase its profits so long as it . . . engages in open and free competition without deception or fraud."[1]

Thus, for example, the manager who makes decisions affecting immediate profit by reducing pollution and increasing minority employment more than present law requires is in effect imposing taxes upon his stockholders and acting without authority as a public legislative body.

Other critics of the doctrine like to point out:

How much easier are the platitudes of virtue than the effective combination of profitable and socially responsive corporate action.

How little experience with social questions businessmen immersed in their narrow ambitions and technology can be expected to have.

How urgent are the pressures of survival in hard times and against competition.

How coercive of individual opinion in an organization is a position on social issues dictated by its management.

How infrequently in the entire population occur the intelligence, compassion, knowledge of issues, and morality required of the manager presumptuous enough to factor social responsibility into his economic decisions.

Given the slow rate at which verbalized good intentions are being converted into action, many critics of the large corporation suspect that for every chief executive announcing pious objectives there are a hundred closet rascals quietly conducting business in the old ways and taking immoral comfort in Friedman's moral support.

The interventionists question the effectiveness of the "invisible hand" of competition as the ethical regulator of great corporations capable of shaping in significant degree their environments. Interventionists think also that regulation by government, while always to some degree essential under imperfect competition, is not sufficiently knowledgeable, subtle, or timely to reconcile the self-interest of corporate entrepreneurship and the needs of the society being sore-tried and well served by economic activity.

The advocates of public responsibility for a so-called "private" enterprise assert that, in an industrial society, corporate power, vast in potential strength, must be brought to bear on certain social problems if the latter are to be solved at all. They argue that corporate executives of the integrity, intelligence, and humanity required to run companies whose revenues often exceed the gross national product of whole nations cannot be expected to confine themselves to economic activity and ignore its consequences, and that henceforth able young men and women coming into business will be sensitive to the social worth of corporate activity.

To reassure those uneasy about the dangers of corporate participation in public affairs, the social interventionists say to the economic isolationists that these hazards can be contained through professional education, government control, and self-regulation.

This is not the place to argue further against Friedman's simplistic faith in the powers of the market to purify self-interest. We must observe, however, that the argument for the active participation of corporations in public affairs, for responsible assessment of the impact of economic activity, and for concern with the quality of corporate purposes is gaining ground, even as uneasiness increases about the existence of corporate power in the hands of managers who (except in cases of crisis) are answerable only to themselves or to boards of directors they have themselves selected.

Criticism of corporate activity is manifest currently in consumerism, in the movement to introduce social legislation into stockholder meetings and to reform board memberships, and (more dangerously) in apathy or antipathy among the young. The most practicable response to this criticism by those holding corporate power is to seek to justify limited government by using power responsibly — the ultimate obligation of free persons in any relatively free society.

We need the large corporation, not for its size but for its capability. Even the vivisectionists of the Justice Department who seek a way to divide IBM into smaller parts presumably have no illusion that the large corporation can or should be eliminated from the world as we know it.

On the assumption, then, that corporate social responsibility is not only here to stay, but must increase in scope and complexity as corporate power increases, I suggest that we look forward to the administrative and organizational consequences of the incursion of private corporations into public responsibility.

## Nature of the Problem

Among the many considerations confronting the executive who would make social responsibility effective, there are some so well known that we can quickly pass them by. Hypocrisy, insincerity, and hollow piety are not really dangerous, for they are easily detected.

In fact, it is much more likely that genuinely good intentions will be thought insincere than that hypocritical protestations of idealism will be mistaken for truth. "Mr. Ford (or Mr. Kaiser or Mr. Rockefeller) doesn't really mean what he says," as an organization refrain is more Mr. Ford's or Mr. Kaiser's or Mr. Rockefeller's problem than what he should say. Cynicism, the by-product of impersonal bureaucracy, remains one of the principal impediments to the communication of corporate social policy.

I would like to set aside also the problem of choice of what social contribution should be attempted — a problem which disparity between the infinite range of social need and the limits of available corporate resources always brings to mind.

### Self-consistent Strategy

The formulation of specific corporate social policy is as much a function of strategic planning as the choice of product and market combinations, the establishment of profit and growth objectives, or the choice of organization structure and systems for accomplishing corporate purposes.

Rather than wholly personal or idiosyncratic contributions (like supporting the museum one's spouse is devoted to) or safe and sound contributions like the standard charities, or faddist entry into fashionable areas, corporate strategic response to societal needs and expectations makes sense when it is closely related to the economic functions of the company or to the peculiar problems of the community in which it operates.

For a paper company, it would seem a strategic necessity to give first priority to eliminating the poisonous effluents from its mills rather than, for example, to support cultural institutions like traveling art exhibits. Similarly, for an oil company it would seem a strategic necessity to look at its refinery stacks, at spillage, and at automobile exhaust.

The fortunate company that is paying the full social cost of its production function can make contributions to problems it does not cause — like juvenile delinquency, illiteracy, and so on — or to other forms of environmental improvement more appropriate to corporate citizenship than directly related to its production processes.

As leaders of business move beyond conventional philanthropic contributions to strategy-related investments in social betterment, they begin to combine the long-run economic interests of their companies with the priorities (as for pollution) becoming evident in public concern, seeking those points where indeed what is good for the country is good for General Motors.

Once the conscious planning which a fully developed corporate strategy requires is understood, the practical alternatives before any company are not impossibly difficult to identify and to rank according to relevance to economic strategy or to organization needs and resources.

The outcome is an integrated self-consistent strategy embodying defined obligations to society relevant to but not confined to its economic purposes. The top management of a large company, once it elects to, can be expected to have less difficulty in articulating such a strategy than in dealing with the problems of organization behavior to which I now turn.

### Organization Behavior

The advance of the doctrine of corporate social responsibility has been the apparent conversion of more and more chief executive officers. Change toward responsible behavior and the formulation of strategic intentions are obviously not possible without their concern, compassion, and conviction.

So long as the organization remains small enough to be directly influenced by the chief executive's leadership, certain results can be traced to his determination that they occur — as in centrally decided investments, specific new ventures, cash contributions to charity, and compensation, promotion, and other personnel policies.

But as an organization grows larger and as operations become more decentralized, the power and influence of the chief executive are reinterpreted and diffused. For example:

If a large company is to be sufficiently decentralized to make worldwide operations feasible, power must be distributed throughout a hierarchy inhabited by persons (a) who may not share their chief executive's determination or fervor, (b) who may not believe (more often) that he means what he says, and (c) who may be impelled to postpone action on such problems as management development, pollution, or employment and advancement of minority representatives.

At this point, the overriding master problem now impeding the further progress of corporate responsibility is the difficulty of making credible and effective, throughout a large organization, the social component of a corporate strategy originating in the moral convictions and values of the chief executive.

**Quantifiable results.** The source of the difficulty is the nature and impact of our systematic planning processes, forms of control, systems of measurement, and pattern of incentives, and the impersonal way all these are administered. The essence of the systematic rational planning we know most about is quantitative information furnished to the process and quantitative measures of results coming out.

Once plans are put into effect, managers are measured, evaluated, promoted, shelved, or discharged according to the relation of their accomplishments against the plan. In the conventions of accounting and the time scale of exact quantification, performance becomes short-run economic or technical results inside the corporation. Evaluation typically gives full marks for current accomplishment, with no estimate of the charges against the future which may have been made in the effort to accomplish the plan.

Since progress in career, dependent on favorable judgments of quantifiable performance, is the central motivation in a large organization, general and functional managers at divisional, regional, district, and local levels are motivated to do well what is best and most measured, to do it now, and to focus their attention on the internal problems that affect immediate results.

In short, the more quantification and the more supervision of variance, the less attention there will be to such intangible topics as the social role of Plant X in Community Y or the quality of corporate life in the office at Sioux City.

The leaner the central staff of a large organization is kept, the more stress there will be on numbers; and, more importantly, the more difficulty there will be in making qualitative evaluation of such long-term processes as individual and management development, the steady augmentation of organizational competence, and the progress of programs for making work meaningful and exciting, and for making more than economic contributions to society.

The small headquarters group supervising the operations of a conglomerate of autonomous organizations hitherto measured by ranking them with respect to return on equity would not expect to have before it proposals from the subsidiaries for important investments in social responsibility. Such investments could only be made by the corporate headquarters, which would not itself be knowledgeable about or much motivated to take action on opportunities existing throughout the subsidiaries.

**Corporate amorality.** One colleague of mine, Joseph L. Bower, has examined the process by which corporate resources are allocated in large organizations.[2] Another, Robert W. Ackerman, has documented through field studies the dilemmas which a financially oriented and present-tense accounting system pose for the forward progress of specific social action, like pollution abatement and provision of minority opportunity.[3] Still a third, Malcolm S. Salter, has studied the impact of compensation systems in multinational corporations.[4]

It appears that the outcome of these and other research studies will establish what we have long suspected — that good works, the results of which are long term and hard to quantify, do not have a chance in an organization using conventional incentives and controls and exerting pressure for ever more impressive results.

It is quite possible then, and indeed quite usual, for a highly moral and humane chief executive to preside over an "amoral organization"[5]—one made so by processes developed before the liberalization of traditional corporate economic objectives. The internal force which stubbornly resists efforts to make the corporation compassionate (and exacting) toward its own people and responsible (as well as economically efficient) in its external relationships is the incentive system forcing attention to short-term quantifiable results.

The sensitivity of upward-oriented career executives at lower and middle levels to what quantitative measures say about them is part of their ambition, their interest in their compensation, and their desire for the recognition and approval of their superiors. When, as they usually do, they learn how to beat the system, the margin of capacity they reserve for a rainy day is hoarded for survival, not expended in strengthening their suborganization's future capability or in part-time participation in corporate good works or responsible citizenship on their own time.

With individuals, as with organizations, survival takes precedence over social concern. All we need do to keep even experienced, capable, and profit-producing managers on the ropes of survival is to focus the spotlight on their day-to-day activities and exhaust their ingenuity in outwitting the system by increasing the level of short-term results they are asked to attain.

The isolationists should be quite content with the amorality of an organization motivated by career-oriented responsiveness to narrowly designed measurement and reward-and-penalty systems. The interventionists are not. They look for solutions in the experience, observation, and research I have been drawing on in describing the set of problems a new breadth of vision reveals to us.

Thus the art of using the two-edged sword of contribution to society and of stimulation to creative achievement within the corporation becomes even more sophisticated when that institution must not only relate to the societies of different countries and cultures but also attract and keep the dedication of men and women with values and desires not typically American.

## Program of Action

Inquiry into the nature of the problem suggests the outlines of a program of action. It begins with the incorporation into strategic and operating plans—of subsidiaries, country or area organizations, or profit centers—of specific objectives in areas of social concerns strategically related to the economic activity and community environment of the organization unit.

Since the executive in New York cannot specify the appropriate social strategy for the company in Brazil or the branch in Oregon, or even know what the people there want to work on, intermediate managers who are aware of the social and organization policy of the company, must elicit (with staff help if necessary) proposals for investment of money, energy, time, or concern in these areas.

The review of plans submitted may result in reduction or increase in commitments in all areas; it is essential that the negotiation include attention to social and organization objectives, with as much quantification as reasonable but with qualitative objectives where appropriate.

The development of such strategic and operating plans turns critically on the initiative of responsible corporate individuals, who must be competent enough to accomplish demanding economic and social tasks and have time as well for their families and private affairs.

Financial, production, and sales requirements may be transmitted down rather than drawn upward in an efficient (though often sterilizing) compaction of the planning process. The top-down promulgation of an imaginative and community-centered social and organization strategy, except in terms so general as to be ineffective, is not only similarly unwise in stifling creativity and commitment but also virtually impossible.

### Qualitative Attention

Once targets and plans have been defined (in the negotiation between organization levels), the measurement system must incorporate in appropriate proportion quantitative and qualitative measures. The bias to short-term results can be corrected by qualitative attention to social and organization programs. The transfer and promotion of managers successful in achieving short-term results is a gamble until their competence in balancing short- and long-term objectives is demonstrated.

Incidentally, rapid rotation virtually guarantees a low level of interest in the particular city through which the manager is following his career; one day it will be seen to be as wasteful as an organization-building and management-development device as it is useful in staffing a growing organization. The alternative—to remain in a given place, to develop fully the company's business in a given city assisted by knowledge and love of the region—needs to become open to executives who do not wish to become president of their companies.

When young middle managers fall short of their targets, inquiry into the reasons and ways to help them achieve assigned goals should precede adverse judgment and penalty. Whenever measurement and control can be directed toward ways to correct problems observed, the shriveling effects of over-emphatic evaluation are postponed. In addition, managers learn that something is important to their superiors other than a single numerical indicator of little significance when detached from the future results to which it relates.

Internal audit. The curse of unquantifiability which hangs over executive action in the areas of corporate responsibility may someday be lifted by the "social audit," now in very early stages of development.[6] In its simplest form, this is a kind of balance sheet and operating statement. On it are listed the dollar values of such corporate investments as training programs, individual development activities, time devoted by individuals to community projects, contributions to pollution abatement, transportation, taxes, and the like. All of these investments call the attention of a company and community to the cumulative dollar worth of corporate functions ancillary to production and sales.

But the further evolvement of the social audit, which one day may develop the conventions that make comparison possible, is not essential to immediate qualitative attention to progress being made by managers at all organizational levels toward their noneconomic goals. Consider, for example:

Internal audit groups, necessarily oriented to examining what the public accounting firm must ultimately certify, can be supplemented by adding to their auditors and accountants permanent or temporary personnel, public relations, or general management persons who are qualified to examine, make comment on, and counsel with managers on their success and difficulties in the areas of social contribution and organization morale.

The role in the community of a local branch office, the morale of the work force, clerical and functional staffs, and the expertise and enthusiasm of the salesmen are all capable of assessment, not in hard numbers but nevertheless in valid and useful judgments.

The public relations and personnel staffs of organizations are all too often assigned to superficial and trivial tasks. The employment of such persons in the internal audit function, especially if they have—without necessarily the qualifications or temperament of high-spirited doers—the experience, perspective, and judgment of long service in the organization, would raise the importance of these functions by increasing their usefulness.

**Maturity of judgment.** Every large corporation develops unintentionally a group of highly experienced but, after a time, uncompulsive managers who are better assigned to jobs requiring maturity of judgment rather than the ability to sprint. The internal qualitative audit, combined with a parallel inquiry by a committee of outside directors, to which I shall allude in a moment, could be an internal counseling, review, and support function epitomizing effective staff support of line operations. It could also provide opportunity for the cadre of older managers no longer motivated by primitive incentives.

People with executive responsibility, including accountants and controllers, often exercise judgment only distantly affected by numbers; this is not a new requirement or experience. To the extent that managers in the hierarchy are capable of interpreting numbers intelligently, they must be capable of relating results produced to those in gestation and of judging the significance of a profit figure (not to be found in the figure itself) at a given point of time.

**Incentive modification.** If measurement of performance is to be broad and knowledgeable enough to encompass progress under a strategy containing social and organizational objectives, then the incentive system in a company or organization unit must reward and penalize accomplishments other than those related to economic efficiency.

Moreover, it must become well known in such an organization that persons can be demoted or discharged for failure to behave responsibly toward their subordinates, for example, even if they are successful in economic terms. Career-oriented middle managers must learn, from the response that their organization leadership and community activities receive, how to appreciate the intrinsic worth and how to estimate the value to their own future of demonstrated responsibility.

### Management Development

Besides liberating the evaluation process by adding qualitative judgment to numbers, the activity which needs expansion in making an organization socially effective and internally healthy is management development—not so much in terms of formal training programs (although I should be the last person to demean the importance of these) as in planned careers.

If organizations elect, as interesting organizations will, high standards of profit and social contribution to be achieved simultaneously, then much is required of the character, general education, and professional competence of managers who must show themselves — whatever their schooling — as liberally educated.

It follows from the argument I am making that, in moderating the amorality of organizations, we must expect executive mid-career education to include exposure to the issues of responsibility raised here and to the invaluable experience of participating in nonprofit community or government organizations. Under short-term pressures, attention to development is easily postponed, either as a cost that should be avoided for now or as a process requiring more attention to persons than is convenient or possible.

The management action so far suggested does not constitute innovation so much as reemphasis: it requires not heroic action but maturity and breadth of perspective. Once the aspiration to reach beyond economic to social and human objectives is seen to require extending conventional incentive and performance measurement systems, it is not difficult to avoid imbalance and the unintended organizational consequences of which I have spoken. Awareness of the problem generates its solution.

### Audit by Directors

But the current move toward revitalization of the board of directors does provide a formal resource to the chief executive who is secure enough and interested enough to avail himself of it. Committees of outside directors are now being formed in a number of companies to meet regularly with the internal audit and outside audit staffs to look closely at the thoroughness and adequacy of the procedures used to ensure that the true condition of the company is reflected in its published accounting statements.

The Penn Central debacle, in the midst of which the board of directors was apparently unaware of approaching disaster, has given considerable impetus to this trend.

If internal audit teams were to extend their counsel, nonpunitive inspection, and recommendations for improvement to social performance and to the quality of organization life as felt by its members, the information they would gather and the problems they would encounter could be summarized for the board committee in the same way as the more conventional subjects of their scrutiny.

In any case, the pervasiveness of the chief executive's posture on social responsibility can be inquired into, and the quality of the management across the organization can be reported on. The board of directors, supposed to provide judgment and experience not available inside the organization, can be — in its proper role of constructive inquiry into the quality of the corporation's management and its support for investment in improving it — a potent force in moderating the management's understandable internal interest in day-to-day achievement.

## Conclusion

Nothing will happen, either inward or outward, to further advance the doctrine of social responsibility unless those in charge of the corporation want it to happen and unless their associates share their values and put their backs into solving the organization's master problem. There must be desire and determination first. It must be embodied in a strategy that makes a consistent

266 of private economic opportunity and public social responsibility, planned

whole of private economic opportunity and public social responsibility, planned to be implemented in an organization which will be humanely and challengingly led and developed.

A few good people cannot change the course of a large corporation by their personal influence, but they can arrange that the systems of implementation are appropriate in scope to the breadth of corporate economic and social purpose. Now that enlightened chief executives have made this commitment, it would be tragic to have their will subverted, their determination doubted, and their energy dissipated by bureaucratic organization.

The giant corporation, which in small numbers does half the work of our economic system, is here to stay. It is the dominant force of our industrial society. In its multinational forms it has no higher sovereignty to which it reports; in its national forms it is granted wide latitude. Thus it is important to all of us that its affairs be responsibly conducted and that limited knowledge of the art of managing a large organization not be permitted to thwart us.

If organizations cannot be made moral, the future of capitalism will be unattractive — to all of us and especially to those young people whose talents we need. It is not the attack of the muckrakers we should fear but the apathy of our corporate citizenry.

### NOTES

1. *Capitalism and Freedom* (Chicago: University of Chicago Press, 1962), p. 133.
2. *Managing the Resource Allocation Process* (Boston: Division of Research, Harvard Business School, 1969).
3. "How Companies Respond to Social Demands," HBR July–August 1973, p. 88 ff.
4. "Tailor Incentive Compensation to Strategy," HBR March–April 1973, p. 94.
5. The phrase is Joseph L. Bower's, from *Technology, the Corporation, and the State*, edited by R. Maris and E.J. Mesthene, published by the Program on Technology and Society at Harvard University.
6. See Raymond A. Bauer and Dan H. Fenn, Jr., "What *Is* a Corporate Social Audit?" HBR January–February 1973, p. 37.

# 5

# Business Leadership and a Creative Society

## ABRAM T. COLLIER

High on the list of tasks facing the business administrator are those relating to the basic attitudes, interests, and objectives of his employees. Meeting antagonism and misunderstanding, as he often does, his immediate reaction is to cry out: "How can I get across to my employees some understanding of the objectives I seek?" Well, that question may be important, but perhaps it should not have such priority. It might be better to ask first: "What, in truth, do I seek? What objectives do I have that my employees can also share?"

Some administrators, of course, have not bothered their heads with such intricate problems, feeling that "only results count" or "actions speak louder than words." But advertising and public relations men have demonstrated how inadequate this view is; words and the things they connote are as much a part of our experience as the things that we perceive immediately and directly. And top-rank administrators such as Chester I. Barnard know also that one of the first and greatest functions of leadership is that the leader express for his group the ideals toward which they all, consciously or unconsciously, strive.

Winston Churchill's powerful "blood, sweat, and tears" speech in 1940 has now become a classic model in the political field of the way in which a leader can express the purpose of the people and rally them to common effort. Businessmen, especially those of us concerned with personnel, productivity, and morale, have come to recognize the need for much the same kind of leadership, convinced that only in this way will employees ever have the satisfaction of really feeling they are identified with the enterprise for which they work.

But in seeking to exert such leadership we have already learned that there are some difficult problems of communication in the way. Take the many attempts that have been made in recent years, following the example of such companies as Du Pont, General Electric, and Republic Steel, to give supervisors and workers in business some understanding of the economic and political society in which we live. The general experience is that the terms "capitalism," "competition," "American way of life," "land of opportunity," and "free private enterprise," through excessive repetition, abuse, or otherwise, have lost much of their capacity to convey the meaning intended.

Moreover, where new symbols have been introduced for the old, they too have missed the mark. The editors of *Fortune*, for example, have characterized our society as the "permanent revolution," but we do not think of ourselves as revolutionaries—at least not of the black-bearded and bomb-carrying kind. Other attempts to call our society "open" or "free" have raised the perplexing questions: Open for what? Free for what?

It seems to me that we businessmen ought to aim at articulating an ideology that, in addition to being an accurate expression of management goals, is a little closer to the personal and even religious aspirations of the people than anything we have espoused in the past. Is it not possible that we have been thinking too much in terms of systems, of economics, of products, of laws? Perhaps these approaches should not have failed as they did; perhaps they can be improved. But in any event it seems to me that the fact of their failure (or, at best, their lack of any great success) should be accepted, and that the most profitable line of inquiry is to turn to a different sort of approach altogether.

## The Creative Ideal

Accordingly, I put forward this simple proposition: that our society is a creative society; that its prime objective, as well as its great genius, is its creativeness; and that, as creative accomplishment is the actual day-to-day goal of modern business, it is also the keystone of our business philosophy.

I am thinking of creativeness in its widest and deepest sense. Thus, business does not exist merely to produce more goods and services, or better goods and services for more people, though that is no small part of its task. Business also, particularly in these days, affords the principal or the only means whereby individual men may gain the satisfaction of accomplishing something more than merely sustaining their own lives. Pleasure, power, and fame appear to be but by-products of the efforts we make to be useful members of society and to leave it with something more than it had when we arrived. Perhaps we leave only the grain of sand that Robert Frost said he wished to leave on the beach of history; but at least, if we do that, we can feel that we have fulfilled our role in living.

What I am suggesting is that the great goals of happiness, freedom, security —even goodness and truth—are values which should be viewed as subordinate to, and resulting from, a new and positive creative ideal. Our people in business and elsewhere seem to be driven by an urge to build; by a longing to explore and reach out; by a desire to realize, through men and for men, such things and experiences as humanity has never known before. In this light, our vaunted freedoms of thought and action, our sought-for freedoms from worry and want, and even our ethical standards of behavior (products as they are of other places and times) are not ends in themselves; rather, they emerge as important values just because they support and make possible a creative society of men.

This is the modern heresy: that it is not enough to be good, to lead a blameless life; we must also be creative.

**The new and the old.** In one sense this ideal is modern in expression only. Wise men in almost every age have been trying to tell us that the greatest individual satisfaction there is comes from a job well done. Samuel Johnson, for example, observed: "Life affords no higher pleasure than that of surmounting difficulties, passing from one step of success to another, forming new wishes and seeing them gratified." And Emerson said: "The *sum* of wisdom is that the time is never lost that is devoted to work."

In another sense, however, this ideal of ours shows some new, significantly new, aspects. Specifically, in American business it is now beginning to be recognized that *everyone* has the capacity for the satisfaction that comes from creative accomplishment. As science unleashes vast new sources of power, it appears possible for the first time in history for men of all types and classes to avoid the toil and suffering of hard labor and to experience the joys of work — a satisfaction which in times past was limited to the few.

Contrast this with the older view. We used to classify as creative only those accomplishments that certain individuals could achieve. The writer, the artist, the composer, the scientist — in other words, the rare people who had the genius to find and express new ideas or new truths — were considered the creative members of our society; the classic examples have been the Newtons, the Beethovens, the Kants, the Michelangelos, the Shakespeares. The magnitude of their work often crushed us by making us feel our own inadequacy.

Today, however, we are beginning to recognize that creative work may be accomplished collectively as well as individually. The great and small organizations that have built and operated our industrial plants, farms, transportation and communication networks, financial systems, and distributive organizations, all are examples of the creative genius which comes from the collective effort of administrators and workers, as well as specialists of all degrees.

**Dimension of the task.** The first task of business leaders, therefore, is to create an environment in which there can flourish not only individual genius but, more important, the collective capacities of other people in the organization. Some difficult and searching questions must be answered if this task is to be accomplished. What are the basic positive forces operating in a creative business society? What generates their power? What keeps them in balance? What conditions their survival? What controls their direction?

To this end, I should like to submit that the creative ideal depends on these concepts:

      1. That the forces in business (and many other types of organization) are nurtured by the existence of *differences between individuals and groups.*

      2. That these forces are kept in control and balance by the process of *individuals understanding each other.*

      3. That a creative society depends for its survival upon the belief that *rights must be matched by obligations.*

      4. That the directing force in a creative society is the *faith* of its members in *individual growth.*

### The Power of Difference

In considering the importance of individual difference, it should first be noted that the goal of many societies — including the goal of communist society today and of almost every Utopia that has ever been conceived, from Plato to Aldous Huxley — has been to compel men to conform. The theory is that if everyone is induced to accept the same ideas of what is good and proper, conflicts between men and groups of men will disappear and humanity will live happily ever after.

By contrast, one of the cornerstones on which the creative society is built is the incontrovertible fact that men are different, that they cherish these differences, that the joy and fascination of life depend on the existence of differences, and that there are great social values in differences.

**Driving force.** Every great ideal has its own theory of the nature of man. The wholly competitive or acquisitive society, which is gone (if it ever in fact existed), assumed that man was motivated only by his own pleasure, that he was egoistic and greedy, and that his wants were insatiable. By assuming that the average man, the economic man, was moved by animal impulses, it was possible to work out satisfactory theoretical explanations of how men acted in the marketplace.

On the other hand, socialists have assumed, following the notions of Rousseau (and possibly the story of Genesis), that man was essentially good, self-sacrificing, considerate, and loving, but was corrupted by social institutions. On this basis they thought that if institutions were changed or destroyed and if nonconforming individuals and classes were eliminated, then all social problems would cease and the state could and would wither away.

But in a creative society neither of these views is adequate. We observe that men are both egoistic and self-sacrificing—and many things more. While men are, taken as a whole, driven by an urge to create and grow, their characteristics vary with their times, experiences, culture, inheritance, and with all the other circumstances in which they find themselves. To illustrate with a simple example:

In the company with which I am associated we are using, as an aid in selection and placement, a test of personality or temperament in which the results are described not in imprecise words but in graphic form. Taking several major behavior characteristics, it plots with a fair degree of accuracy where a given individual falls on each of several temperament spectra. For instance, there is a spectrum of gregariousness in which the extreme extrovert falls at one end and the extreme introvert at the other; in between are those having various needs for sociability or a capacity to live within themselves.

Thousands upon thousands of tests of this type have been made, and it is fair to say that in no two cases have the results—the combinations of characteristics on the several spectra—been exactly the same. Similarity of types may be observed, but every man and every woman is found to be unique. Furthermore, research into personality shows that men change their personalities, usually extremely slowly but sometimes dramatically. It also shows that behavior is not wholly a matter for the individual alone but depends in large part on the situation in which he finds himself. That is, the set of values according to which he makes his decision may vary with his external circumstances.

The driving force of difference—in individuals and in groups—seems well illustrated by the history of the United States and Canada (in contrast to some other countries). While no doubt we have strong forces in many companies, labor unions, churches, and schools which are trying to enforce a high degree of conformity to some particular viewpoint, practice, or belief, nevertheless those forces have been observably less dominant than the forces of individual integrity. In our business world, if a man has felt that he could do a job better than someone else, he has been free to try; indeed, the fact that he saw things differently has given him both the opportunity and the courage to try.

Moreover, there is good reason to believe that the differences between groups of people in the United States and Canada with respect to cultural, racial, and religious backgrounds have been a factor in the dynamic development of these countries. What does it mean that never before in history have so many diverse religious groups been able to live together with so little disharmony? Has our society progressed *in spite of* differences or *because of* them? Possibly the very existence of differences among various people and groups has given people the courage to disagree with prevailing opinions. Every discovery, every invention, every new industry, every new idea has come about because some person or some group of people has had the courage as well as the insight to disagree with the majority or do what the majority has not thought of doing before.

This is perhaps part of what David McCord Wright had in mind when he pointed out: "Our dilemma . . . is that if we make men 'free,' they will become creative and from their creations will spring the probability of growth and the certainty of trouble."[1]

**Diversity rather than conflict.** Differences do, of course, lead to trouble—to misunderstanding and conflict. Yet conflict is essential to constructive work. More than a generation ago Mary Parker Follett, a woman who has since become recognized for her many profound insights into the nature of business organizations, wrote:

> What people often mean by getting rid of conflict is getting rid of diversity, and it is of the utmost importance that these should not be considered the same. We may wish to abolish conflict, but we cannot get rid of diversity. We must face life as it is and understand that diversity is its most essential feature. . . . Fear of difference is dread of life itself. It is possible to conceive of conflict as not necessarily a wasteful outbreak of incompatibilities but a *normal* process by which socially valuable differences register themselves for the enrichment of all concerned.[2]

Creativeness in an organization depends to a large extent on people who are not too ready to agree. In our own experience, most of us abhor the attitude of "Well, if you're going to argue about it, let's do it your way." We have found that we must have diversity of opinion, firmly as well as fairly expressed, if our business is to make the wise decisions that will enable it to develop and grow.

If we accept difference, it necessarily follows that we are not sure we are right ourselves; we accept the notion that our conclusions about people and society must be treated only as working hypotheses and that there are realities beyond those of our immediate perceptions. It is sometimes forgotten how highly we esteem this concept in the physical sciences. The entire atomic world of neutrons and electrons has never been perceived directly; despite Hiroshima and Nagasaki, it is still a theory or a working hypothesis. The same hypothetical character pertains to all of our knowledge about genes—the transmission of traits from organisms to their offspring.

But if it is necessary to trust to more than our immediate perceptions in the physical sciences, it would seem even more important to do so in social, ethical, and political matters that deal with human beings. The observation of Yale's F.C.S. Northrop, that the ability to live in a world of both immediate perceptions and unperceived hypotheses is the essence of the genius of the West, would apply no less to our industrial and political society than to our scientific progress.

This means that we must subject our old concepts of right and wrong, of good and bad, to a radical change; things are no longer so black and white. Judge Learned Hand, philosopher as well as judge, has described the spirit of liberty as "the spirit that is not too sure that it is right." Tolerance for difference, for the viewpoint that we do not agree with, implies that we are not so sure of our own. We accept our principles of action as working hypotheses, realizing that something may happen to lead us to revise these opinions. While it often sounds as though some of our friends would never change their opinions (particularly on matters of ethics or politics), our great genius lies in the fact that we may talk loudly but, when the chips are down, we seem to act on the basis that all general rules of what is right and wrong must be tempered by common sense.

It can be reasonably contended that the great upheavals of modern history — its wars and its revolutions — are not so much the result of differences between people as of the feeling of a nation or a class that its capacity for creative expression is in some way threatened or thwarted. This was one cause of the Russian revolt of 1917, although the revolutionaries themselves later made the great and historic blunder of seeking to abolish conflict by abolishing difference rather than by accepting difference and in that way removing the barriers to creative work.

Nations such as ours, that have insisted on the freedom of their people to be different, have had to fight and may well fight again to preserve their right to disagree with one another. Yet, if the principle of difference is one of the cornerstones of creativeness, our society has little to fear *in the long run* from the Stalins who deny the privilege of difference to their own people.

### Process of Understanding

If diversity is the first condition of the creative society, then understanding is the second. The Bible's exhortation, "with all thy getting, get understanding," is particularly appropriate for modern industry. If for their dynamic creative power our businesses depend on continuing differences in viewpoint, for balance and braking power they must equally depend on understanding, on the felt necessity for securing agreement and cooperation.

In the sense that I am using the term, understanding refers both to self-understanding and understanding of others. Self-awareness as a desirable personal attribute is certainly not newer than the Socratic injunction, "Know thyself"; but what is new in our time is the fact that thoughtful social scientists and hard-headed businessmen are coming to see that self-awareness or self-understanding is directly related to an individual's capacity to do creative work with other people. Businessmen are beginning to think not only of the logics of business but also of what Pareto described as the nonlogics or the sentiments of people. They are beginning to see that their own behavior is a factor which influences the behavior of others, and that they are personally involved in more roles than one in every situation in which they play a part.

Let me illustrate from my own personal experience.

For a short time, some years ago, I engaged in the general practice of law. Later I was employed as a lawyer by an insurance company. As a lawyer I found that my clients' problems were not mine; and no matter how hard I tried to solve them, I stood outside of the situation and was not involved in it. But when later I took an administrative position, I found that this detachment was no longer possible, even if I wanted it. I was personally involved in every important decision, and my behavior was affecting others. The shock of being forced to examine my own behavior was by no means small. What I needed to do, however, was no less than what all successful administrators are doing daily in every business.

In addition to self-awareness there is the need for understanding others. What we are learning today is not just that it is a "good thing to see the other fellow's point of view," but also what it is that often makes it difficult to do so. We are learning that we cannot really understand another if we agree with him, nor can we understand him if we disagree! When we feel either love or hate, we lose our power to see the world as others see it. We blur our own perceptions, and we cut off the normal flow of words which help us see into another's mind.

**Communication gateways.** This conclusion has tremendous significance. If understanding the needs and desires of others is an essential for collective creative effort, it means that we can no longer be quick to evaluate people or their opinions as either good or bad. During the understanding process at least, we must throw our ethical judgments out the window.

Carl R. Rogers and F.J. Roethlisberger made this same point when in essence they said that the great barrier to communication is our tendency to evaluate, to approve or disapprove the statements that other people make.[3] For example:

If you say to me, "I prefer Englishmen to the French," there is almost an overwhelming urge for me to say either "So do I" or "No, I think they are stuffy." We may then talk for hours without a meeting of the minds. If, on the other hand, I want to find out whether we really agree or disagree about this matter, if I want to listen intelligently and to understand what you mean, thus opening the gateway to communication, then I must restrain my natural inclination to presume what you mean and instead make an effort to draw you out. I might ask something like, "Do you mean Englishmen are more to be admired?" You may reply, "Yes, they are really facing up to their economic problems better than the French." And if I continue in that way, rephrasing your comments in question form to test out what you are *trying* to tell me, there is a much better chance that we can have a fruitful discussion.

This brief explanation of a gateway to understanding, of receiving communications, of listening, may sound extremely obvious and somewhat simple. We spend most of our time learning to express ourselves, which is difficult enough but still easier than listening. Indeed, it is fair to say that listening is one of the most difficult things in the world to do. When someone charges into your office and criticizes some action that you have taken, it is not easy to find out what is really on his mind when your first impulse is to tell him to "go to hell." Or take the case where somebody asks you for your advice because he cannot make up his mind about a personal problem; most of us are inclined to comply with such a request without knowing what the real problem is, or without realizing that the decision will be sound only if it is made by the troubled person himself.

It takes real insight to be able to express in words what someone else is trying to tell us. It also takes great effort and even courage. If we put ourselves in someone else's position, if we try to express adequately his point of view, we may find that our own views become changed in the process. Professor Rogers says, "The risk of being changed is one of the most frightening prospects many of us can face."[4]

There are, of course, many other ways of securing understanding; some of them have been outlined by Stuart Chase in his recent popularization of social science, *Roads to Agreement*.[5] One is particularly worth mentioning:

This way is modeled on the long-established custom of the Quaker business meeting. Quakers as a class are great individualists, but in handling the business affairs of their churches they act only with unanimity. They have no formal voting, no sense of a majority imposing its will on a reluctant minority. If a problem cannot be settled by unanimous agreement, they invoke periods of silence or put over the question until some future meeting. Some solution is usually forthcoming.

This rule of unanimity, it seems, is now being practiced by boards of directors and executive committees in businesses throughout the land. What a far cry this is from deciding what is the greatest good for the greatest number by a mechanical counting of hands! Where difference is accepted, it is possible also to accept the notion that a minority may be right.

**Integration versus compromise.** The concept of integration as opposed to compromise is also achieving a wider recognition. Integration may be called the means of solving a conflict of opinion in such a way that both sides prevail. The idea behind it is that the basic interests underlying many disputes are not inconsistent. For example:

If two people in an office want to use the same desk, it may appear at first that a major conflict is in the making, which can be solved only if one or the other wins the decision. On investigation, however, it may appear that one of the persons wants the desk in order to have better light, whereas the other wants it in order to be near some friend. If these facts come out, it will be apparent that neither wants the desk as such and that it may well be possible to satisfy the basic interests of both.

In order to achieve integration, says Miss Follett, we should

never, if possible, allow an either/or situation to be created. . . . There are almost always more than two alternatives in a situation and our job is to analyze the situation carefully enough for as many as possible to appear. A yes-or-no question is in itself a prejudgment.[6]

May there not be some relationship between these methods of reaching understanding and the spirit which is not too sure that it is right? Is there not some connection between these techniques of agreement and our capacity for collective creativeness? Can it not be said that in a creative society we must have both conflict and agreement?

### Rights and Obligations

A third standard of a creative society, and an essential ingredient in our workaday world, has been foreshadowed by the previous discussion of difference and of understanding. It is the belief that human relationships are two-way matters and that rights are matched by obligations.

**The "*double plus*".** Karl Marx predicted that in Western society it was inevitable that the rich would become richer and the poor would become poorer. This increasing division between the classes would, as he saw it, accelerate class warfare and the revolution. If our society had indeed been basically competitive and acquisitive, instead of creative and cooperative, Marx might well have been proved right. But the fact is that today, through our collective creativeness, the poor have become richer. Our society has been able to create wealth at a vastly greater rate than it has increased its population.

By and large, we have been able to maintain the viewpoint that our economic and political problem is not so much to redistribute the wealth that exists as to create more wealth for all. As the eminent economist, Kenneth Boulding, has written, "Economic life is not a 'zero-sum' poker game in which a fixed volume of wealth is circulated among the players, but a 'positive-sum' enterprise in which the accumulation of each person represents something he brings to the 'pot' rather than something he takes out."[7] In other words, we are engaged in a creative task of producing more and better things. We recognize that we share as we contribute, that no society can long give something for nothing (to the poor *or* the rich), and that we cannot do great work unless *everyone* shares both in the work and in its results.

This concept has been called by many names. Mutuality is one; give-and-take is another. Professor Charles I. Gragg of the Harvard Business School calls it the "double plus." As he sees it, business transactions and other relationships can be described in one of three ways:

1. There is first the kind of a transaction in which the plus is all on my side, leaving a big minus for you. If I take all the profit, however, through my power or my cleverness, then I have really lost the bargain, because you will come to distrust me and will refuse to do business with me for long.

2. The reverse situation is equally disastrous. If I, through an excess of altruism or with misguided notions of humanity, permit you to take the entire profit, with nothing for myself, I put you in the unhappy role of being a recipient of my charity; moreover, I leave myself unable to do further business with anyone.

3. But there is still another and more satisfactory form. Only if you profit moderately and I profit moderately, only if there is a plus for you and a plus for me — a double plus — can we continue to deal with one another steadily and with confidence.

In our business lives we are beginning to see that by consciously fashioning our relationships with our employees, with our suppliers, with our customers — and, indeed, even with our competitors — we are not making suspicious and careful deals so much as common-sense arrangements that are carried on in this spirit of mutual give-and-take. That does not mean anything petty like back-scratching; every service and every kindness is not to be immediately returned, nor is every service to be performed in the hope of return. The correct attitude, rather, is a healthy respect for the well-being and personal integrity of the other fellow.

**Profit for all.** What does all this imply? Only in an atmosphere of profit (in the broad sense) to all parties can we meet the creative objectives that our society sets. If, in times past, we erred on the side of taking too much for ourselves, it is equally essential that we do not err in the future on the side of trying to do too much for others. A too-literal application of the Sermon on the Mount — the turn of the cheek — does small damage to us but great damage to him who strikes the blow.

Why is it, otherwise, that the problem of providing for the aged worker has once more raised its head, when we thought a few years ago that we had safely tucked it away with compulsory retirement and pensioning at age 65? From the point of view of sympathy for the aged and of convenience in administering our business enterprises, the practice is as desirable today as it was 15 years ago. We have discovered, however, that many individual men who retire are hurt because they lose their sense of being creative, of being useful members of society. Moreover, when we contemplate that 11% of our population will be over 65 in another 20 years, we begin to realize that the real economic cost of compulsory retirement is not the money that goes into pensions but the lost productivity of these older people.

It seems that people, individually and in groups, must continue to be creative; if they are not, the individual or society, or both, will suffer. If we do not intend to keep people over 65 in business, some other way must be found to permit them to continue active membership in the world's work.

The same kind of thinking underlies our concern for other noncontributors to society. Society has been doing an increasingly successful job of minimizing sickness of almost all kinds, not so much out of solicitude for the feelings of persons who are ill as out of its own self-interest in having the benefit of their contribution. Programs undertaken with this motive quickly earn common respect, for the galling part of illness to the sufferer is the necessity of having to depend on others, of not being able to contribute his share.

We are concerned for similar reasons about the criminal and the indolent. It is true that we have not as yet learned enough to be confident of our ability to rehabilitate these people. But we have at least learned that it is no answer to judge them or to punish them; our first task is to understand them. We consider them "cured" only when they join the majority of their fellows, contributing commensurately to what they receive.

Why do businessmen fight against the welfare state? Are businessmen actually heartless and callous? Don't they recognize that the sick and the poor need the aid of the rest who are well and able? Of course they do. But their experience says to them that doctors do not give pills to everyone because a few are sick; that when a man is given something for which he has not worked, he feels degraded; that a man who is well and able wants to earn what he receives.

Businessmen, who have learned from experience that paternalism has failed, hope that government will learn from their mistakes. Businessmen have good reason for believing that government will not really serve the poor and sick until it stops regarding them as "little people" and undertakes instead the harder job of giving them an honest chance to do useful and creative work.

### Faith in Men's Growth

The fourth and last condition of maintaining and strengthening a creative society, the force that provides direction and control, is a clear faith in the growth and development of men. The machine age poses a great challenge to our willingness to demonstrate this faith. All of the new wealth we can produce with modern technology is of little avail if in the process men are reduced to the levels of the machines they tend. But fortunately we are not confronted with a Hobson's choice between wealth and men. We have found that the more we are able to train and develop men as individuals, leaving repetitive work to machines, the greater satisfactions they obtain and the more productive (in a material sense) they become.

Take a business with a large content of routine clerical work, e.g., life insurance. In this business we stand on the threshold of a new era in adapting electronics to office workers' problems. When any business reaches this point, to be sure, management is bound to face the problem of securing the cooperation of people who may prefer things as they are. It may even have to face a problem of technological unemployment. But however real and thorny these difficulties are, they are insignificant compared to the human values that are gained. Instead of a business in which, say, 75% of the employees are engaged in routine tasks, the modern machine makes it possible for 75% to be engaged in tasks requiring skill and judgment. The machine eliminates human toil; but, much more important, it also provides opportunities for men to do only those tasks men alone can do.

**New concept of organization.** The development of the machine economy has numerous important implications for management. For one thing, it is fast bringing about a new concept of business organization. No longer can the boss know all the details and the intricacies of the operation he supervises. He is being forced more and more to rely on his subordinates, to consult with them, to be guided by their joint conclusions — in short, to permit them to share and to grow in breadth of vision.

This in turn means, of course, a gradual abandonment of authoritarian principles. Administrators have begun to conceive of their role not as manipulators of labor but as coordinators of functions. Re-examining themselves and their jobs, they have discovered that they have no special claim to superior wisdom, no vested authority over the work and lives of others. They have found, rather, that they have a function to perform: to plan ahead, to coordinate the others, to secure their interest and cooperation.

Society will not, as a result, tend to become classless in any Marxian sense. Far from it. We may reasonably anticipate, however, that members of future "elites" will come to occupy positions of status and power less because of wealth, position, or birth and more because of the kind of contributions they make or because of the kind of functions they fulfill. Key positions will tend more and more to be occupied by those who are best able to conceive new ideas and the application of old ones, who are best able to communicate ideas and events, and who are best able to pull together people and things to achieve creative ends. Today's inheritance tax and management's increased interest in personnel development are fast speeding this process along.

**Administrators as teachers.** In an important sense the role of the administrator seems destined to become more and more that of the instructor — the kind of teacher who understands his pupils, accepts their differences, commands their respect, and inspires them to creative work of every kind. In such a role, administrators will have less of a problem of discipline to the degree that they are able to develop an environment for creative experience and to lead their students (their workers) to savor the satisfying taste of personal accomplishment. In so doing they will have gone far to eliminate the distinction between "schooling" and "education" which Mark Twain quite properly made when he quipped, "I have never let my schooling interfere with my education."

In their new role as teachers, administrators are learning that attitudes and viewpoints which affect behavior can frequently be communicated effectively only if they are reduced to concrete terms. In their efforts at training and development, particularly, they are recognizing the need to start from real case situations. Witness the growing attention to discussions of actual business problems rather than the oft-repeated clichés on general principles of management.

Abstract ideas, however, are not to be discarded simply because they so often fail to influence behavior. Indeed, as the mark of civilized men they are necessary tools of communication which are quite adequate *if* both writer and reader start from the same premises. They are easily accepted, in other words, if they seem meaningful in relation to one's own experience. Aneurin Bevan's autobiography affords an example of this:

Bevan's life as a young Welsh miner was filled with frustrations. Then he read Karl Marx. This experience "had all the impact of divine revelation. Everything fell in place. The dark places were lighted up and the difficult ways made easy."[8] Marx is most abstract, but nevertheless his words have had a great effect on people whose experience has led them to feel like chained and exploited men.

The moral of this fact has not been lost on businessmen and statesmen, who know that the only real and lasting bulwark against Marxism is in the experience of the large body of our workers and our citizens. If that experience is basically creative and satisfying—and it is management's task to see that it is so—the stultifying conformities of the socialist state will always be bitter to their taste.

But businessmen and statesmen, while often seeing what is the best *defense* against Marxism, have not been so quick to see what needs to be done in a *positive* way. Like Marxians, we too must have an appropriate body of abstract ideas— ideas that can constitute a simple article of faith but are also capable of profound extension, ideas that are consistent with experience but are also adaptable to new insights and new truths.

Perhaps this discussion will stimulate others to work out such ideas—each in his own way, as a part of our individual differences, but all toward the same goal, in the spirit of mutuality. What I have written can be no more than a preface.

## Conclusion

The problems of production, distribution, and finance are usually foreign to a worker's experience and interests. It is therefore just as silly for top management to hope that workers will be anxious to understand the problems of the business as it would be to fear that they are interested in gaining control of the business. What workers do appear to want is a chance to increase their usefulness and creativeness, a chance to develop their full potential as individuals within the scope of their environment and experience. It has become part of management's function to see not only that they have that chance but that the philosophy behind it is made articulate.

But the creative society is based on more than the relationship between management and workers, indispensable though that is in our industrial age. It depends on close relationships between all fields of human endeavor. Business is not "just business." The Chinese wall between business and the home, the community, the school, and the church has long since been stormed. Business is all people, places, and things; it is physics, economics, politics, sociology, psychology, philosophy, ethics, and aesthetics.

In the same broad sense, business is also religion. One of the recurring themes in most religions is that God is viewed as the Creator and that creativeness is one of His essential attributes. Another recurring theme is that man's spirit, his conscious "self," his unique ability to transcend his material and animal limitations, is the essence of God in man. To suggest that creativeness may be a basic attribute of men in society is thus merely to relate these two ageless insights.

Moreover, it seems that a religious sense of wonder, humility, and faith helps us to see the vision of a boundless future built by the inherent capacities of men from all walks of life and of all races, creeds, natures, and backgrounds. It is a vision of cooperation, togetherness, and sharing the great adventure. It is a vision of independence and courage that explores the far reaches of the universe and probes deep into the essence of what we call man. It is, in short, a vision of a changing, growing, and infinitely exciting world which depends for its existence on the spirit that is not too sure it is right, on a deep-seated desire to open our minds and our hearts to the lives of others, on the practical sense of give-and-take, on our faith in the growth and development of ourselves and our fellow men.

### APPENDIX

The author of an article which is exhumed some 15 years after publication [January–February 1953] has mixed feelings. In some ways he feels as though he were seeing a ghost. In other ways he feels like a father of a foundling who hears that the boy has grown up and won a prize at school: as a father he is proud, but his pride is limited by the knowledge that his own contribution was made in the very distant past.

Reviewing the results of these distant events, I believe I would not write the article much differently if I were to write it today. The events of 15 years, I think, have not proved me wrong.

I still believe that the business of business is discovery, innovation, and creativity. I still believe the job of management is to maintain creativity with order —and order with creativity. I still believe creativity without order breeds chaos, and that order without creativity is a living death.

There is one aspect of the article, however, to which I might want to give greater emphasis if I were writing today—namely, the role of time. As the article suggests, difference, understanding, and mutuality are essential elements in a creative enterprise and should be accorded adequate time so they can be fully operative. Today I am perhaps more aware of the fact that everything has a price in time. Sometimes the price is too high. Sometimes diversity and understanding must be sacrificed to competitive pressures and other dangers.

I continue to believe that most things *can* be done—given sufficient time. The administrator can control, to a considerable extent, the rate of change within his own organization, but he finds it immeasurably more difficult to affect the rate of social change for a society as a whole. This latter rate continues to be agonizingly slow as race riots at home and the war in Vietnam so amply illustrate.

Nothing I say today, however, can change what I left on the HBR doorstep many years ago. If the foundling has survived, he speaks on his own. And if, gentle reader, you should disagree, please take it up with him, not me.

—A.T.C.

### NOTES

1. *The Impact of the Union* (New York: Harcourt, Brace, 1951), p. 274.
2. *Creative Experiences* (New York: Longmans, Green, 1924), pp. 300–301.
3. "Barriers and Gateways to Communication," HBR July–August 1952, p. 46.
4. Ibid., p. 48.
5. New York: Harper, 1951, p. 45 ff.
6. *Dynamic Administration — The Collected Papers of Mary Parker Follett* (New York: Harper, 1940), pp. 219–220.
7. "Religious Foundations of Economic Progress," HBR May–June 1952, p. 36.
8. *In Place of Fear* (New York: Simon and Schuster, 1952), p. 19.

# Epilogue

As a former editor of the *Harvard Business Review*, I am acutely aware of how difficult it is to persuade business people to write or speak about corporate ethics. I am myself not comfortable in doing so. To generalize the ethical aspects of a business decision, leaving aside the particulars that make it real, is too often to sermonize, to simplify, or to rationalize away the plain fact that many instances of competing ethical claims have no satisfactory solution. When important and incontestable breaches of conduct are made known, however, we also hear little comment from business leaders of high integrity. Their public silence suggests to cynics that they are not offended by the most outrageous breaches of trust. This, I have become convinced, is a misconception. They are instead acutely aware that some day they may be betrayed by someone in their own organizations. A sense of immanent vulnerability, leading to diffidence in prescribing moral behavior to others, is the ultimate silencer.

The impediments to explicit discussion of ethics in business and professional schools of management—and in many other arenas as well—are many. They stem from the complexity of business ethics as a continuing stubborn problem. Moral exhortation and oral piety are offensive, especially when attended by hypocrisy or real vulnerability to criticism. Any successful or energetic person will encounter in a mean quarter a question about methods and motives, for even well-intentioned behavior may be judged unethical from some point of view. The need for cooperation among persons of differing religious belief diminishes discussion of religion and related ethical issues. The jargon and imputed impracticability of philosophers more interested in theory than in its application have already drawn my prolonged complaint. That persons with management responsibility must find their own approaches to conflicting ethical claims in their own minds and hearts is an unwelcome discovery. Most of us keep quiet about it.

In such an environment of inhibition, I no longer feel apologetic about the unassuming array of articles presented here. The ideas they develop or imply go a long way to put in any manager's hands and head the means to deal with an ethical problem once identified. Recognition is the more difficult achievement, but once it is realized that every important business decision has an ethical dimension, we need only ask ourselves and others to take its measure.

The other major ideas in this book and my reflections on them are in summary quite simple. Perhaps the most important is that total loyalty to maximization of profit as the theoretical center of management practice is the principal obstacle to higher standards of ethical practice. The exclusively economic definition of the purpose of the corporation is a deadly oversimplification, allowing over-emphasis on self-interest at the expense of consideration of others. That no school of philosophy or dogmatic form of thought is capable of a formulistic solution to conflicting ethical claims is a minor disappointment to those already aware that the practice of management requires a prolonged play of judgment. Executives must find in their own will, experience, and intelligence the principles for balancing conflicting claims. They will do well to submit their views for corroboration by others, for openness in the discussion of problems will reveal previously unsuspected ethical aspects and develop the variety of points of view that should be taken into account. Ultimately, however, in the instance of infinitely debatable issues, executives must decide, relying on their own judgment and points of view. The selection of executives, therefore, should include inquiry into character—a process that should go on all through the course of executive development within the corporation.

And so it goes. That much and that little. The encouraging outcome of this consideration is that the promulgation and institutionalizing of ethical policy is not so difficult as, for example, escaping the compulsion of greed or the obsolete theory that makes ethical inquiry repugnant. Once undertaken, the process can be as straightforward as the articulation and implementation of policy in any other sphere. Any company has the opportunity to develop a unique corporate strategy summarizing its major purposes and policies. That strategy can encompass not only the economic role it will play with its product lines in its national and international markets but also the kind of company it will be as a human organization in relation to its employees, customers, shareholders, and communities. It will embrace as well, though perhaps not publicly, the nature and scope of the leadership to which the company is to be entrusted.

This strategy is necessarily an expression of the creativity, energy, desire, and commitment of the company's membership. Commitment is not long sustained by economically or ethically unsound strategic decisions.

I am indebted to the original authors for their willingness to write about corporate ethics. I thank the staff of the *Harvard Business Review* (especially during the ten years when I was first its chairman and then its editor) for the solicitation and development of the stream of articles from which the present collection is taken.

This volume has found its form with the help of Eliza Collins, once executive editor of the *Review* and now an editor of the Harvard Business School Press. I appreciate Professor Kenneth Goodpaster's work in developing a practical perspective on applied ethics and his permission to include here his Ruffin lecture at the University of Virginia. Rachael Daitch prepared the text of my introductions with characteristic cheerfulness and competence, for which I am continuously grateful.

# About the Contributors

## Kenneth R. Andrews

Kenneth Andrews retired in 1986 after a forty-year career at the Harvard Business School. Professor Emeritus Andrews devoted his attention to business policy, management development, and executive education. He served as editor of the *Harvard Business Review* from 1979 to 1985. He is the author of the well-known book, *The Concept of Corporate Strategy* (Dow Jones Irwin, 1971; revised 1980; third edition 1987).

## Timothy Blodgett

Timothy Blodgett is executive editor of the *Harvard Business Review*, where he has worked since 1966. Mr. Blodgett has edited several collections of HBR articles.

## Steven N. Brenner

Steven Brenner is professor of business administration at Portland State University and holds a sponsored professorship in business ethics and corporate social responsibility.

## Sir Adrian Cadbury

Sir Adrian Cadbury has been chairman of Cadbury, Schweppes since 1975 and a director of the Bank of England since 1970. He is active in the civic and educational councils in Birmingham, the headquarters of Cadbury, as well as in the councils of the food and drink industry in England.

## Albert Z. Carr

The late Albert Z. Carr was a consultant and author of *Business as a Game* (New American Library, 1968). During World War II he was assistant to the chairman, War Production Board, and later a special assistant to President Harry S Truman.

## Joanne B. Ciulla

Joanne B. Ciulla is a senior fellow at the Wharton School, University of Pennsylvania, where she teaches business ethics in the M.B.A. and executive education programs. She is completing a book on the meaning of work to be published by Random House.

Robert Coles

Robert Coles is professor of psychiatry and medical humanities at Harvard Medical School and teaches moral inquiry in many parts of Harvard University. During his distinguished career, he has been active in civic and political affairs. His recent works include *The Moral Life of Children* (Atlantic Monthly Press, 1986) and *Harvard Diary: Reflections on the Sacred and the Secular* (The Crossroad Publishing Company, 1988).

Abram T. Collier

Abram Collier is the retired chairman and chief executive officer of New England Mutual Life Insurance Company. In 1978 he received the Harvard Business School Statesman of the Year Award.

Arch R. Dooley

Arch Dooley is Jesse Philips Professor of Manufacturing at the Harvard Business School. Professor Dooley has taught in many executive education programs worldwide. His current research interests include entrepreneurship and management of smaller enterprises.

David W. Ewing

David Ewing, former managing editor of the *Harvard Business Review*, is the author of several books, including *Freedom Inside the Organization: Bringing Civil Liberties to the Workplace* (McGraw-Hill, 1978), *Do It My Way or You're Fired* (John Wiley, 1983), and the forthcoming *Justice in the Workplace* (Harvard Business School Press, 1989).

Saul W. Gellerman

Saul W. Gellerman is dean of the Graduate School of Management, University of Dallas. An industrial psychologist, he formerly headed his own consulting firm. His most recent *Harvard Business Review* article is "Cyanamid's New Take on Performance Appraisal" (May–June 1988).

Kenneth E. Goodpaster

Kenneth Goodpaster is associate professor of general management at the Harvard Business School, where he teaches a popular course on business and ethics. His work in progress includes a book on management and moral philosophy entitled *The Moral Agenda of Corporate Leadership* (Ballinger, 1989).

Robert Jackall

Robert Jackall chairs the Department of Anthropology and Sociology at Williams College, where he has taught since 1976. His latest book is *Moral Mazes: The World of Corporate Managers* (Oxford University Press, 1988).

Robert L. Katz

Robert L. Katz is president of Robert L. Katz and Associates, a consulting firm specializing in corporate strategy. He has taught at the graduate schools of business at Dartmouth, Harvard, and Stanford, and has written three textbooks.

## Paul R. Lawrence

Paul R. Lawrence is Wallace Brett Donham Professor of Organizational Behavior at the Harvard Business School, where he has taught since 1947. He is the author of numerous articles and books including, with Davis Dyer, *Renewing American Industry* (Free Press, 1983).

## Edmund P. Learned

Edmund P. Learned is Charles Edward Wilson Professor of Business Policy, Emeritus, at the Harvard Business School, where he taught for 40 years. His teaching and research interests included business policy, planning, and control. Mr. Learned pioneered the use of statistics in management.

## Bowen H. McCoy

Bowen McCoy is managing director of Morgan Stanley & Company, Inc., Western Region. He serves as an overseer of Stanford University's Hoover Library and is an ordained ruling elder of the Presbyterian Church (U.S.A.).

## John B. Matthews, Jr.

John Matthews is Joseph C. Wilson Professor of Business Administration at the Harvard Business School. Professor Matthews has served on the board of directors of many companies and has written five books and numerous articles.

## Earl A. Molander

Earl Molander is professor of business administration at Portland State University where he chairs the Department of Management. His article "A Paradigm for Design, Promulgation, and Enforcement of Ethical Codes" appeared in the *Journal of Business Ethics*, vol. 6, 1987. Mr. Molander also owns a golden retriever.

## Laura L. Nash

Laura Nash heads Nash Associates, a consulting firm for executive training in business ethics. She is also a fellow at Boston University's Institute for the Study of Economic Culture.

## Louis William Norris

The late Louis Norris was president of Albion College from 1960 until 1970, when he was appointed to the National Council for the Humanities. A minister of the Evangelical Congregational Church, Mr. Norris wrote two books, including *Polarity: A Philosophy of Tensions Among Values* (H. Regnery, 1956).

## O.A. Ohmann

O.A. Ohmann was assistant to the president of the Standard Oil Company of Ohio. After he retired, Mr. Ohmann consulted with organizations on management development and was director of The Church Executive Development Board in New York.

Douglas S. Sherwin

Douglas S. Sherwin is a retired executive of Phillips Petroleum Company, having served as president and a director of its wholly owned subsidiary, Phillips Products, Inc. He currently is a partner in Sherwin, Davison and Associates, an investment and acquisition partnership. Mr. Sherwin is also chairman of the board of Canada Cordage, Inc. in Ontario, a director of Canada Western Cordage in Vancouver, and an owner and director of Real American Actionwear, Inc.

Jeffrey Sonnenfeld

Jeffrey Sonnenfeld is associate professor of business administration at the Harvard Business School. His latest book is *The Hero's Farewell: Retirement and Renewal for Chief Executives* (Oxford University Press, 1988).

# Index